THE
GOSPEL
OF
WELLNESS

THE

GOSPEL

OF

WELLNESS

GYMS, GURUS, GOOP AND THE FALSE
PROMISE OF SELF-CARE

Rina Raphael

SOUVENIR
PRESS

First published in Great Britain in 2023 by
Souvenir Press,
an imprint of Profile Books Ltd
29 Cloth Fair
London
EC1A 7JQ
www.souvenirpress.co.uk

First published in the United States of America in 2022 by
Henry Holt and Company, Macmillan Publishing Group, LLC.

Portions of this book originally appeared, though sometimes slightly different,
in the following publications: *Fast Company*, the *Los Angeles Times*, and
Medium's *Elemental*.

Designed by Omar Chapa

The names and identifying characteristics of some persons described
in this book have been changed.

1 3 5 7 9 10 8 6 4 2

Printed and bound in Great Britain by Clays Ltd, Elcograf S.p.A.

The moral right of the author has been asserted.

A CIP catalogue record for this book is available from the British Library.

ISBN 978 1 78816 823 6
eISBN 978 1 78283 860 9

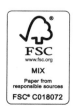

FSC
www.fsc.org
MIX
Paper from
responsible sources
FSC® C018072

Contents

Introduction

Santa Monica, California

It's a sunny spring day in Southern California. Two thousand women are gathered on the wooden planks of the famous Santa Monica Pier. Seagulls are squawking overhead, but the women pay them no mind. They're busy saluting the sun from a rainbow of colored yoga mats in perfectly spaced rows, spread out over a half mile of the pier. A yoga instructor's commands blare at them from a stage's loudspeakers: "The universe is calling and your right leg is going to answer." The women extend their legs in unison, with military precision.

Usually, after a yoga class, everyone grabs their stuff and walks to their car, maybe chatting it up a bit with fellow classmates. But not here. The loudspeakers switch to club music, and the yoga class morphs into a rave. Women bounce up and down and headbang to Robyn. Their stainless steel water bottles become percussion instruments. Nobody is drunk, or high, or rolling—the only thing they've consumed recently is complimentary kombucha. Also: it's eleven o'clock in the morning.[1]

This is Wanderlust, a traveling wellness festival that bills itself as an "all-out celebration of mindful living." It goes from town to town, setting up pop-up outdoor fitness events like revival tents, drawing women together to bond, set personal goals, meditate, and revel in collective namaste vibes. Wanderlust is Coachella for healthy living, and like the famous desert concert, Wanderlust sells both tickets and sponsorships.

On the far side of the pier is an Adidas-sponsored lounge with an interactive art installation where you're invited to post a mantra to their website. A blond woman wearing Tory Burch workout gear offers her own: "To feel whole again." She then slips her Chanel handbag over her arm and proceeds to the yoga shopping fair.

New York, New York

The scents of bergamot and frankincense flow through a minimalist spa. White walls, light birchwood floors, soft gray furniture. Succulents in sparse pots. WTHN is not an East Coast radio station—it's a word that's pronounced "within," and it's the name of this soothing spa. Though "spa" isn't exactly the right word for this place. WTHN is the Drybar of acupuncture.

Traditional Chinese medicine is now as chic and as easy to book as a blowout. I've been afraid of needles all my life, but WTHN has made this ancient practice into a modern luxury experience, with women lining up to be pricked and prodded by a copious number of them. While a pampering acupuncture session for "mind + body relief" is the main item on the menu, WTHN also offers a blend of Chinese herbs to prevent stress and boost energy so you can "keep calm and rock on."

Several thirtysomething women crowd WTHN's bustling lobby. It's a weekday afternoon in January. Some are dressed in work attire, others wear stylish black wool coats. "I mean, *who isn't* exhausted?" says one woman, running her freshly manicured hands through her honey-highlighted hair. Several ailments brought her here: constant headaches, groggy mornings, and pervasive anxiety. An attendant calls her name, and she stands up, excited.

As the staff lead her to her own private cubicle, her voice echoes down the hallway. "I'm off to be relaxed!" The rest of us, waiting for our turn, are left to browse the impressive display of supplements.

Palm Desert, California

It's early fall and I'm at Ganja Goddess Getaway, a women-only weed retreat about a half hour outside Palm Springs. This self-described "stoner girl slumber party" is held on a rented equestrian estate where the event organizers expect you to be high the whole time. Most of the guests sleep in tents on the grounds; I get to sleep in a horse stall in the stable. (Don't worry—it's furnished like a hotel room.)

Weed is available, in large quantities and in many appetizing forms. There are cannabis-infused cotton candy machines, waitstaff holding trays of pre-rolled joints, cookies and brownies, and something you use for "dabbing." There is also an open snack bar in case you get the munchies.

It's a diverse crowd. At night, by the campfire, a young Black mom in her thirties trades parenting advice with a retired white trucker in her fifties. A twentysomething Latina decked out in athleisurewear talks politics with a sixtysomething former hippie. At dinner, I mention to a twenty-five-year-old at my table how refreshing it is to hang out with older women. "Yeah," she says, exhaling pot smoke. "They're chill." Then someone else excuses herself from the meal, explaining "My edible just kicked in." Everyone else nods in solidarity.[2]

At one point a soothing voice comes over the public address system. "The belly dancing class will start on the great lawn in five minutes." Then the voice adds, "I love you." A pair of millennials in bright tank tops sway lazily down to the lawn with a gray-haired woman in a floral housedress. Several women have crowns of flowers in their hair. One middle-aged mom gives up early and retires to lie down in the grass, where she sprawls and looks up at the sky in amazement.

"I feel like we live in a society that requires a lot of charging ahead, getting things done, and going on autopilot in order to accomplish a lot of tasks," the co-founder of Ganja Goddess Getaway told me. "We need this kind of a moment where you slow things down and really just focus on yourself."

. . .

These women—from the designer-attired Wanderlust participant to the cannabis campers—are just a few examples of the millions of women contributing to the $4.4 trillion global wellness economy. Far beyond yoga classes and veganism, they are modeling their entire lives—from where they live to whom they socialize with and how they parent—on the wellness lifestyle du jour.

What is "wellness," exactly? At its most basic level, it's the active pursuit of well-being outside the realm of medicine. It's more than just avoiding sickness; it encompasses prevention and maintenance: nutrition, fitness, sleep, community support, and stress management. It's the choices we make to feel better physically, mentally, socially, and spiritually.

Does it all sound a bit general and vague? That's because it is. There is no agreed-upon definition of what "well" is, and it's one reason why the wellness industry has grown so big. Plenty of companies have their own idea of how to get there—what you need to do, buy, or think—which is why the term "wellness" has devolved into an ambiguous marketing term that can just as easily mean activated charcoal toothpaste as it does mindfulness. Wellness can mean almost anything.

In many ways, wellness is whatever you need for your health. There's no one right path; wellness requires awareness of the uniqueness of your experience. It's about what you, the individual, can do for yourself to get through this thing we call life.

In Western countries like the UK, Australia and across Europe, entire industries have suddenly popped up around the desire to get healthier and live longer, but this has happened on a particularly large scale in the US. Small boutique fitness studios now comprise 40 percent of the gym market and have become *the place* for women to exercise and hang out. Sales of organic food top $60 billion a year. Once a fringe practice, meditation has seeped into mainstream American culture (to create a multibillion-dollar industry). Two-thirds of American women devote half of their closets to athleisurewear, and in the UK athleisure market is on track to be worth £6.7 billion in a few years.[3][4]

Wellness has taken over beauty, tech, and even housing and alcohol. Vitamin IV drip services are wait-listing customers; nightclubs serve booze-free herbal tonics; spiritual healers sell out workshops; real estate developers rush to build "wellness communities"; and Silicon Valley is pushing psychedelics as a mental health therapeutic. Even our language has changed. People say things like "I need this for my self-care," "I'm on a cleanse," or "I'm practicing gratitude." These slogans weren't around fifteen years ago. Now they're repeated by celebrities, business founders, suburban moms, and many a Gen Zer.

Of course, people have always bought things to help their well-being, but what we're witnessing today is an unprecedented cultural and historical moment. Wellness is a movement now. According to *NielsenIQ*, health and wellness was "the single most powerful consumer force of 2021."[5] Never before have we seen this level of focus on self-improvement, with U.S. millennials labeled the most "health-conscious generation."[6] We have become a self-care nation, though arguably one that still lacks the fundamentals of well-being.

Being "healthy" once meant going to the doctor regularly. Now it means you should rarely need to see a doctor. Wellness, in its current form, is almost an aspirational obsession for some and close to religious dogma for others. The average wellness devotee believes adherence to popularized methods can overcome sickness, unhappiness, and even death. A strict overhaul of diet, movement, and thoughts is hailed as the new messiah. In wellness, it seems, we trust.

• • •

When athleisure seized fashion in 2014, it coincided with other lifestyle trends of its time, like the proliferation of boutique fitness studios and cold-pressed juice bars. Back then, I was a thirty-one-year-old digital news producer at NBC News in New York City. I had an inkling that a cultural phenomenon was coming into place, which I chalked up to holed-up, tech-addicted millennials craving physical movement. But by 2017, when I began to cover the wellness industry full time as a business magazine reporter in L.A., I saw the emergence of far more trends—clean eating, "forest bathing," meditation retreats—with more age groups joining the fold. Suddenly, it wasn't just your New Age pal in Venice Beach raving about bone broth. It was most of your friends too. Sometimes it was your mom. Or your boss.

Women flocked to these trends with urgency and intensity. They went fully organic, bought ClassPass subscriptions, and replaced dairy milk with soaked almond water. This wasn't just something they did, but something that soon came to define them. All these new habits and products made them believe they could change things. In their minds, things weren't good—and they hadn't been in a while.

I know. Because, you see . . . I am one of these women.

I mean, who doesn't want a bit of aspiration in their lives? I know I did. I wasn't any more immune to the industry's charm than any other adherent. My life was consumed by wellness. It determined how I spent my weekends, picked where I vacationed, dictated which restaurants I frequented, and prescribed my "natural" medications. I spent, on average, hundreds of dollars a month bolstering my health—a good chunk of it on expensive boutique fitness classes.

My pantry, meanwhile, was stocked with "natural" wine. My diet incorporated "superfoods" and organic vegetables. These items elbowed for room in the fridge alongside sparkling cannabis beverages and egg-free Vegenaise. Even my dog was on the trend: I sprinkled his dry food with canine-approved bone broth. (In my defense, it was on sale.)

Today I own five crystals, an interactive smart home gym called a

Mirror, and an entire shoebox of skin care facial masks. Twelve pairs of yoga leggings—half of them accompanied by matching sports bras. Two aromatherapy devices. And six different kinds of bath salts. (I don't even own a bathtub. I used to bring them with me on vacations, filtering hotels according to tub availability.) It's all a bit odd because, by all accounts, I was never technically sick: I have no chronic diseases or disabilities, and I receive a clean bill of health every time I visit my general practitioner. So why all these rituals? Why all this stuff?

Because at the time I started down this path I didn't *feel* good.

Rewind to thirty-one-year-old me in New York City circa 2014. From afar, it sounded like the dream: single, living in a big city, and working for the *Today* show, the number one morning show in America. It was the kind of thing you could tell people at a cocktail party and they were often excited to hear more. "Do you get to meet every celebrity?" they'd always ask.

The truth of it was less than intriguing. I worked long, fast-paced workweeks tied to a desk in a windowless office with no real lunch break. By early evening, I was utterly depleted. At one point during my seven-year tenure, I had to undergo four months of physical therapy for a painful bout of tendinitis (which I feared would cost me my job). Typing nonstop for eight to ten hours a day left my wrists in agony, to the point where I could no longer massage shampoo into my hair.

Exhausted by stressful workdays in a 24/7 news environment, I'd order Thai food to my poorly heated studio apartment, then cuddle up on the couch to watch *Downton Abbey*. Most nights I was too tired to see friends, let alone make new ones. Loneliness became as routine as a bum radiator. I was also in my thirties, getting older, and increasingly nervous about my vanity, or more like, nervous about what losing my looks and figure *meant*. I saw how both higher-weight individuals and the aging were treated in the media industry and dating scene—and it was far from kind.

Ageism, unfortunately, is prevalent within journalism. I was at the

Today show when it booted a tearful Ann Curry as co-host to make room for a peppy Savannah Guthrie, fifteen years her junior. It was eerily quiet in the newsroom that morning, the producers fearful to talk lest they say something they'd regret. Then came the commands to start scrubbing Curry from the website. Photo albums, talent holiday recaps . . . it was as if she'd never existed.

Not too long after, my boss and mentor was forced out after her maternity leave and replaced by a younger, less experienced manager who was promoted while subbing for her. Although it seemed like blatant discrimination, she was told by her attorney she would have no luck with a lawsuit. The rest of us got the message: Don't age. Stay young. Keep your job.

It was a brutal blood sport, and one I wasn't prepared to engage in. Probably because I was so tired.

And what did wellness offer? Solutions.

Wellness promised me food that could deliver more energy *and* keep me thin. Supplements dangled better sleep when I lay awake wondering whether I'd die alone. A fitness class hinted I didn't need to make plans to see friends—*they'd just be there.* Meditation advertised a silencing of all the "dying" journalism industry woes clogging my brain. Wellness said it could fix me, like a toy that was not so much broken as in need of new batteries. And I wanted to believe it.

It would be dishonest to say that I was wooed by wellness as much as I was searching for remedies. Too many things in my life started to feel diseased. I couldn't always put my finger on it, but I started to suspect there was something fundamentally unhealthy about the way I was living. The work stress, the greasy takeout food, the endless, soul-crushing dating . . . I was actively looking to manage all of it. I was open to alternatives. And wellness brands spoke my language; they understood full well there were real issues impacting people just like me. People who felt depleted, frustrated, isolated, and nervous. People who needed a boost.

My conversion didn't happen overnight. I fought this culture for so long. I rolled my eyes and teased pals about trends like mushroom coffee, yet soon enough I found myself at the cash register, admitting defeat. That's because it was no longer countercultural—*it was the culture*. As they say, it happened slowly at first, and then all at once. I increasingly became further consumed with my health, like some sort of lab rat awaiting testing. It was fun and seemingly vital: yoga felt good, but it was also a *very important* mental health tool. Could a fitness tracker help me move more? Let's try! Cupping reportedly relieved muscle tension, and heck, everyone else was doing it. Surely there's something there?

In 2015, I moved from New York to L.A. for simple reasons: I wanted warmer weather and I envied what looked like a healthier, chiller lifestyle. On the West Coast, I saw people jogging outside year-round. They gulped green juice the way my New York pals downed tequila at after-work happy hours. On weekends, Angelenos favored hikes in Runyon Canyon over shopping and brunching. (If they did shop, it was at Whole Foods.) It seemed, at the time, like a promised land where everyone felt better.

A little over a year later, I was writing full time for *Fast Company*, a progressive business magazine centered on innovation in tech, leadership, and design. I mostly wrote about fashion and food, but the more I got into the L.A. lifestyle, the more my pitches reflected my metamorphosis. So that same year, my editor agreed to let me cover the sector entirely, going so far as to let me launch a newsletter about the latest developments in wellness.

"Why is everyone guzzling kombucha, buying DNA kits, and downloading meditation apps now?" I wrote in the announcement for my newsletter, *Well To Do*. "Are these inventions and new pursuits actually helping people? Do they even work?" These are questions I would spend the next four years answering. Not only for *Fast Company*, but for outlets like the *L.A. Times*, the *New York Times*, Medium's *Elemental*, and wellness research institutes. I wanted to know why there were so many women just like me, looking to exhale.

Over the years, I tried out innovative ideas like a texting therapy bot. I investigated Facebook's war on alternative health groups. I profiled beauty brands selling "athleisure makeup," that is, mascara and foundation designed to be worn in the gym. I also tested out the more ridiculous— including a "sleep robot" (which was more like a faceless Teddy Ruxpin for insomniacs) and, no joke, sleep-friendly ice cream. My job took me to brain optimization labs and to the flotation tank studios expanding across the country.

I got to know a lot of communities. In a remote ski resort in Utah, I got to spend time with the tech elite building the exclusive wellness community of the future. In rural Alabama, I spent a weekend at a utopian commune for women only. Another time, I attended an "overcoming death" conference where scientists and hopeful senior citizens believed they could crack the code on immortality (and which honestly felt like the sequel to *Get Out*).

I interviewed Gwyneth Paltrow, biohacking icon Dave Asprey, Peloton founder John Foley, and also femtech founders fighting to discover new medical solutions. I watched as their influence quickly grew to reach beyond America to keen audiences in the UK, Australia and elsewhere. I also spoke with women across the country who were suddenly doing things like shunning dairy, but they weren't exactly sure why. Others felt they had a new lease on life as soon as they found a gym they loved.

But a funny thing happened a few years in: my thoughts on the industry changed. Quite dramatically. What had first begun as fitness, nutrition, and stress relief increasingly gave way to muddy waters: crystal-infused water bottles, "detox cleanses," and shady workplace wellness programs. After interviewing countless founders and trying out every trend under the sun, I grew skeptical. Out of curiosity, but also out of journalistic duty, I started doing my homework. By then, I had left the hamster wheel of digital news production and was afforded more time to dive deeper into the issues that wellness brands raised.

I called up medical professionals to investigate health claims. I checked chemical concerns with scientists. I started asking everyone just how their CBD collection was working out. I read the fine print.

I began realizing I couldn't take many of these companies at face value. Their marketing promises didn't align with science. The evidence was paltry or, at times, wildly exaggerated. Influencers with market growth agendas jumped to fearmongering conclusions far too fast. More than that, they were instituting their own pressures on women. The wellness industry isn't quite what we are led to believe. And surprise, surprise, many of the "facts" we take for granted about what's healthy and what isn't aren't true.

That's because wellness is often treated a lot more like fashion in the media. It's not always pressed upon reporters to investigate wellness companies' claims.

It's easy to fall into the marketing over accurate science trap: so much of what a wellness company's PR department puts out *sounds* right. And I was working for *Fast Company*, not *Scientific American* magazine. My readers cared about investor funding. Market share. Creative campaigns. Forward-thinking design. The science wasn't ignored, rather it was just secondary.

But at some point, there was a more general reckoning with the mission statements of VC-funded brands out there to "change the world," and the founders we'd previously revered to godly proportions. The *Wall Street Journal* released its groundbreaking investigative report on the now defunct company Theranos and its deceptive practices, and we all began examining Silicon Valley leaders' claims more closely.

I'll level with you: you might not like some of the stuff I unearthed throughout this process. I say that because I too was hesitant. It can all be quite jarring if you've only ever been exposed to one side of an equation. I didn't want to admit what became increasingly obvious: we've been conditioned to accept certain wellness beliefs, cemented as conventional wisdom because they're ubiquitous. We're bombarded by wellness propaganda—in our magazines, social media feeds, and Sephora stores. Marketing has a far stronger power than scientific proof. Few of us follow scientists, but we sure as hell follow celebrities, influencers, and brands that are in no way health experts but sure act like them.

The more I learned, the more alarmed I became. As a reporter, I had to admit the obvious: the wellness industry isn't well.

• • •

In this book, I examine how and why Western women were led down the kale-covered path of wellness, looking to America as the starting point for an industry swiftly replicated in wealthy countries around the globe. Part investigative report and part sociological analysis, this book dives deep into this booming movement, going inside the sprawling landscape of wellness to explore how and why it grew to be the behemoth it is today. I analyze the solutions it offers, and the dangers—but also the possible promise—it holds for the future of our health. Many people assume wellness is simply the desire to be thin or to purify our lives, and while there are aspects of that, such a simplistic interpretation would be naive. There are far more facets to this movement, each demonstrating long-simmering discontent and hopes.

This book is about commodified wellness: the big business of selling you health. The marketing of wellness has inspired a religious fervor—and not in a good way. This industry communicates the idea that with enough devotion, we can manifest only goodness and manage what feels unruly or threatening in our lives—an idea that works almost like a divine principle. This book's title is rather tongue-in-cheek, but it does allude to how health has emerged as a regulatory framework, much like religion, telling us *how to live*. Sometimes these comparisons are subtle, but at times blatant. But make no mistake: the gospel of wellness has its own commandments, its own morality, its own community, and its own rituals.

It also has its own false idols. These golden calves indoctrinate women with false beliefs: pseudoscience, distrust of medicine, and unnecessary pressures robbing them of time and energy. And we need to combat these beliefs before they devolve into a full-blown cult. In wellness, the cure occasionally becomes worse than the disease.

The gospel of wellness spans multiple sectors and draws on a complex web of cultural and political forces for its sustenance. This book could have been a multivolume set—there is that much to talk about. Many of my examples focus on the biggest pillars of wellness, including nutrition, exercise, stress management, and spirituality. But know that any of the specific examples I delve into from one area teach lessons that can be applied elsewhere.

It's a lot of ground to cover. While I understand wellness is a fast-growing sector now spreading to multiple communities and income brackets, the majority of this book focuses on the groups most adoptive of commodified wellness—namely women. This is not to say men aren't also participating, just that women are more heavily represented, for reasons such as gender equity gaps and the specific roles of women in society. Naturally, not every reason discussed will apply to every woman—wellness is a massive, vague umbrella term with numerous sectors, so some might be more relevant than others to any individual woman. But if it doesn't reflect you, I bet it sums up someone you know.

This book traces not only the many segments of the industry and how they got here, but also the historic trends that planted the seeds of what was to come. You'll see sidebars that delve into a related historic episode in line with each chapter's theme. History shows that so many of these issues and solutions aren't anything new: we've been dealing with the same problems (and like-minded gurus) for centuries. Everything that seems innovative today possesses a long, rich history.

Here's what we do know: Wellness—in all its many forms and bizarre rituals—springs from universal truths. Everyone just wants to feel good, and that's becoming harder and harder as modern life becomes more chaotic. Too much feels out of control: a poorly constructed medical system, tech overload, a tumultuous news cycle, lack of community, *you name it*. We live lives that demand too much of us. Wellness, which spans both real, groundbreaking solutions and total bunk, is the direct response to genuine complaints in this country. Something is rotten in the state of Denmark, and wellness, we believe, might heal it. The question is whether what we're being sold is delivering. Can wellness truly solve these issues?

At the end of the day, I come neither to bury nor to praise the wellness industry. My goal is to help sort the wheat from the chaff, to distinguish the legitimate benefits from the marketing copy, and to identify those which only add more stress or sickness. In the quest to minimize what bothers us, wellness has both empowered and enslaved women. The more effectively we can disentangle the good from the bad, the more promising a future we can create for the movement—and for our well-being.

This is more than a book about a rapidly growing industry. It's a book about women's search for a cure to all that ails them—and their journey to regain something they believe they've lost. They've discovered a new agency to chart different paths and search for better solutions. They are reimagining community, medicine, even faith. They are standing up to say, *The status quo isn't acceptable.* There must be a better way through.

Chapter 1

Why the Hell Is the Advice Always Yoga?

Can you remember the last time you felt *free?* Do you recall a time in which you weren't consumed by text notifications, computer install updates, grocery lists, school pick-ups and drop-offs, work emails, the news, and shedding "those last ten pounds"? Remember giving less of a shit? Being psychologically unburdened? And relaxed?

Neither do many other women. Modern life, for all its comforts and privileges, can feel wildly overwhelming. To be a woman today is to be stuck in a loop of unrelenting maintance.

I am, by all accounts, not a chill person. Type A is a more accurate description. My husband likes to motion for me "to take it down a notch" whenever I'm riled up by politics, line cutters, or nonsensical fashion. This is partially due to my own makeup but partially bred out of a chaotic career existence. And yes, let me preface all this by saying that I am overall a very fortunate person who is housed, fed, and not stuck in a war-torn country. I am lucky, 100 percent.

But by my midthirties, I'd become loaded with stress, even for Type A me. I worked as a full-time reporter at *Fast Company* with set hours and was expected to participate in Slack channels, conferences, news shifts, and company-wide initiatives. I even had my own newsletter and represented the outlet at industry conferences. But I wasn't granted any benefits, health insurance, or paid time off. For years I wasn't technically on staff even though I functionally was. Like many others, I'd become a gig worker with none of the "freedom" of a freelancer and none of the assurances of a staff employee. A permalancer. I had a contract stipulating a specific number of stories, but it could be canceled within two weeks' notice. This put me and my fellow writers in a perpetual state of job insecurity, of having to constantly prove ourselves to our "employer."

As a gig worker, taking a vacation or sick leave is out of the question. You aren't paid for any days you aren't working. Thinking about having kids? Forget it. If you can barely afford two weeks off, who is going to pay for your maternity leave?

Mind you, I wasn't about to start complaining, because by 2017, the journalism industry was in free fall as advertising money dried up. I was coming off previous positions where I saw budgets slashed, reasonable freelance wages disappear, and entire teams decimated. Site traffic—not necessarily quality—reigned supreme. Aggregation replaced original reporting. Ad sponsorship commitments steered content decisions. The sensational trumped the meaningful. *Be more like BuzzFeed*, we were told. *Churn, churn, churn.*

At those previous jobs, fewer bodies meant more work. It meant you had to be trendspotter, writer, editor, newsletter aficionado, sponsorship deal creative, contributor manager, media partner liaison, social media savant . . . an entire team in one body. And as digital journalism became more competitive, we had to follow our beats as soon as the "workday" ended. If I wasn't at my desk, I was on Twitter or on blogs trying to keep up with a twenty-four-hour news cycle. Sometimes I'd do my after-hours "research" while I was at the gym—one sweaty, slipping hand on the elliptical machine, the other scrolling my phone—trying to ensure that neither my career nor my body would fall by the wayside.

You couldn't complain. You were told you were fortunate just to have a job in journalism.

I was burned out at this point in my career. The stress was building, the anxiety seeping out sideways into other areas of my life. This was on top of everything else I worried about. As a Jew, I was anxious about rising rates of anti-Semitism. (By 2017, Jews were targeted in 58 percent of all religious-based hate crime incidents despite being just *2 percent* of the U.S. population.)[1] Then there was concern over reproductive rights, the growing political divide, and so on and so on.

It all kept me up at night. It was in my thirties that I'd stopped sleeping and shortly thereafter began suffering from anxiety. Which is how I found myself looking for stress relief—and major emotional release. Mind you, I was already dipping my toes in wellness at the time. This just heightened my need for it.

I found it one day tucked away on the third floor of a small and unremarkable brick building in Tribeca. Soothing neutral palettes and a wall of mirrors filled this airy fitness studio. Below one's feet, the wood floor rested atop a layer of rose quartz crystals. (Even if clients don't see the crystals, the hope is that they feel the "vibrational energy.") Right outside the studio doors, a bathroom boasted marble counters, modern gold-plated fixtures, and Chanel bath products. Inspirational tunes by Florence and the Machine set the pace for this class called The Class.

Thirty toned women in Lululemon sports bras and leggings stood silent, their flat tummies on display. Eyes closed, they placed their right hands firmly on their hearts. In this pose, they patiently awaited the command of their instructor, the fitness guru Taryn Toomey, who would lead them through a "meditation, just with your body."

This self-described "cathartic mind-body experience" serves as an unorthodox therapy session. Here, women are encouraged to yell, shout, scream, and express themselves while also doing challenging cardio moves. At other points, they're told to stand still and quiet the mind. The

Class centers around emotional management, which is why class names echo women's late-night venting sessions: I Love My Kids Just Not Right Now (give me a break!), F*CK Everything (when everyone and everything seems like the absolute worst), and the I Don't Wanna Workout (don't make me work out!).

Toomey, a blond, lithe, statuesque figure with the raspy voice of a Kathleen Turner, addressed the room while perched on a window ledge overlooking the Lower Manhattan skyline. "We're out of our bodies most of the day," Toomey said. "It's time for a reunion." The crowd nodded in agreement. Some looked genuinely touched.

Together, the crowd furiously squatted and shook, all while repeatedly shouting "Huh!" in tribal chorus. From there, the women contorted themselves into winged positions, their arms outstretched. They breathed heavily as their leader urged them to "rise up."

Midway through a medley of jumping jacks, lunges, and burpees, Toomey's voice intensified, taking on new gravitas. "What are your blinders?" Toomey demanded. "Your blocks—what are they?" Her voice got even louder, like a commanding priest. "What are they? What are they?!" As if hitting the crescendo at an opera, she shouted with gusto, "Feel! Feel! Feel!"

The room lost it. The session devolved into a rave as the Prodigy's electronic music anthem "Firestarter" roared over the speakers. Some class members moaned like birthing animals, while others shook their limbs with the spastic fervor of inflatable air dancers outside used car dealerships. One jumped wildly in place, tears rolling down her cheeks, as she yelled. Others frantically thrust their arms into the air, their $4,450 Cartier Love bracelets jangling. Rage, grief, and frustration were suspended in the sweat-mixed-with-Chanel-moistened air.

"This is a safe space," Toomey whispered.

Toomey at times can come across as a therapeutic healer, a cross between Deepak Chopra and Jane Fonda. "You start to realize that most of what's going on [in the body] is in the mind," Toomey told me. "And you know that you actually have a choice, and you can reroute it—that's what we do in The Class: we practice the ability to do that." That type of thinking is part of Toomey's appeal: a splash of the woo-woo grounded in the practical, incorporating her self-help messages within tried-and-true elements of mainstream fitness. She is completely aware that metaphysical and spiritual practices can seem foreign, and she makes the effort to render them more accessible to consumers without alienating her more Goopy fans. Her studio's crystal-embedded floors, for example, are alleged to "cleanse" bad energy. Despite spending thousands of dollars on them, Toomey will quickly label herself as a "pretty big skeptic." When asked whether she believes in crystals' supposed healing properties, she says she believes the most important healing element is the "power of intention."

Toomey created this new kind of workout after realizing she loved the meditative component of yoga as a way of connecting with her breathing but also craved the endorphin rush of cardio routines. The result is a mix of quiet reflection with bursts of fast movement. Sound is another component. She noticed that whether or not she vocalized what was bottled up inside made a difference in how she felt. Getting loud—*really* loud—was a catharsis of sorts.

Toomey built a cult following around this unique, visceral form of exercise—if you could even call it strictly exercise. Is it meditation? Athletic vocalization? Calorie-burning primal scream therapy? Celebrities like Naomi Watts swear by the $35 sessions. Ask New Yorkers to describe The Class, and they'll call it "a brain-body release," "an emotional workout," and "a spiritually orgasmic exercise." One participant simply explained it by saying, "Sometimes you just need to yell, ya know?"[2]

I definitely did know.

For almost two years, I was a regular at the L.A. outpost of The Class, surrounded by several dozen women who, by all accounts, seemed to have it together.

During one session, The Class took it up a notch. It was the Sunday following the Supreme Court confirmation of Brett Kavanaugh, who had earlier been accused of sexual misconduct by a former classmate, California professor Christine Blasey Ford. Liberal-leaning women tended to view the proceedings in a certain way: they saw a woman take the stand, be doubted by the public, then be torn apart. Acknowledging the week's news, the instructor led the entire room in a sing-along of the 4 Non Blondes song "What's Up." Participants thrust their arms forward and back—rowing without an oar—as the lyrics demanded,

And I scream from the top of my lungs
What's going on?

The room erupted in song, women shouting at the top of their lungs, turning their faces to the ceiling as if to summon the heavens to rescue them. Some pounded their fists in the air as though they were punching ghosts. "I pray every single day for revolution," they bellowed along with the 1993 hit single. The emotion was palpable. It was unlike anything I had ever seen, perhaps only rivaled by the kind of Christian revival faith healings I've seen depicted in movies.

After the class, I approached a few of the women about the intensity we had just witnessed. The Class skews older millennial—women in their thirties and forties, many of them moms or midcareer professionals. The atmosphere felt unreal, certainly not the norm for a nine a.m. workout class. "[The confirmation was] the last straw," said one woman in line at the studio's café. "We are broken camels."

How could it be, I wondered, that so many "privileged" women were so exasperated? What *was* going on? This was much larger than just my own anxiety. A simmering cauldron of frustration had come to a boiling point, and somehow it was exploding on a pastel-colored yoga mat. It couldn't just be the political situation inspiring such an outpouring. These women had evidently come to class to express their grievances, and no amount of sage was going to clear up that kind of toxic energy. But when and why did squats and burpees, among other wellness activities, become therapy?

Drowning in Stress: Not Enough Time or Support to "Have it All"

Women are overwhelmed. I hear it over and over and over again from folks across the country, on all sides of the political and social divide. They can be stressed by PTA meetings and ever-rising childcare costs or by a never-ending stream of work coupled with growing piles of laundry. They can be single, drowning in student loan debts and unbelievable housing prices. They might be college students, 40 percent of whom report being so stressed and depressed that "it's difficult to function," according to the American College Health Association. Or perhaps they're graduates hitting LinkedIn's virtual pavement (with little success) or moms struggling to find the time to "sneak in" a shower. Expectations continue to mount, yet they're barely able to tread the rough waters.

Of course, men are also overstretched, but women experience a particular strain of stress, and if recent surveys are to be believed, experience far more of it. Almost half of American women say their stress levels increased over the past five years (compared to 39 percent of men) and that anxiety keeps them up at night. And despite the benefits of coupledom, the legally bound seem to carry a heavier load: more than one-third of married women report managing "a great deal of stress" versus 22 percent of unattached women.[3]

The home is one of the bigger battlegrounds in the war between the sexes. The average woman spends two more hours each day than the average man cooking, cleaning, and caretaking,[4] and nearly two-thirds of women say they bear the responsibility for most of the chores.[5] They are constantly multitasking, holding a laptop with one hand and a Swiffer in the other. That unequal distribution of work affects them in multiple ways. Women have less time to focus on their careers, get involved in politics, kvetch to their friends, or heck, go to therapy. In one survey, 60 percent said the one person they never had enough time for was *themselves*.[6]

Stressed as they are at home, work, at least anecdotally, appears to also be one of women's chief complaints. Americans work the longest hours of all the industrialized nations, with the average workweek clocking in at forty-seven hours.[7] Germany, in comparison, averages thirty-five hours. The land of the free is also the only advanced economy that doesn't guarantee workers paid time off, whereas European Union members mandate at least twenty days of paid leave.[8] Three out of four women suffer from burnout, defined as emotional, physical, and mental exhaustion caused by excessive stress. Just how bad is it? One survey discovered that 48 percent of employees have cried at work, and while women are more inclined to break down in tears over stress, 36 percent of men also acknowledged crying on the job.[9] That's because day-to-day work is an exhausting obstacle course of stressors. Further, the stress often doesn't end once you leave the office: an "always-on" environment encourages bosses to email you at any time. Knowing a ping of anxiety could be incoming at all hours, there is no real end to the workday.

One might tell women to just find other jobs if their workplaces don't support them, but in this economy? It's not so easy. Few options are available in what's become a cutthroat race for well-paying, full-time employment with solid benefits. Job insecurity and a growing gig economy put the American dream ever-teetering on a pinnacle, always on the verge of tipping over. We're not hustling to get ahead as much as to just stay put and pay off our student loan debt—or the mortgage.

A wide cross section of women battle stress, though their wounds differ. Caretaking responsibilities within the office—organizing birthday celebrations, mentoring new hires, mediating disputes between co-workers—often fall to female managers with little acknowledgment. Childless women complain they're routinely expected to work longer hours than caregiving peers, and they feel insulted that management assumes they have no life after six o'clock. Maybe they too would like to leave at a reasonable hour so that they could tend to personal matters or just do whatever it is that fulfills them? Maybe they have a date?

Not that dating necessarily generates stress relief: many singles report they need to compete in a *Hunger Games*–like scene where individuals "swipe" their way through an endless supply of mates, where chasing "something better on the horizon" is as easy as ordering a pizza. Those wading through the dating circuit can get caught up in a shallow hookup culture, which some researchers link to lowered self-esteem. (Almost 50 percent of women report a negative reaction after a fling, versus 26 percent of men.) However you identify—gay, straight, whatever—casual sex may not always be as fun and carefree as *Sex and the City* would have us believe. While some do enjoy a buffet of one-night stands, others might experience depressive symptoms and loneliness.[10]

As for parents, the storm of stress elevates to a Category 5 hurricane: the average mom claims an 8.5 out of 10 on a scale of stress, positioning them somewhere between a Cathy cartoon and a ticking time bomb. A leading cause of stress is time. Sixty percent of moms say they simply can't squeeze in everything on their to-do list, which usually amounts to planning a nutritious dinner, helping with children's homework, organizing the social calendar, and oh, also staying fit and attractive. In addition to all that, 72 percent of moms are stressed about how stressed they are.[11]

Delving into why the American woman is about to burn down her white picket fence would undoubtedly fill volumes. But suffice it to say that one major reason is that she is in no way living the utopian dream envisioned by feminists past. Women are not equal in status nor immune from sexism, and they are still burdened by the domestic assumptions made by society. Our foremothers burned their bras and filed for divorce en masse, but that didn't release Betty Draper from pot roast duty. College girls dreamed of being Tina Fey or Ruth Bader Ginsburg, then found themselves soothing male egos in the boardroom or arguing with their spouse over whose turn it was to carpool.

While middle- to upper-middle-class women are technically liberated, for many their situation feels like further imprisonment: now they need to be both *Working Girl* and June Cleaver. Their life is nonstop emails and baby tantrums; they have two jobs but the respect of one. This is what the renowned sociologist Arlie Hochschild in 1989 termed "the second shift," by which Western women inherit a double-career life. They'll work a full day at the office, commute in traffic back home, hang up their coat, then run into the phone booth to transform into Superhousewife. The current hyperproductive and performative nature of American life is likely to blame. We're on a constant treadmill of doing way more than a normal human would have aspired to do until recently: attain career success, birth two kids, achieve a slamming body, cook like Ina Garten . . . You get the idea.

Futher compounding the issue, the days of living off a single income are long gone; as the cost of living increases and wages stagnate, both partners need to bring home the Beyond Meat bacon.

But again, there's the rub: as the average American increasingly needs to work long and sometimes unpredictable hours at demanding jobs, who is going to manage caregiving? When the workday doesn't end until six, who fixes dinner? How can you make partner at the law firm when you need to scuttle out at a reasonable hour? *Someone* needs to hold down the fort. Someone needs to take care of the kids. Not everyone has relatives nearby who can pitch in and provide free babysitting. And not everyone can afford paid childcare. This is not a predicament exclusive to women raising children with men. Same-sex couples also deal with one partner who inevitably needs to pick up the slack at home.

We may have fought the good fight for women's careers, but as Hochschild observed, "The workplace they go into and the men they come home to have changed less rapidly, or not at all. Nor has the government given them policies that would ease the way, like paid parental leave, paid family medical leave, or subsidized child care—the state-of-the-art child care, that too is stalled."[12] In essence, women changed, but many men, employers, and the government simply put up their feet. They see women struggle to scoot out of the office before children's bedtimes. They hear the exhaustion of those pumping breast milk in their cubicle. But bosses just put another meeting on their calendars. In 2019, a Pew Research survey confirmed what everyone already knew: half of employed moms say being a working parent makes it harder for them to get ahead professionally.[13]

The COVID-19 pandemic only intensified this workload, exposing deep cracks in the system. With schools closed, moms quickly found themselves juggling work Zooms while trying to help their first-grader log in to class. Mothers scrambled to monitor the kids, keep up with double or triple the dirty dishes, and then somehow appear alert during department meetings. In between all of that, they had to stave off a virus that kept them away from friends and family. A significant portion also had to manage eldercare for their aging parents. Their lives, like their wardrobes, began unraveling. They wiped their hands on their sweatpants, looked all around, and asked, *How?*

We might have hit a breaking point. By the fall of 2020, not even one year into the pandemic, 865,000 U.S. women surrendered and handed in their resignation.[14] The number was roughly four times more than the number of men, thereby further contributing to a gender disparity in corporate America. One mom, a friend of a friend, wrote on Facebook, "I've basically abandoned my career that I've worked for 15 years to build in order to care for my kids and give them an education. It's crazy."

An obvious fact that needs to be stated: some groups have it way harder than others, dealing with a wide array of stressors on top of the average American experience. One 2020 survey found that Latino and Black adults have experienced twice as much economic hardship as white adults during the pandemic. They also face more discrimination and greater mental health issues, and they do so with fewer resources.[15] As one co-founder of a meditation program for Black communities once told me: "We joke that [mainstream outlets] always try to get you to calm down in your commute. Our communities are dealing with a lot more things than just a hard commute."

Worn out by the daily grind and greater injustices, women seek solutions. During the last few years, breath work instructor Jay Bradley has drawn in far more female than male clients, many of them high-achievers who say they've tried everything to relax—pharmaceuticals, therapy, or "spiritual work"—but nothing's worked in the long term. These women are, by his account, depleted, demoralized, and discouraged. They are driven but feel unable to "accomplish it all." Bradley's clients are afraid if they let go *just a little*, everything will all fall apart. They express an "underlying unworthiness," says Bradley, who believes it stems from unhealthy boundaries surrounding work or family in addition to self-imposed expectations. This ongoing struggle leaves them "feeling powerful one day and then feeling powerless [the next]."

In his group sessions, Bradley acknowledges how well participants take care of everyone else. "Women, in particular, give, give, give," Bradley tells his class. He encourages clients to spend the session to truly focus on one person and one person only: themselves. Through breath work, they can hopefully release whatever worries occupy their headspace, maybe even practice some self-compassion. At the same time, says Bradley, they are "ready for something that will permanently shift them out of that fight-or-flight mode."

Women often voice that they need some time out, a Sabbath, a rest (though preferably not in a corporate nap room). They instinctively feel the urge to pull away and indulge in some self-care—a term that hit record Google searches in 2020. Some decide to waste a few minutes checking their Instagram, only to face an onslaught of clean kitchens and photoshopped bodies. What should have been a break turns into additional pressure. The same technology that was supposed to ease our lives is now arguably ruling them. Indeed, Americans who check their phones most frequently report the highest levels of anxiety. As soon as they wake up, they're assaulted by a barrage of texts, then spend eight hours or more staring at a work computer screen, followed by incoming emails and breaking news alerts in the evenings. It never ends. What's more, tech companies increasingly add more addictive features and design infinite ways to keep us hooked or "bingeing." I once heard Netflix CEO Reed Hastings deliver a conference speech in which he flat-out said he was competing not with HBO, FX, or Amazon, but with . . . sleep. "And we're winning!" he exclaimed to rapturous applause.

Well, guess what sleep deprivation causes? Fatigue, irritability, and stress.

Women are looking for *less* in their life. Less noise, fewer tasks, and reduced pressure. Self-care is marketed as the exit strategy. It's become so popular that the Instagram hashtag #selfcare grew to 60 million posts, and self-care is one of the top downloaded app categories. But what exactly are we being sold? And to what extent are these practices helpful?

Flashback: Running Free: "Exercise Is the Best Tranquilizer"

James Fixx had settled into the sedentary American lifestyle by 1967. The magazine editor took public transportation to work, where he was stuck in an office all day working long, stressful hours. To blow off steam, he smoked two packs of cigarettes a day. By his midthirties, he was unhappy with his weight and his habits.

Recognizing he was out of shape, Fixx tried running, and to his amazement, it made him feel significantly better. Running on an empty road became a therapeutic nirvana: quiet time to think, go at your preferred pace, and be free of distractions. In a domineering society, in which one is constantly being told what to do, wear, or think, running became an appealing way to assert some autonomy, to symbolically run away from "the chains of civilization."[16]

In speaking with runners across the country, Fixx noticed that many reported that anxiety, depression, and ruminating thoughts melted away as they hit mile after mile. Divorced men claimed it worked as "an ideal antidepressant." Women reportedly said they were "less cranky and bitchy." Fixx quoted one doctor who stated, "exercise is the best tranquilizer."

Fixx felt called to share his miracle cure, no doubt the work of endorphins and exercise's ability to reduce stress hormones. Soon enough, he inspired Americans to do something they'd never done before: jog. Before then, running constituted a gym class chore or an army requirement. In the late sixties, the activity was so unusual that police would stop running "freaks" for disturbing the suburban peace.[17] Bemused pedestrians hurled insults, and sometimes trash.

James Fixx changed all that. Considered the father of recreational running, his bestseller *The Complete Book of Running* became the bible of newly minted joggers. The handbook sparked a jogging revolution, prompting *People* magazine to label it a "craze" on a 1977 cover featuring Farrah Fawcett in gym shorts.

Was it just the stress relief and freedom of the road? Or something more?

Some historians have a different theory: Americans turn to fitness during stressful times.[18] They took up exercising in greater numbers during the Great Depression, throughout the tumultuous seventies, after 9/11, and during the COVID-19 pandemic.[19] Starting in 2002, boutique gyms exploded in popularity. Some industry experts believe the World Trade Center terrorist attacks spurred Americans into an existential crisis overnight. They wondered: Could being reminded of one's mortality inspire a desire to want to live longer, better? Does caring for our health make us feel more grounded? I've heard this idea from several researchers (as well as crystal sellers, who saw sales soar after 9/11).

Rhythmic exercise routines are indeed calming. Intentional repetitive actions can redirect focus away from anxious and depressive thoughts, lulling us into a relaxing trance. Researchers have also found that repetitive, ritualistic behavior can increase people's belief that they can manage situations that are otherwise out of their hands.[20]

In addition, as your body image improves, so do your confidence and sense of mastery. For women, this often also correlates with societal body size pressures. (Historically, women didn't have control over many aspects of their lives, but they could determine their size.) Perhaps it's a false sense of control, but people will grasp at whatever tools they have at their disposal.

"I felt more in control of my life," Fixx said. "I was less easily rattled by unexpected frustrations. I had a sense of quiet power, and if at any time I felt this power slipping away I could easily call it back by going out and running."[21]

Just Sweat Off the Stress?

"Your mobile phone is ringing. Your boss wants to talk to you. And your partner wants to know what's for dinner," reads the Mayo Clinic website. "Stress and anxiety are everywhere. If they're getting the best of you, you might want to hit the mat and give yoga a try."

The esteemed institution praises yoga's ability to help lower blood pressure, manage lower back pain, and "quiet your mind." The Mayo Clinic joins a wide array of outlets vouching for the workout's ability to modulate stress response systems. (Of the many different types of yoga, I am sticking to the mainstream American adaptation for the purposes of this book.) The wellness site *Well+Good* reports that when it comes to stress, "one thing that works *without fail* for almost anyone is yoga." The *New York Times* published a guide on "How to Use Yoga to Destress."

If you haven't read the dozens of headlines extolling yoga, then you've likely heard celebrities swearing by it. Reese Witherspoon relies on it before the chaos of award show season. Miranda Kerr says the daily practice keeps her grounded and calm. Lady Gaga does it in a thong. Yoga has become so popular that almost 37 million Americans hit the mat regularly, and of those, 72 percent are women.[22] They come across soothing fitness gurus like Adriene Mishler of the hit YouTube channel *Yoga with Adriene* and like what they hear. Instead of body transformation talk, all the approachable yogi asks is that you love yourself, find what feels good, and—like catnip to women—"make space." The space can be physical, mental, or emotional, but whichever kind it is, schedule in time for yourself, away from frenetic energies that consume us.

In fact, when Mishler asked her nearly seven hundred thousand Facebook fans what theme they wanted to honor for December 2020, she received an overwhelming response: "Myself."

Yoga has grown so very popular because it emphasizes emotional health in the context of mind-body union. In a society where we feel so disconnected from our bodies (and confined to a sedentary lifestyle), we need outlets that let us explore that union. Some also see it as a less competitive discipline that lets them go at their own pace, in stark contrast to hard-hitting cardio; slow, gentle movements act as a restful cushion from the rat race.

Of course, movement has long been recommended to release stress. Strong evidence shows that regular exercise is associated with lower levels of anxiety, and even just a twenty-minute stroll has been shown to clear the mind.

Frequent exercise is also an American tradition, albeit one historically more afforded to men. While nineteenth-century women prone to "hysteria" were prescribed bed rest or hysterectomies, men were handed a horse and told to head to the wilderness. At the time, "neurasthenia" became a catchall term for elite men's weakness of nerves caused by overly civilized life.[23] The cure for spending too much time working indoors was returning to the rugged outdoors. Teddy Roosevelt advocated a "West Cure": vigorous treks into the wild to build muscles while roping cattle, hunting wildlife, and exploring nature. Manly cowboy activities, he believed, could restore nerves sapped by an effeminate, coddling culture. (Some historians assert that the national parks owe their existence to the popularity of Roosevelt's therapies.)[24]

Today we have far more options than a fainting couch or a cowboy expedition. A host of self-care modalities promises to get you back on the Zen track, filling whatever gap you need filled: massages (touch), facial masks and manicures (pampering), meditation (being present), cardio fitness (movement), cannabis (relaxation), and so on.

To be honest, anything can be self-care provided it makes you feel better (although no real money can be made by telling people to go take a walk outside). Two prominent desires for women are the need to escape stress and the need to release stress. Sometimes one, sometimes the other, but often both. Fans of indoor cycling studios, for example, compare pedaling in place to a vacation from life. They speak of mentally transporting themselves to something more akin to a nightclub than the perceived hell they're living in. One SoulCycle devotee wrote, "I can shut out the world and my own thoughts for a while. There's no beep from my notifications, no expectations, no deadlines, no rules."[25]

With exercise, your worries completely shut off. Your brain is so intently focused on following the prescribed moves that you don't have time to fathom if you potentially chose the wrong career. You are jumping so hard that your shitty ex melts into the abyss. The absorbing repetitive motions occupy the space previously afforded to a ticking biological clock. Nothing else exists, for you have one task and one task only: complete the burpee. You are, for once, *present*.

Some use running quite literally as therapy. Jogging therapy is a combination of talk therapy with mindful movement. The unique workout has gained a small following in Silicon Beach, the L.A. region home to more than five hundred technology companies. Start-up professionals lace up their sneakers to join psychotherapists-slash-trainers who run beside them as they complain about their demanding boss or nagging parent. One jogging therapist's office has all the trappings of a Freudian experience—mid-century couch, end table topped with a tissue box—but also foam rollers, hand-sized FIJI water bottles, hair ties, and energy bars. A mini-gym of sorts.

"You're literally moving forward, *together*," the psychotherapist Sepideh Saremi, founder of Run Walk Talk, told me as I gasped for air while trying to vent and run at the same time. "That is a powerful experience for people to have when they feel really stuck in their lives."[26] (But only for those who can manage to talk while running.)

Solo runs prove equally powerful. One writer explained that she runs to break free of bad thoughts and to metaphorically pound frustration into the pavement. "There's a point during my run when I get this invincible I-could-run-forever feeling, as long as I keep running forward," Patricia Haefeli wrote for *Women's Running*. "But my runs are always large loops, and as I round the bend to head back, I'm reminded that you *can* run away from your problems—at least temporarily."[27]

Temporarily. That's a key point. We are briefly excusing ourselves from our lives and engaging in spurts of stress release before jumping back on the hamster wheel. And what you do, therefore, is sometimes less important than just separating time for yourself. Self-care can be snuggling puppies, watching *30 Rock* reruns, or stretching on a yoga mat because what often matters most is the disengagement from [fill in the blank].

As long as your mind is preoccupied with anything other than what would spur a meltdown, you're golden. But what happens when self-care doesn't cut it, or worse, is weaponized against us?

Stress *Is* Your *Problem*

Beatrice* graduated from nursing school at one of the most challenging times for healthcare workers. The upstate New Yorker was fast-tracked through her last semester of school so she could help with the COVID-19 relief efforts. In 2020, she found herself working full time at a frantic hospital, shuffling from one heartbreaking death to another. Any free hours were spent educating herself about the latest pandemic policies or visiting patients in the ICU, holding vigil under harsh fluorescent lights. Beatrice didn't complain. She knew full well these were extraordinary times that required extraordinary sacrifices.

As a healthcare worker in a short-staffed environment, Beatrice felt overstretched, though she knew her work was crucial in the "horribly stressful, grim" situation. At one point, she had a full-blown breakdown as she felt completely hopeless after "trying to follow every order to a T and people still died." It was defeating.

Following the holiday season, when COVID-19 deaths hit a new peak, Beatrice was summoned to a Zoom meeting with her team and supervisor. The nurses had been working massive amounts of overtime and were in desperate need of a break. They had voiced their need for backup support so they could take a little time off, or at the very least get some extra compensation to take care of all the errands piling up at home.

But Beatrice's boss didn't offer that kind of relief. Rather, the staff supervisor gave a presentation about employees' need to engage in self-care activities, asking them, "What are *you* doing to take care of yourself?" The suggested solutions were yoga, running, and drinking more water.

Beatrice was at first perplexed, and then furious. Why was the onus

---

* Throughout the chapters, you will notice that some people are referred to by their first name only. These are people who preferred to speak anonymously or whom I interviewed in a specific setting, not necessarily for this book—and as such, they are not fully identified or go by a pseudonym.

on *her* to fix a situation the hospital had put her in? Even a monetary bonus toward her student loans would have been more meaningful. When would the staff be able to exercise amid twelve-hour-plus shifts? How would sipping more water ease her anxiety? "It's patronizing that during a pandemic you're asking service workers to do so much more than they've ever been asked to do and then their employer doesn't absorb any of the responsibility . . . it's victim blaming," said Beatrice. "At a certain point, employers are morally responsible for what's going to [psychologically and physically] happen to their staff."

To Beatrice, the suggestions came across as taking further advantage of a gendered profession, since 90 percent of nurses are women. She felt they targeted what little energy women—forever society's caretakers—had left. "[Our employer] knows we would never go on strike," she fumed, "they know we care too much about our patients."

If you can't take the heat, the saying goes, then get out of the kitchen. But what if the kitchen is on fire? Telling overworked nurses to do yoga is similar to walking into a sweatshop and informing the employees they really ought to do something about all that stress. *Maybe they shouldn't be working insane hours.* Employers can dangle workplace wellness initiatives to offset the stress they create in part because we've accepted the concept en masse: it's *our* job to fix what's "wrong" with us. Consequently, employers are always suggesting more ways to get well, yet never offering less work or more substantial help.

My pet peeve is when companies offer "wellness days" but don't readjust the workload so that we can actually take advantage of them. Employees secretly work anyway, then resent their employers who pat themselves on the back for accommodating "work-life balance."

Or worse, companies offer nothing more than empty virtue signaling for press attention. In 2021, Nike publicly announced it was closing its corporate offices for a week in the name of mental health. Employees were told to "destress" and spend time with loved ones—a move rattled off in self-congratulatory statements shuffled out to reporters and applauded in

LinkedIn posts. But guess who reportedly didn't get time off? Warehouse and retail employees, proving that only white-collar workers matter to management. And you can be sure the company's burnout "break" didn't extend to all those hushed-about subcontracted factory workers abroad. The same goes for the athleisure darling Lululemon, which partnered with the United Nations Foundation to promote mental health for humanitarian aid workers and posts Instagram statements like "Everyone has the right to be well." That is, save for their outsourced Bangladesh factory's female workers who, in 2019, reported that they were beaten, overworked, verbally abused, and denied sick leave. These women said their paltry pay wasn't enough to survive on. They allegedly made roughly $112 a month, just $6 shy of being able to afford a pair of the very leggings they produced.[28] But you won't see that scrawled on Lululemon's feel-good mantra–covered tote bags.

I'm all for learning stress management techniques to aid us throughout day-to-day chaos. This is not a case against yoga. My point is that we should take a step back to analyze the root issues. Stress is rarely a matter of a broken brain or a poor "lifestyle choice" but often a symptom of the structural issues facing society. At times, wellness can serve as a disciplinary power whenever our emotions are unruly, or as horse blinders to keep us on track. We're instructed to revel in feel-good escapism, thereby tuning out the untouched problems. Instead of pointing the finger at management, we absolve them of guilt; we use self-care to become mentally bulletproof, the better to serve corporate needs. Mastering your stress, it would seem, helps toe the company's bottom line.

"[Burnout] is not a disease. It's not a medical condition," says Christina Maslach, a professor at the University of California, Berkeley, and a pioneer of burnout research. She created the Maslach Burnout Inventory (MBI), the most widely used instrument for measuring work-related stress. "To treat it as such means it's inside the person and the individual has more responsibility to take care of it on their own. It really misses a whole other part of what's going on in life, which is that there are stressors out there." Maslach is not opposed to relaxation tools, but there's a balance that's since been distorted. We believe our feelings are supposed to change while an imperfect system should remain as is.

The wellness industry stepped in to fill a void created by the unreasonable expectations that torment us. Self-care promised salvation, deliverance from the evils of stress. But if it's a toxic workplace, a meditation program isn't going to fix it. A fitness app won't solve the uneven distribution of housework within your marriage; CBD gummies will not enforce better childcare policies; bath salts won't stop late-night work emails. Buy whatever makes you feel good, but realize that these are short-term mental Band-Aids that do not ensure long-term redemption. Wellness remedies help, but the problem is that they're sold to the public as miraculous cure-alls.

We've somewhat butchered what "self-care" means. Historically, it stems from far more radical, activist roots. Marginalized groups in the 1960s adapted the medical term in response to the lack of adequate attention from mainstream medicine. Health care, they proclaimed, is a civil right—one that should be available to all, no matter one's skin color, ethnicity, or income. And if the powers that be failed to provide it, individuals would take it into their own hands.

In time, community members themselves took it upon themselves to serve their own. Hispanic civil rights groups set up programs to combat the lack of access to affordable health care; the Brown Berets, a Chicano activist group, founded the El Barrio Free Clinic in East Los Angeles. Likewise, the Black Panthers created and operated more than a dozen health clinics in underserved areas. These community-focused care centers offered a host of free services, ranging from food pantries to blood pressure screenings. Many centers were stationed in trailers or run out of storefronts and staffed by volunteers. But they all had a strong message: together we can take health into our own hands.

The Black activist and writer Audre Lorde expanded on the concept of self-care, viewing it as a radical vehicle for personal health in order to address larger societal issues. She wrote in 1988, "Self-care is not self-

indulgence, it is self-preservation, and that is an act of political warfare."
At the time, Lorde was battling cancer. Self-care meant survival—so that
she could continue to fight against racism, sexism, and homophobia.

Taking care of oneself was acknowledging your needs so you could
adequately push back against a system of social inequality. It caused one to
ask, "How can I fight injustice or overcome adversity if my tank is empty?"
Self-care meant standing up for yourself to declare, "I need more." I need
to protect my mental and physical health so that I can right what's wrong
not just for myself but for others too.

Self-care *today* is far more inward-looking—and dependent on a purchase. Not only that, but it hands the problem back to the sufferer, repackaged and tied up in rugged individualism. America has always treasured
the lone soldier who relies solely on grit and perseverance. But it seems
like we're giving up on communal change to cocoon ourselves, building
our own Noah's ark in place of petitioning God to spare the fate of our
fellow man. That's the new American way.

In this regard, we prioritize our inner private response over our potential ability to change situations via collective effort. By reimagining stress
as something that can be overcome individually—separate from social,
political, and economic influence—we are barring it from actual strategies
to fix it.

To be fair, we obviously can't tackle the root problems of all our stressors.
That mentality doesn't get us too far when we're stuck in traffic. But escapism
and consumption do not promise real change. Actual progress only comes
from engaging in whatever was responsible for the stress in the first place.
Self-care should move you toward a life you don't need to run away from.

Maybe We Should Use Stress to Get (Politically) Moving

One could say we need to jump off the Peloton and fight for change, which
is, of course, easier said than done. Structural transformations such as subsidized childcare or extended paid parental leave require complicated fights

that most American women can't afford to consider for many reasons—financial, emotional, and more. But certainly nothing will change if we lose sight of the real issues.

What would happen if we mobilized even just a little instead of performing so many downward dogs? Could we use all that energy to demand smaller but still worthwhile longer-term solutions? Wouldn't that be preferable to shoving issues under the frayed rug?

Not that everyone suffers from soul-crushing burnout; some simply battle everyday chronic stressors that add up over time. Changes like organizing your own hours or taking adequate lunch breaks might not sound significant or sexy, but they might eventually lessen the stress weighing you down.

I've been in workplaces where the women came together to demand extended maternity leave. I've witnessed managers give Friday afternoons off after several employees complained of burnout. I've been in a newsroom where the staff stood up and organized a union. We can collectively treat some structural issues: a human resources department can dismiss your individual request, but what about when it's a whole group—or a whole department—that's asking? That's a lot harder to ignore.

With more flexibility and fewer hours tied to a Herman Miller chair, mothers could make it back home for bedtime. Women could have time for physical movement in their daily schedule. Perhaps if we implemented these changes, we wouldn't be constantly exhausted and "sneaking" an hour of solo time. We could enjoy our friends and family and look after ourselves.

In other words, we'd have a life.

In a way, there's been a sliver of a silver lining to the pandemic, which inadvertently sparked a backlash to workaholism. Whereas in the past we may have believed stress is a good thing that builds character or resilience, now we're (hopefully) leaning into a healthier work-life balance. While we once battled employers who insisted corporate life had to be a certain way, social distancing regulations proved that we *could* do things differently.

Suddenly we discovered society wouldn't fall apart if we worked from home instead of commuting long hours and rarely seeing the kids. The office, we learned, wasn't essential.

We all came to the realization that many of our previous workplace mandates were unnecessary or burdensome or just plain dumb. We began insisting on better alternatives moving forward.

• • •

In a sick way, we're sedating women with consumerist self-care—or worse, silencing them instead of encouraging them to vocalize their grievances. I want to see headlines that read STRESSED? HERE'S HOW TO CRAFT A LETTER TO YOUR BOSS STATING YOU WILL NO LONGER CHECK EMAIL AFTER WORK HOURS or FIVE WAYS TO TELL YOUR PARTNER TO DO THE DISHES SO YOU CAN TAKE A SHOWER or HOW TO ORGANIZE YOUR WORKPLACE TO DEMAND BETTER BENEFITS. Why the hell is the advice always yoga? Weirdly, wellness is becoming almost as prescriptive as the medical industry. If we criticize some doctors for simply treating symptoms, why are we repeating the same mistakes with wellness?

The Class gave me the space to briefly reconnect and reset. But a few years into taking The Class, along with buying a host of other self-care products, I started questioning what was becoming a very expensive lifestyle. I had to ask myself: Was I significantly less stressed? How come the effect wore off shortly after? What else could help?

I also worry about how gendered this entire messaging has become. I spoke to one mother of a high school student who, along with her classmates, was resisting an elective offering. The curriculum mandated that boys would get to play team sports, while the girls would learn "how to relax" with a wellness course focused on yoga, meditation, and spa activities. Students complained that boys would learn team building skills, leadership abilities, and strength training exercises while the school presumed girls were so fragile that they needed a less demanding, soothing alternative. The mother described how the girls were required to buy "soft, pretty things." The boys just needed to show up in shorts.

In the nineteenth century, "hysterical" women were sent to an asylum. In the twentieth century, they were put on Valium or Xanax. Today, they're directed to a wellness app.

Stress exists for a reason: it's a mental state informing us that something is wrong. And yet we're constantly told this is something we should bury away. When women furiously pedal away on a Peloton to "silence their mind," you begin to ask: *Why should we silence our mind?*

Maybe my mind has legitimate complaints.

Chapter 2

The House Always Wins

Nearly every single lifestyle interview with a female celebrity sounds the same, as if they all rolled off the same conveyor belt. When asked about their daily routine, you get something like this: *I get at least eight hours of sleep because rest is so important. When I first wake up, I meditate before reaching for my phone (to practice gratitude, which keeps me grounded). I make sure to drink eight glasses of water (gotta hydrate!), then do yoga at least three times a week. And I always make sure to eat clean!*

It's like a game of health buzzword bingo, where at some point, the actress in question will comply and rattle off the revitalizing effects of whole foods. The questions might differ a bit, but answers remain the same: pure, unprocessed, *untainted*. Drew Barrymore eats "really clean and healthy" (along with doing an hour of Pilates four days a week).[1] Zoe Saldaña prefers "superclean" and "fresh" foods. And former vegan Olivia Wilde said she tries her best to eat healthfully but admits to the occasional Coca-Cola.[2] It should be noted that a decade ago, before the wellness revolution, magazines rarely asked celebrities to list their hour-by-hour health habits. Now it's standard practice.

"Clean eating" has become shorthand for eating as healthfully as possible, ascending to the crown jewel of the wellness industry's nutritional advice. Though lacking a clear definition, you're encouraged to fully recognize and pronounce every ingredient you put in your mouth—the consumption of food in its most natural state. That means whole foods such as vegetables and fruits, but no (or minimal) dairy, gluten, added sugars, or processed foods. It's a trend that's gained traction over time: In a 2015 Nielsen survey, more than a third of respondents reported they were choosing to consume fresher, more minimally processed foods.[3] By 2019, "clean eating" was the most widely cited food regimen, according to the International Food Information Council. The hashtag #eatclean has been used more than 60 million times alone on Instagram.

Clean eating is alluring because it is full of promises. Liquefied celery and various juicing programs assure you a sexy body, more energy, glowing skin, improved digestion, and the Tesla of immune systems. Heck, it may even be "the key" to balancing hormones and stabilizing mood swings. "Everyone's toolbox for optimal wellness looks different," Gwyneth Paltrow writes in the introduction to her cookbook, *The Clean Plate*. "For me, the most powerful reset button is food. I don't know any magic bullets, but eating clean comes close . . . There's a marked difference, for the better, in how I feel, and to a lesser degree how I look, when I'm eating at least fairly clean."[4]

I'm not surprised that many women and celebrities bask in the glow of turmeric-infused ginger shots, convinced that clean is the better way to eat. I've dabbled in it myself. It sparked my interest as a good way to get healthier and reverse a decade of ordering *pad see ew* for dinner. If I was constantly drawn to salty takeout, I reasoned, then I'd need a strict protocol to ensure I didn't drop dead from noodle overdose. In a way, clean eating felt like a protective barricade. With only lettuce and farm-fresh eggs permitted, I could seclude myself from oh so many greasy temptations.

I was intrigued when a functional medicine nutritionist wrote we only needed to shift our mindset to eat clean, *to feel our best*. "Food is medicine, and your mind is the cure," she wrote. Should we cave and give into mac 'n' cheese, it's because we use food "as a distraction, a reward, or to placate an emotion." Hence we needed to "dismantle" our reptilian brain's desire for a cookie at the end of the workday. That is, if we want "the vitality, clarity, and radiance that comes from consistently eating a clean diet."[5]

I did want vitality, clarity, and radiance. I wanted whatever Olivia Wilde was having.

Health was one part of the attraction. But if I was being completely honest, health took a backseat to another more pressing intention. Clean eating, like many other trendy food philosophies, hides ulterior motives—bad aims I wouldn't have necessarily noticed because they were hidden under glowing press coverage that made the idea sound so very appetizing.

But the hidden agenda is there. And it's as old as the diet it embraces. For clean eating isn't even all that new. Nor is Gwyneth Paltrow the first clean food influencer; she's heir to a long tradition—from the Atkins, South Beach, and Mediterranean diets to even more far-flung ancestors.

Flashback: The Moralistic Origins of the Graham Cracker

The mob of Boston business owners headed straight for the Marlborough Hotel front door, shouting and clamoring for blood as carriages rolled by. Butchers carried cleavers, bakers clutched rolling pins as their stained aprons flapped in the fall wind. Brawling their way forward, they came to collect the one who made that year, 1837, their poorest-performing one yet. Bread sales were down, and chunks of beef piled up in display windows. Their shops were on the verge of closing, and they knew who was to blame: a Presbyterian minister by the name of Sylvester Graham.

Barricaded in the hotel dining room, Graham and his supporters thought quickly. They ran into the kitchen, then dashed up the stairs to the rooftop. Staring down upon the crowd, they began pelting the rabble with bagfuls of limes, one after another.[6] The mob soon dispersed. Graham's life was spared.

What had caused such a literal food fight? How did a minister turn bakers into sworn enemies? Graham said something unremarkably common by today's standards but which back then constituted heresy: he told people not to eat certain things. And Americans, especially women, ate it up.

In the 1800s, Graham captivated a public terrified of the cholera pandemic. By Graham's account, sickness stemmed from an unsuitable way of life in which Americans consumed a heavy amount of meat and "unnatural" store-bought foods. A gifted orator, Graham lambasted American gluttony, claiming that overindulgence corrupted both body and soul. Salvation, he claimed, lay with rest, exercise, and a bland diet. (Flavorful condiments like mustard and ketchup, for example, could cause insanity.) He advocated "food in its natural state" not only to stay healthy but to reduce sexual tendencies.[7] It was clean eating with an added dose of repression. And like many fads to come, it mixed spirituality with pseudoscience.

Graham jump-started the idea that people can't fully trust that which is produced out of sight. At the time, some shops and bakeries packed their mass-produced products with fillers like chalk and clay, or what Graham described as "the most miserable trash that can be imagined." Homemade food was ideal, he advocated, as it ensured the purity of whole grains and fresh ingredients. Graham explained how to use unsifted whole wheat flour to bake plain, simple (or flavorless) bread. And hence the graham cracker was born, though far from anything Nabisco's Honey Maid produces today.

But Graham's philosophy also centered on how to attain a certain body size. "Grahamites" weighed themselves to assure they *weren't* losing weight because, at the time, a voluptuous body was fashionable. Some historians consider this diet the first to connect eating with weight, whereas before, food restrictions centered on spirituality or indigestion.[8]

The minister gained such a huge following that an entire collection of brand extensions popped up in the 1840s, like Graham hotels and boardinghouses. His popularity soon became an actual threat to the food industry. The press, however, was less than impressed, calling Graham "the philosopher of sawdust pudding." Ralph Waldo Emerson dismissed him as the "poet of bran and pumpkins."[9]

Graham passed away at the age of fifty-seven from, ironically, complications from several opium enemas. And Grahamism, like all fad diets, petered out. But a preoccupation with unwanted ingredients and "pure" food—a knee-jerk reaction to industrialization—would repeat itself in time.

Is Clean Eating a Front?

Today, a parade of wellness influencers—a substantial number of them lacking any nutrition science or medical credentials—have amassed millions of followers with their meticulous food regimens, seemingly existing on a strict diet of grapefruit and homemade nut milk. Almost every single wellness guru claims an identical origin story: they didn't feel well, realized they ate too many processed foods and swam in chemical-laden products, then repented. Like messianic messengers, they saw the light around "clean" and are now healed, which is why their lives are now so fabulous.

Unlike in previous eras, these crusaders have far more influence: social media allows for the rapid proliferation of clickbait in a way *Prevention* magazine or a best-selling diet book never could. They reach their fans every single day, sometimes multiple times on any given day. They do not live on your nightstand, waiting for a free, quiet moment to be read. They are in your pocket, ready to interact at all hours. Just click on the Instagram icon.

Their success isn't merely due to the ease of their availability, however. Like their counterparts from much earlier eras, what these influencers are selling goes directly to the heart of our aspirational selves. Because sure, I thought health was nice, I guess. But you know what I thought was even nicer? Looking good. Having a svelte body. For in 2015, I finally met a kind, honest, and intelligent man. We got engaged a little over a year later and I breathed a sigh of relief: I could get off the dating carousel and rest on the solid matrimonial bench. But as one stressor melted away, another quickly took root in its place. I felt I needed to shed a few pounds to squeeze into a tight Johanna Ortiz ensemble for my wedding in 2017. (It had sequined palazzo pants—it was really something.)

Clean eating, level one of wellness food regimens, looked like the ticket to ride. And I didn't make the connection between clean eating and thinness all on my own. It was served up on a biodegradable platter by everyone who professed concern for healthier living. For all the flowery language of "nourishing" your body with broccoli salad, influencers hinted at something almost every American woman wants: an "acceptable" weight.

It's not just that clean leaders were all thin. They also pushed thin ideals. Some posted "before" photos of themselves, back when they were eating processed foods, juxtaposed with "after" photos of their impeccable physiques from clean eating (often, right next to a $600 Vitamix blender). Successful entrepreneurs like Amanda Chantal Bacon, founder of the cult supplement brand Moon Juice, gushed about a mostly sugar-, wheat-, and dairy-free diet that emphasized whole foods. "I'm heavily rotating the watermelon rind and aloe juice," she generously shared.[10] Simultaneously, she sold us on $49 supplement bottles that, among other lofty ambitions, promised to control "stress-related weight gain."

Almost everyone would sooner or later mention, *By the way, you'll lose weight*, either subtly or overtly. They were right: the clean eating regimen itself is so very limiting that you're nearly guaranteed to shed some pounds. Because you're forbidden processed food, you inevitably end up staring at an arugula salad. When Nabisco cookies are supposedly toxic, you resort to cauliflower. It's as simple as that.

Mass media and brand marketing also play the disguise-diets-as-health game. If in decades past, women were told to slim down to get a "beach-ready body," now slimming down is couched in a new mandate: to "be nutritious." Instead of counting calories, you're weighing kale intake. Magazines will claim that they're anti-diet, utilizing positive self-love language, but then promote the clean eating "lifestyle," the paleo "philosophy," or how to be "keto-friendly" alongside photos of thin models. It's all the same concept, just different outfits. By invoking health (who can debate the importance of health?) the media masks what is actually involved—namely hard work and a restrictive lifestyle.

What had begun as a legitimate concern over more nutritious food has devolved into a more PC reincarnation of diet culture. For everyone talking endlessly about "health," what a portion is truly saying is, *I want a specific body shape and size.* Not all, of course (we'll get to that in a later chapter), but a good chunk.

Perhaps there's no better indicator of this than Weight Watchers officially changing its company name. When I profiled the company's "lifestyle rebrand" in 2017, their executive team told me that Weight Watchers, which usually sees a spike at the start of a new calendar year, saw a new low in 2015. When they commissioned a survey, they found that what once worked with generations past now felt old-fashioned and reactive. In this newfound era of feel-good campaigns, Weight Watchers learned that the term "diet" was rife with negative connotations, not in line with the growing body positivity movement. The general response, as one senior vice president told me, was: "You are a diet brand, and frankly, we are no longer willing to diet."[11] So the brand ditched the word "weight" to simply go by WW. Their new tagline? "Wellness that works."

Updating the terminology isn't just about conflating thinness with health. Far from it. It isn't necessarily about health at all. It's about money. A lot of money. Because here's the dirty secret of most diets: *they don't work.* The house, as we know in gambling, always wins. The majority of people quit their overly restrictive diets after three weeks, reports the *Shatter the Yoyo* author and clinical psychologist Candice Seti, who works with chronic dieters. "And then all of the impacts of that diet play out: the restriction effect, the overeating, the frustration, the self-confidence drop . . . all of these things that come from the deprivation take hold and we end up feeling like a failure," Seti told me. It's estimated that between 80 to 95 percent of dieters regain the weight within a few years, propelling them to try another and another and another.[12]

You'll see friends utterly devoted to a diet, be it Atkins, paleo, Whole30, or intermittent fasting. The next year, they moved on to something else, having entirely forgotten just how religiously they once protested a certain food group. You're tempted to remind them, Hey, remember when I needed to change my entire dinner menu to accommodate your adherence to the keto diet? This constant revolving door of hot new eating regimens is what makes diets hugely profitable.

The same goes for "detoxes" and "cleanses," short-term dietary regimens which claim to remove "toxin" buildup from human organs. These scams are everywhere. You can pick up "detox" kits at your local Whole Foods or just scan any wellness influencer's Instagram page for hawked products that essentially amount to water, lemon juice, honey, and pepper. It's an appealing idea: eat crap and party hard, then purify the buildup to "reset" the system. Spring cleaning for the body! You'll often hear how it worked for the influencer or brand spokesperson, ergo, we are to presume it will work for us.

If only science confirmed such a convenient process. The thing is, we already have an efficient detoxification system in place: a liver, kidneys, skin, and lungs. "You cannot detox, period," states Ada McVean, a science communicator with the McGill Office for Science and Society. "There is nothing you can do to remove more toxins from your body short of eating and drinking and taking in nutrients to support your liver and kidney function."

Our biological systems aren't perfect (otherwise, we'd never get drunk or poisoned). But popularized detox kits won't do much of anything except maybe extra hydration. These products don't help organs work better or help one recover faster.

That doesn't stop peddlers from peddling. Goop favorite Dr. Alejandro Junger sells a $475 three-week Clean detox program that gets raves from Gwyneth Paltrow, who claims it left her feeling "pure and happy and much lighter."[13] In reality, some of the detox reviews on the Clean Program website and other sites note that any weight loss program's mileage will vary by customer and might even pose dangers to those for whom the change is radical to their system. While some buyers express great enthusiasm after achieving desired weight loss, others attest to headaches, nausea, hunger, fever-like chills, and plain old disgust.[14] Dissatisfied customers are unable to make it through a few days of the strenuous diet, the deserted pills proof of hunger's victory.

I have met very few women who have done a "cleanse" out of serious concern for their liver. More often than not, detoxes are crash diets with heftier price tags and better cultural clout.

It's gotten to the point where it's hard to tell the difference between health and diet culture anymore. Wellness brands infuse body pressures into their messaging—a blur so successful that women often don't even think about whether something is being sold to them for health reasons or to play into their desire to look like an unattainable ideal. When consumers do catch on, brands defensively feign ignorance.

Take Rae, a trendy line of wellness supplements found in stores like Target and touted in women's lifestyle publications. "We believe nurturing your mind and body isn't just essential—it's your power," reads their website. In March 2020, the brand announced it was pulling one of its products off the shelves after "obsessed" teen girls popularized it on TikTok as a weight loss aid. The specific item? "Metabolism-boosting" tincture drops. The brand claimed it was for health, but it's hard to believe anyone wants to enhance their metabolism except for dropping pounds. Rae paused sales of the product because "it was the right thing to do" and because they wanted to "remind young girls that they are strong and beautiful just as they are." But that was only after *Vice* published a report on teen use and the product's ineffective ingredients.

Why do we keep falling for these pseudo-health scams? Perhaps because we are a pathologically optimistic nation, forever clinging to hope and exceptionalism in the face of crude reality. We just keep holding out for this rumored "perfect diet," always out of reach. But also, because we've been force-fed diet culture from every which angle: TV, magazines, social media, and targeted ads. Detox ads follow me from Facebook to Instagram to Google search results like some sort of virtual stalker. We're bombarded, even at the supermarket. We're sold on gimmicky "cleanses" and extreme regimens that only benefit the $192 billion diet industry.[15]

"What you have to remember is that it's not science dictating what's popular," says Bill Sukala, "but marketing." Sukala is a clinical exercise physiologist and nutritionist who regularly exposes wellness pseudoscience and deceptive marketing. He warns that we're getting used to the white noise of nonsense. We forget that health has been commoditized with ambiguous terminology and meaningless jargon. And what sells, swells.

Sukala is almost nostalgic for the good old days when all we had to worry about was a few fad diets. "Now the gloves are off and it's become an MMA fight for eyeballs and dollars. Wellness marketers have gotten brasher." If we once bought NutriSlim cans, now we scoop up "detox" kits. It's as if we traded one addiction for another.

While we might laugh off the Orwellian coded language games of "wellness" brands and media sites, disingenuous marketing practices have deeper ramifications. Sukala likens it to a single drop of water. One drop doesn't do much. But if you leave the leaky faucet unfixed long enough, eventually it carves out a big enough hole in the side of a mountain. The constant slow drip systematically erodes people's ability to separate fact from fiction. Or, worse, their sense of self. "Marketing zeroes in on your pain points—every emotional, mental, physical vulnerability that you have," says Sukala. The irony, of course, is that these wellness companies and outlets are supposedly trying to make people healthier, "but in many cases, they're just shooting everyone in the foot."

The tsunami of misinformation has gotten so big that science communicators worry whether the genie can ever be shoved back inside the bottle. The landscape has changed. Competing against an avalanche of overnight influencers and Internet echo chambers takes more resources than are available. "The gatekeeper has been chloroformed," says Sukala. "There are no gatekeepers anymore. The inmates are running the jail and anybody can say anything."

But even with all these inmates running amok, some influencers attempt to push back against the nonsense. More than a few previously healthy women are openly discussing the damaging effects of extreme wellness-dieting tactics. They speak from personal experience.

Taking It Too Far: Clean Eating Extremism

"In the last few weeks it's become clear to me how silly it is that I am so afraid to share this on the blog and in my life," began the post. "It's not healthy to feel guilt for listening to your own body—I should be thanking myself, not telling myself I've done something wrong. I have 'sinned.'"[16]

In 2014, a successful wellness blogger named Jordan Younger decided to publicly break up with clean eating. The blond, blue-eyed, svelte influencer, who went by the moniker The Blonde Vegan, broke ranks with devotees of the wellness creed. On her blog, she recanted her "entirely vegan, entirely plant-based, entirely gluten-free, oil-free, refined-sugar-free, flour-free, dressing/sauce-free, etc." diet.

The eating regimen that propelled her to Internet stardom had left her worse off. Her so-called "bubble of restriction" had devolved into an 800-calorie-a-day intake. Some days she had a green smoothie for breakfast, kale salad for lunch, and roasted veggies with quinoa for dinner. Other days, she'd live off juice cleanses. At age twenty-three, she suffered near panic attacks over restaurant menus, fearing one bad choice would "throw off" her system. Even juice bars made her anxious if their beverages had more than a tiny bit of apple, fearing the sugar would set her back.

One time, Younger ordered oatmeal in a restaurant only to realize it was cooked with cow's milk. She "freaked out" and threw a tantrum.[17] Occasionally she was so starved of energy she would binge on dates, one of her only sources of sugar. Then she'd beat herself up for going off-script. "I was so sick and upset with myself, the only answer was to skip the next meal and have a juice instead," she recalled in her memoir.[18]

As the months progressed, the blogger wasted away to a mere 101 pounds. In time, Younger's nutrient-starved body began rebelling. Her hair was falling out in clumps and her periods had stopped. Her skin was turning orange from eating too many carrots and sweet potatoes. These were foods she had promoted to her audience of seventy thousand followers with the hashtag #eatclean, alongside selling copies of her detox cleanse program. Younger (who has since changed her brand's name to The Balanced Blonde) feared the heresy of abandoning that which she had so wholeheartedly advanced. "I felt the pressure to remain vegan—it's what my readers and followers lived for," she later told the *Today* show. "I was worried my whole business would come crashing down."

In a blog post to fans, Younger finally admitted she could no longer abide by clean veganism, stating, "It's time to advocate a lifestyle that doesn't involve restriction, labeling or putting ourselves into a box . . . I ask for your support and acceptance." Her request was denied: Younger lost hordes of followers and received countless angry emails, including a few death threats. Irate customers demanded refunds for her hawked apparel, namely $32 T-shirts emblazoned with the words OH KALE YES!

Some expressed their disappointment that she lacked the dedication to be "clean." Others discredited her entire journey, skeptical as to whether she actually ate whole foods. Some went so far as to doubt whether she was even really blond. "You weren't eating enough fruit!" they launched from their laptops. "Now you're just boring," another added. "No wonder you're so ugly." A few seemed genuinely offended, protesting, "You're putting down the **best** diet on Earth!"[19]

That Younger was not a nutritionist seemed lost on a group who so willingly abided by her advice. The heretic was sentenced to excommunication, her influencing powers revoked. She had unknowingly joined the religion of health, never foreseeing she would be burned at the stake. Later, she would reflect on "this cult-like mentality"[20] that simply couldn't handle a defector, an affront to the holy consumption they so valiantly upheld. Fanaticism, she decided, just wasn't worth the toll.

An unhealthy obsession with healthy eating has a medical name: orthorexia. It's food pickiness on steroids, or more like nutrition taken to an extreme degree. And it's what Jordan Younger had suffered from. How widespread is orthorexia? Hard to tell. Those who take to clean eating seem most susceptible. As it's so new, it's believed that less than 1 percent of the U.S. population engages in orthorexic behavior, although small studies attest to its growth among younger women.

In fact, eating disorders as a whole are on the rise: a 2019 study published in the *American Journal of Clinical Nutrition* found that the prevalence of eating disorders doubled between 2000 and 2018.[21]

When reporters asked Younger how it all started, she answered innocently enough: she wanted to be healthy. Younger just wanted to feel good and look good, so she adopted the *en vogue* wellness trend of the day.* She hoped to lose a few pounds but she was also searching "for something more in her life,"[22] and a restrictive eating regimen gave

---

* A survey of more than 1,200 Americans between the ages of fourteen and twenty-four found that over half learned about "clean eating" through social media, online sources, and their peers.[23]

her, not surprisingly, purpose. The willpower (or more like starvation) made her feel extraordinary. It gave her an identity. But she was likely also impacted by our society's lopsided views on women's health and appearance.

"We are told from all different kinds of sources, that we are a body first and maybe a human second," says Katherine Metzelaar, a "non-diet" registered dietitian and nutrition therapist. Before becoming a nutritionist, she battled orthorexia from age twenty-two to twenty-seven. Metzelaar had cut out whole food groups, including gluten, meat, eggs, and dairy. Over time, her diet grew more and more restrictive, excluding "anything that wasn't directly from the ground." She consumed only vegetables, nuts, legumes, and very little fruit, though she was also spending a ton of money on costly supplement powders. "I was deeply afraid of foods causing me some kind of harm, but the irony was that undereating and restrictive eating was harming me significantly. All I did was think about food," recalls Metzelaar. All the while, multiple friends and family members showered her with compliments and exalted her discipline. They'd say she was amazing or "so strong" and ask her for advice. In reality, she was "quite sick."

Clean eating doesn't automatically lead to eating disorders, but the way we discuss and treat food can lead to an unhealthy fixation with what we consume. Your average clean eater may not go to the same extremes as Jordan Younger or Katherine Metzelaar, yet the thinking baked into the message given to an ordinary dieter has a disturbing amount in common with the extreme thinking of orthorexics. It's a slippery slope, and one that needs plenty more guardrails.

Promoting Promises Your Body Can't Keep

Like restrictions of yore, clean eating moralizes our daily choices. Certain foods are deemed "good" and "natural," serving as a "detox" of all the bad foods clogging our arteries (and supposedly stretching our swimsuits). Celebrities list their "guilty" indulgences or "cheat day" menus. Influencers refer to cauliflower bowls as "plant-based goodness" and call sugar-laden cereal "poison." This type of language taints daily decisions with unnecessary virtues and vices.

Christy Harrison, the registered dietitian and host of the popular podcast *Food Psych*, lambastes this new culture that's more about "performing a rarefied, perfectionistic, discriminatory idea of what health is supposed to look like." Nutrition matters, but the notion that food is medicine (or poison) can twist people into all sorts of knots. "It suggests that consistently making the 'right' food choices will heal or prevent all ills and that eating certain kinds of food will inevitably harm our health," she writes. "Putting too much emphasis on our day-to-day food choices doesn't lead to improved health at all, but to a preoccupation with food and panic about our health."[24]

Constant deprivation proves anxiety-inducing and can lead to overindulgence, inspiring more shame cycles. As Judith Matz, the co-author of *The Diet Survivor's Handbook: 60 Lessons in Eating, Acceptance and Self-Care*, explains, even the thought that something's going to be taken away is enough to lead to people bingeing on it. If someone says starting tomorrow, you can never have ice cream again, what would you do? You'd hold the local Baskin-Robbins hostage. Psychologically, we want what we can't have. "There's nothing wrong with that—it's normal," Matz told me. "And abundance makes us calm down when we know something's available. Like water, you don't have to think about it."

Absolutist guidelines and cutting out whole food groups can also lead to nutrient deficiency. Low-carb followers, for example, might experience low energy and brain fog, since carbohydrates provide the body with energy. Or, as in the case of clean eating, dietary convictions can increasingly take on more and more militancy. The boundaries keep tightening: more food groups get the axe, potentially jump-starting compulsion. First, the enemy is highly processed foods, then it becomes meat and fish (making protein harder to come by), then dairy (potentially endangering calcium requirements), then all sugar . . . until you're left with cabbage and a grumbling tummy.

A pursuit of perfection is praised, even though many people on ultra-restrictive diets are practicing disordered eating. But pressure is to be expected when women's bodies are scrutinized from a young age, thereby making them more susceptible to messaging about food as they grow older. One can just look at how the media obsessed over Selena Gomez's weight fluctuation or the late Princess Diana's body (since she was nineteen!) to understand that women's size matters.

Also, we're influenced by cruel messaging consumed with individual responsibility. We're made to believe that should someone get sick or gain weight, it's because they did something wrong. They didn't try hard enough. "Bad eaters" of today are yesterday's smokers: *Maybe you deserve this.*

There's nothing wrong with wanting to eat healthier. The issue is when diets gobble up too much headspace. WW (formerly Weight Watchers) alludes to this preoccupation in a 2021 ad starring spokesman James Corden. After the TV host says that *just by looking at his body* you can tell he's a "bad boy," he admits his head is bombarded with SmartPoints, the brand's food tracking system. "All the time I'm thinking about points: How many points is that, I'm scanning points, I'm over points, I'm under points, I've got my free points," he rattles off to a clinical psychologist. "And I've realized I don't know what a point is. What are points?"[25] The comedian has been driven mad by an imaginary calorie calculator he never even fully comprehended.

Again, WW calls itself a "wellness" company, though that word has more or less become a synonym for diet. The title of this video—"How Has James Corden Lost 20 Lbs?"—makes its true subject, weight loss, clear. And in it we once again see a successful "wellness" company's triumph of marketing the thing that we'll continuously consume and which requires significant mental energy. Lost in the *Beautiful Mind* math of counting points, we forgo time spent on the pursuits of a healthy life. We'd almost certainly be better off using the headspace to finish a long-term project, join a book club, or be more present with our children. But if the company sold us that, who in their camp, as the saying goes, would benefit?

The Skinny on Fat Myths

Clean eating doesn't just moralize our daily food choices, it moralizes our weight, period.

We're conditioned to look to weight as *the* telltale sign of health. But you can't predict medical outcomes just by looking at someone. Some higher-weight individuals are completely healthy, while some size 4 women harbor all kinds of illnesses. And vice versa.

The reality is that an individual's size is not the sole or even leading determinant or predictor of health.

This is not to say that weight doesn't play any role, but rather that weight is overemphasized in our skinny-obsessed culture. In conversations focusing on obesity, there is often a glaring omission of other elements that may lead to future sickness: genetics, poverty, stress, pollution, nutrition, and limited access to health care, physical activity, adequate sleep, or social support. If you live with ongoing poverty, wouldn't chronic stress impact your health? If doctors discriminate against your size, would you be more reluctant to seek medical care or go to checkups?

We don't know the effects of all these factors, and yet some health aficionados automatically, instinctively, jump to weight, partially because it's measurable. How can you, for example, quantify stress?

It seems we're constantly lectured about body size, specifically: how to shrink it. The diet industry, wellness gurus, "war on obesity" . . . they all disproportionately zero in on weight as an independent causal factor. The discourse is counterproductive, explains Paul Campos, the author of *The Obesity Myth: Why America's Obsession with Weight Is Hazardous to Your Health*. We have not figured out a way for people to successfully lose and keep the weight off, "at least not at a statistically significant level," says Campos.

One study of 22,000 adults who followed one of fourteen popular diet programs such as Atkins found that most weight loss is regained within one year.[26] Weight loss might not be achievable for a number of reasons. Maybe it's genetic. Maybe people don't have access to healthy food. Maybe they don't have a support system. Or maybe they need professional advice tailored to their unique situation. Also, human biology is not wired to shed pounds easily.

There are, of course, people who lose and keep off the weight, "but you can't focus social policy around outliers," says Campos. Society constantly scolds people that they *should* be thinner, but we've seen that they often *can't* be thinner. It's like telling teens from underprivileged backgrounds they ought to go to Princeton; it's easy to say, right? So too, the vast majority of people who are in the "overweight" category of the BMI (body mass index)—which is nearly one-third of all American adults—are being told to aim for a BMI range between 18.5 to 24.9, which is unrealistic. By setting people up to fail, we inevitably cause tremendous psychological damage.

"The emphasis on weight instead of health actually makes people sicker," notes Harriet Brown, the author of *Body of Truth: How Science, History, and Culture Drive Our Obsession with Weight—and What We Can Do About It.* "The level of shaming and stigma that is directed is a deterrent, not an encourager for better health behaviors."

And what about the physical health of these chronic dieters? After all, it's bad enough spinning through bouts of self-loathing, fearful eating habits, and stress—all of which have long-term consequences. But the news gets worse. Far from optimal health, research indicates that yo-yo dieting (also called weight cycling) has negative effects: chronic deprivation and fluctuating weight gain are associated with increased risk of heart conditions,[27] strokes, increased insulin resistance, and, naturally, feeling shitty when you just want a damn sandwich.

Despite all the "thin glamour," it's sometimes better to forgo struggling to hit a "normal" weight, experts note. "Each time you lose and gain weight, you double the risk of diabetes," says Dr. Kamyar Kalantar-Zadeh, a professor of medicine at the University of California, Irvine, who has led a study on obesity's impact on kidney disease. Dr. Kalantar-Zadeh will advise patients to change their eating patterns if, say, they have high blood sugar levels. But in general, he encourages patients to focus on healthier habits and weight stability, noting, "massive weight loss and weight gain [are] usually detrimental."

Dr. Kalantar-Zadeh joins other medical researchers in reexamining our de facto strategies. UCLA researchers analyzed thirty-one long-term diet studies, only to conclude that most dieters "would have been better off not going on the diet at all. Their weight would be pretty much the same, and their bodies would not suffer the wear and tear from losing weight and gaining it all back."[28]

Dr. Fatima Cody Stanford is an obesity medicine physician, scientist, and policy maker at Massachusetts General Hospital and Harvard Medical School. She believes in encouraging better nutrition choices without dictating restrictive diet rules or suggesting a target weight. "I never ask my patients the number of calories that they are eating," Dr. Stanford told me. "It has minimal importance when compared to the quality of what they're eating."

Throughout all this discourse, we continue to rely on the BMI as a measure for what's "overweight." The BMI is an outdated height-to-weight ratio tool that many researchers have called out for overly simplistic calculations. It does not account for muscle mass, bone density, genetic makeup, age, or body composition and variation. Not to mention that it was based on white European men and does not account for racial or ethnic diversity (as different populations can have different body compositions). It's ludicrous to assume such a one-size-fits-all measurement method can dictate an "ideal" body weight.

"This hyperfocus that we are all the same human, and we all have the same target, is just flawed," says Dr. Stanford, who prefers a personalized approach to nutrition. The BMI was never intended to measure individual health, and yet it's used to judge millions. To give you an idea of how faulty the BMI is, celebrities who are technically "overweight" include Matt Damon, Will Smith, and Tom Cruise. As Keith Devlin, director of the Stanford Mathematics Outreach Project, has concluded, BMI ratios are "mathematical snake oil."[29]

But the more people are labeled "overweight," the more we can churn out diet consumers. That's more opportunities for diet programs, "detox" hawkers, and wellness gurus. And, historically, for insurance companies to charge higher rates for individuals with a high BMI.

I don't want to give the impression that there isn't a valid debate about body size. Researchers are certainly divided about weight's exact role in medical outcomes. And yes, studies have shown that individuals with severe obesity do have a higher risk of health complications like diabetes and heart disease.[†] Extreme weight—at both the high *and low* ends—is associated with medical issues. But the focus should be on encouraging healthier, sustainable habits.

Bottom line: it's clear that the relationship between weight and health is highly individual. A question we need to ask is, Even if we agree obesity carries risks, why do we think restrictive dieting is the answer? The evidence suggests that not only does it not work, it often causes harm.

Maybe it's to be expected in a country that proclaims a "war" on obesity not by targeting the culprits (stress, financial constraints, lack of time, sugary drink advertising) but by pointing the finger at individuals. People are responsible for fighting an uphill battle to eat nutritiously in our society, then shamed for a lack of "discipline."

Anti-fatness is woven into our cultural fabric, and by some reports it is slow to remedy. A Harvard University study analyzed millions of Americans' implicit and explicit biases, spanning sexual orientation, race, age, and other factors. In 2019, researchers discovered that overall, the country was demonstrating progress toward a less bigoted society. (An anti-gay

---

[†] While restrictive diets can be problematic, that doesn't mean all weight loss attempts should be shunned, especially if medically necessary. "Often, weight loss is required to reduce harmful fat storages," explained Bram Berntzen, a postdoctoral researcher at the University of Helsinki who studies lifestyle factors and their effect on obesity and related metabolic disorders. "However, we don't yet know how to do this effectively [on a large population scale]."

bias, for example, decreased by 33 percent in a ten-year period.) That is, save for attitudes directed at higher-weight individuals. Implicit weight bias—that is, pro-thin, anti-fat—increased 40 percent between 2004 and 2010. "We think the increasing attention to the health benefits of lower body weight and concerns about the obesity epidemic may be responsible for the increase in bias," writes the *Harvard Business Review*. "Additionally, the perception that body weight is always under one's own control (race, sexual orientation, age, and disability, on the other hand, are not) may lead to harsher attitudes toward those who are overweight."[30]

I am the first to admit I have internalized thinness culture and that I have been working on reversing its damaging effects for years now. But at the very least, let's not kid ourselves that ongoing rounds of dieting constitutes healthy behavior or that cleanse after cleanse is real wellness. Because the research just simply doesn't support it. This is the commodified wellness-diet complex, subsisting off skewed marketing to distort real principles of health. We may prefer a specific size, but as Candice Seti notes, just be mindful as to whether it impairs your mental well-being: Does it cause dysfunction? Does it in any way interfere with your personal or professional life? Does it cause extra stress?

These are questions I wish I could answer with a straight-faced "no." And I know I am not alone in that.

Combating the Guilt-Driven and Exploitive Dieting Psychology

Food can quickly become a guilt-generating machine. Too many blame themselves when they can't hit the goal, especially once weight factors in. "Good" eating then becomes less of a choice and more of a reflection of self-worth. And with that, we strip food of its original purpose—not just sustenance, but pleasure. Gosh, remember that? Remember *enjoying* food?

Professionals such as Matz and Metzelaar work to unpack clients' Santa sack–worth of food guidelines collected over a lifetime. Although clients don't follow a fraction of them, the weight of it all subconsciously affects their relationship with food. It's just as much about unlearning as it is about learning. Clients often mourn the loss of dieting culture and ask themselves: Who am I without this preoccupation? How can I be in a better relationship with my body? How else can I connect with women in a way more meaningful than debating almond butter brands?

An anti-diet philosophy called intuitive eating has gained traction as we've come to learn more about the harmful effects of cyclical dieting. The buzzed-about approach advocates listening to internal signals of hunger and fullness to guide eating choices, rather than subscribing to rigid rules. The idea is that humans have all the answers inside them once they unburden themselves of food anxiety. Peeling back the layers of harmful "good or bad" ideas that infiltrate one's relationship with food can help us reconnect to it without guilt or negativity. You don't need to eat "perfectly" to be in good health, as no one food will kill or heal you. You can have that damn cookie.

Elyse Resch, the co-creator and co-author of *Intuitive Eating*, points to the political climate, which has exhausted women to the point of seeking a more freeing lifestyle. They feel disconnected from their bodies, yearning for a more natural connection to their appetites. "[They are] really tired of being told how they should eat, how they should look, and are rebelling against that kind of oppression," she told me in 2021. (Of course, intuitive eating became such a popular idea that Gwyneth Paltrow co-opted the terminology to suit her empire: in 2021, the Goop guru began promoting "intuitive fasting," which is just structured starvation.)

Intuitive eating doesn't mean people don't overeat or choose McDonald's every so often, especially when stressed. Rather, it means food doesn't possess any moral significance: you don't beat yourself up for foods our culture demonizes, like pizza (which, while high in fat and sodium, is also actually quite nutrient-rich). "Having a healthy relationship with food is different than only eating healthy foods," clarifies Matz. "A healthy relationship with food allows you to eat all types of foods in a way that supports your body." This approach also accounts for the fact that each body differs in how it metabolizes food and nutrients, owing to factors varying from genetics to exercise levels.

Intuitive eating is not without its critics. Some assume it's only about hunger and fullness cues, while others argue that because it gives you free rein to eat whatever you want, it potentially will lead you down a path of overindulgence. This is an incorrect interpretation of intuitive eating, which does touch upon balanced nutrition in its ten principles (not rules). The criticism leveled at this movement is also quite telling: it assumes that as soon as you take your eyes off the prize—the scale, that is—you will devolve into a bonbon-munching maniac. (Our bodies seem to require constant vigilance and self-surveillance.)

But the nutritionists I spoke to say that's not the case. People will usually self-regulate once they pull away from a fear-based relationship with food, which triggers an avalanche of "taboo" cravings and overeating. In time, they choose a balance of nutritious foods, along with some "play foods," simply for the pleasure they provide. "It's about listening to what your body needs, listening to how your body feels based on what you choose to eat," clarifies Resch.

While intuitive eating may not be the right approach for everyone (and is certainly not an overnight process), experts say it's a good step for some in overcoming a fraught relationship with food. And unlike plans hawking shakes or products, there's not much to buy here—you can read about it for free online—nor are there promises reminiscent of exploitive diet culture. It's at least one potential way to escape bad habits.

• • •

More moderate solutions are surely welcome. As it turns out, clean eating ends up being remarkably difficult unless you're a forest rabbit. There are only so many roasted cauliflowers and salads you can eat before wanting to burn down a vegetable patch. In my clean eating days, I hallucinated Pepperidge Farm cookies. Rage became as familiar as hunger. I hated my husband for enjoying a frozen pizza in my presence. I was hungry.

It became so difficult to prepare appetizing "clean" meals that I did something nuts. I was reporting on the upsurge of fresh baby food delivery start-ups—imagine HelloFresh for rug rats. Companies sent me samples of pureed squash with spirulina and quinoa or mashed red peppers with black beans, avocado oil, cumin, and cilantro (all very highbrow for a baby). But I didn't just test them. I started living off them. I would empty several baggies of soupy pulverized beets for lunch. It was just way easier than cooking all those vegetables myself.

It all came to a head when my husband stumbled upon my newfound snacking habit. Every afternoon, I would buy a pack of Sour Patch Kids. But I wouldn't eat them. I would only permit myself to lick the sugar off, leaving a heap of sticky gelatin carcasses. That's how desperate I was for sugar. I lost five pounds and quit the regimen shortly thereafter, but my husband still speaks of the time his partner lost her damn mind. "Women do some *weird shit*," he'll remark while looking right at me.

I wasn't the only one throwing in the towel after succumbing to tempting wellness marketing. Even celebrities come around after having been around the hungry block. Olivia Wilde certainly had her own revelation. One day, just like Jordan Younger, the actress/director gave up being a "hardcore" vegan. Following a stressful period in her life, Wilde was done. "Fear of carbs, of gluten, of everything—we've distanced ourselves from the beauty of food, the art of it," Wilde told *Allure*, adding, "it makes me sad when people say, 'Oh, I don't eat gluten. I don't eat cheese. I don't eat this. So I eat cardboard.'"[31] Wilde's life was too hectic—and short—to shun food. If she craved chocolate or onion rings, she was going to help herself to it. She, like many women, had just about had it with denying herself what she wanted.

And what we want is quite simple: to eat in peace.

Chapter 3

Is My Face Wash Trying to Kill Me?

On a chilly March morning in 2018, one hundred women—two from each state—marched up the steps of the Capitol Building. Clad in sleek power suits and designer sunglasses, they topped off their look with bold red lipstick. Balancing handbags in one hand while taking selfies with each other, they laughed and posed for loved ones back home. The side of one of their charter buses was emblazoned with the motto THIS TIME, IT'S PERSONAL.[1] Their palpable energy was like that of an army before battle. Or teens exiting a limo on prom night.

These women represented the billion-dollar "clean beauty" company Beautycounter. And they were on a mission: lobby Congress to nix harmful chemicals from personal care products. Specifically, these women came to support the Personal Care Products Safety Act, a bipartisan bill to promote industry transparency and strengthen cosmetic regulations. They were there to educate politicians on "clean beauty," a relatively new (and shifting) term that refers to products free of any proven or suspected "toxic" ingredients. They wanted to remove "bad" ingredients—be they synthetic or "natural."

These women were representative of many more. Beautycounter counts more than sixty thousand independent salespeople—called "brand advocates"—who are drawn to the company's mission. Beautycounter employs a direct retail marketing model (or what some might call multilevel marketing) that could be described as an activist twist on Avon. Consultants sell the products online and peer-to-peer within their communities, persuading others to buy a face wash and also telling them why they need clean beauty. The latter is what inspires many women to get involved. Their mission feels important, as if the power to prevent sickness (or impact legislative change) lies in their ability to off-load an eye shadow palette. It gives them a sense of pride. As one Alabama-based brand advocate—or salesperson—explained, "The example I am setting for my children is immeasurable. When I returned home from D.C., the first thing out of my daughter's mouth was, 'Mommy, did you change the world?'"[2]

"Empowerment" is a word thrown around a lot with this group. The more I learned about these consultants, I could see why. Show up at your neighbor's door hawking Mary Kay cosmetics, and they presume you've merely found a new side hustle. But show up with a whole awareness campaign on women's health, and suddenly you're Maria Shriver. Blurring the lines between advocacy and salesmanship, Willy Loman got a socially conscious makeover.

Beautycounter founder Gregg Renfrew led this battalion of concerned women who had little or no political experience. Renfrew, with her honey highlights, minimalist jewelry, and understated makeup, exudes effortless professionalism. Think jeans and a striped T-shirt topped with an open blazer. With a high-wattage smile, she rattles off stats and political facts at breakneck speed, made digestible by her ease and optimism. Laughter comes easily to her. She's enthusiastic, but not too enthusiastic. The kind of entrepreneur young women of that era aspired to become.

Beautycounter hopes to change the landscape through activism, deploying an arsenal of charcoal facial masks and lipsticks as a Trojan horse for personal care product reform. "It was never about getting beauty products into the hands of everyone," Renfrew told me. "It was about getting *safer* products into the hands of everyone."

Which brings us back to that energized morning in D.C. As a reward of sorts, Beautycounter flew in a hundred of their top-performing brand advocates to enjoy a weekend of fine dining, champagne, and socializing. They enjoyed a dinner at the National Portrait Gallery before knocking on politicians' doors. They regaled elected officials with moving personal anecdotes, cancer recovery stories, and hopes for their children's health—their passion rubbing off like red lipstick on a shirt collar. Just as the sign on their bus proclaimed, their mission was *personal*. "[Our community] believes in being part of something bigger than they are as individuals," says Renfrew. "Given all that's transpired [since 2016], women have woken up to the fact that maybe our voices haven't been heard as loudly as we would like."

Now their voices *are* being heard. The fight to guarantee beauty product safety has gained momentum on a national, state, and even local level. Shoppers want to know what's in their moisturizer just as they want to know what's in their Goldfish crackers. I see it everywhere. Facebook friends post on how to banish parabens and sulfates from bathroom cabinets. Acquaintances declare they want to "feel good" about what's seeping into their skin, "the largest organ in the body." Friends imagine a *Psycho* shower scene of a shampoo bottle stabbing us with invisible chemicals. Many of their concerns could have come straight from a Beautycounter ad.

But Beautycounter isn't the only firm selling us "clean" and raising an alarm about chemical exposure. If you've read any women's magazine in the last decade, you've likely come across the following stats: Some studies suggest these chemicals play a significant role in early puberty, obesity, cancer, and infertility. Activists say thousands of personal care products contain synthetic chemicals known as endocrine disruptors, which mimic and therefore confuse the body's natural hormones.

That's in addition to all the publicized lawsuits. In 2019, Johnson & Johnson recalled 33,000 bottles of baby powder due to accusations centered on traces of carcinogenic asbestos. Claire's pulled makeup products after the FDA indicated the possible presence of asbestos fibers.[3] WEN Hair Care settled a class action lawsuit after they received thousands of complaints, some from people who claimed their hair came out in clumps. Headlines like these left me skeptical of the government's ability to regulate chemical safety. Was it Big Tobacco all over again?

By the time Beautycounter went to Capitol Hill, I too was "aware." In the Sephora beauty aisle, I began checking out the "clean" skin care products and second-guessing my Pantene conditioner. When I received a bottle of a Bath & Body Works shower gel as a holiday gift, it sat in the corner of my bathroom for months. Finally, I emptied it into the guest bathroom hand soap dispenser, rationalizing, *Visitors will only use it once or twice a year. How much chemical damage could it do?* My husband watched from afar, not fully comprehending the switch-and-bait occurring within what had now become a soap caste system. He freely and merrily continued using his Kiehl's soap and Mitchum deodorant. "I really don't think about that stuff," he shrugged.

I started writing articles about how and why millennials were flocking to "chemical-free" alternatives. I named Beautycounter as one of *Fast Company*'s Most Innovative Companies of the Year. I also started shopping. A lot. Suddenly, my bathroom shelf exploded into a mini apothecary of Goop-approved products. If I was already spending money, I thought, why not drop a bit more cash and get the *better* option. Why take the risk of convenience store sushi when you can go to Nobu?

Renfrew had been ahead of many of the other corporate players now crowding the clean beauty space. Starting the company wasn't Renfrew's first rodeo. The serial entrepreneur had previously found success with her bridal registry company, The Wedding List, which she sold to Martha Stewart Living Omnimedia in 2001. She was itching for a new project when she watched *An Inconvenient Truth*, Al Gore's documentary on global warming, in 2006. "It was really jarring," reflects Renfrew. "A real wake-up call. It was the first time that I began to contemplate my own life and how it was impacting the earth."

Many of Renfrew's friends were dealing with fertility issues and diagnosed with different types of cancer in their thirties. Others had given birth to children who had health problems or couldn't leave the house without an EpiPen. Reading up on the links between substances that are harmful to the earth and also to human health, she zeroed in on toxic chemicals in everyday products. She started washing her floors with water and vinegar. Nonstick cookware was thrown out in favor of stainless steel replacements. Plastic containers got the boot to make way for glass.[4] But when it came to purging her beauty cabinet, she was hesitant: Could anything less "toxic" really meet her high bar for skin care products? Where was the Clinique for Whole Foods shoppers?

Renfrew didn't just want to build a beauty company. She aimed to address the alleged systemic issues at play. "This isn't just shopping your way out of the problem," says Renfrew. And so the company continues to lobby Washington each year and to date has conducted more than 2,000 meetings, made 16,000 calls, and sent 200,000 emails to lawmakers. Renfrew hobnobs at political parties while her consultants host meetings with congressmen in their hometowns.

Beautycounter is fighting for the whole beauty sector, because without regulatory support from the government, clean beauty is still very much out of reach for the average consumer. Clean beauty basics generally cost quadruple the price of a drugstore equivalent. A Beautycounter foaming cleanser runs $35, in comparison to Neutrogena's mass competitor at $5.29. Beautycounter's red lipstick—the same one worn by the Capitol Hill marchers—costs a cool $34. Their aluminum-free deodorant, beloved by Jennifer Garner, goes for a whopping $28. You won't find these at your local Food 4 Less. Hence, Renfrew hopes to represent all consumers in the marketplace through the company's efforts. "Safer products should be a reality for everyone," says the founder. "This is about all people."

Indeed. Though presumably we want to be sure we're steering people in the right direction.

Flashback: Women as House Managers: Foot Soldiers for Health

Boston, Massachusetts, 1870. The faculty at MIT were at a standstill. The chorus of mustachioed men, dressed in varying hues of gray and black suits, were huddled to debate the admittance of a female student. One by one, they addressed the potential issues. Could the applicant keep up? Would this compromise the institute's standing? Did women even have the intellectual capacity to study science?

The student in question was Ellen Swallow (later Richards), a Massachusetts farm girl with a bachelor's degree from Vassar College and a passion for sanitary chemistry. Despite the initial discrimination, Richards prevailed to become the first woman admitted to MIT. A true trailblazer, Richards studied popular packaged foods of her day, in which she found sugar mixed with chloride or cinnamon powder full of sawdust and sand—a discovery that would later inspire the Pure Food and Drug Act of 1906, which prohibited the mislabeling of food and medicines.

At the time, Americans faced a rapidly changing environment: new diseases, new technology, and new public health challenges. Before the advent of advanced sewage systems, illnesses like typhoid fever killed 20 percent of those infected. As germ theory seeped into the national consciousness, how to limit disease in an easily contaminated environment was a popular topic.

As a fierce consumer advocate, Richards acknowledged the need for government and industry oversight of commercial products, but she also encouraged homemakers (and their domestic servants) to oversee their surroundings. She instructed women how to wipe down floors, purify water, and safeguard food. To Richards, chores were "a fine action, a sort of religion, a step in the conquering of evil, for dirt is sin."[5] The man would come home from the factory dripping in evil germs, and the woman's job was to scrub them all away. This art of protection was deemed "domestic science," which we now know as home economics.

Richards believed that a successful housewife "was constantly asking herself what could be better, healthier, cleaner, or more effective in her home."[6] Under this newly intense scrutiny, home-care grew fraught with anxiety. It was up to women to ensure that their children were not carried out in tiny caskets. Then companies began to realize they could capitalize on the fear. A slew of brands marketed a wide range of disinfectants under the guise of sanitary adherence. Women who had been lured to professionally study the science of sanitation with hopes of educating their peers soon found themselves hired to market the latest household appliance or cleaning agent—some of them fraudulent or unnecessary.[7]

What did their tactics look like? To sell iceboxes (nonmechanical refrigerators) in the 1920s, they emphasized the importance of fresh food while invoking gendered and exaggerated fears. Cold storage meant less contamination and thus fewer children's deaths, they claimed. As one fridge pamphlet warned: "When a baby's health hangs in the balance the intelligent mother will see to it that the ice supply never runs too low."[8] Women had become both corporate foot soldiers for health and household safety leaders who couldn't afford *not* to rely on consumerism.

Marketing to Women: "Shopping Right Will Set You Free"

Fear is a potent marketing tool. Today, as much as at the birth of domestic science, women are frightened into taking responsibility for family safety. "Asbestos. Formaldehyde. Lead. Not exactly the words you think of when you're purchasing your favorite personal care products," reads the website of the Environmental Working Group (EWG), an advocacy group popular within wellness circles. "Sadly," the EWG notes, "toxic chemicals in our cosmetics, sunscreens and skin care products have gone unregulated as far back as the Great Depression."[9] The EWG's solution for such paltry regulations? Becoming your very own inspector, supplied with lists of chemicals to avoid and a guide for interpreting product labels.

This practice is called precautionary consumption. As with housewives of yore, the goal is proactive oversight. It falls to you, the consumer, to vigilantly protect yourself and your loved ones from chemical dangers.[10] When you shop at the market, you are expected to recall all the restrictions to ensure safety. If you need a new bodywash, you must scout for a list of "dirty" ingredients. When buying a new moisturizer, you calculate, *Will this product cause cancer?* Each time you see an organic chicken sitting alongside a normal one in the meat section, you are forced to reckon, *How much am I willing to pay to keep my family healthy?* All the small decisions add up.

There's a lot we're told to to worry about. Women on average use twelve personal care products a day, exposing themselves, according to brand marketers, to 168 unique chemical ingredients. The average man, in comparison, uses six personal care products a day. A Beautycounter brand ambassador on Facebook assures: "With all the craziness surrounding us, it's nice to know that the products I'm using are significantly safer . . . giving me one less thing to worry about." By purchasing the right facial cleanser, one brings structure and order to a chaotic world.

The media joins the circus by asking women to evaluate every nook and cranny in their home and handbag. *Women's Health* tells readers to "green your beauty routine with these 5 natural makeup swaps" and warns that toxins are everywhere. Even our nether regions require vigilance: WARNING: YOUR VIBRATOR COULD BE MADE WITH HARMFUL CHEMICALS, one headline proclaims. In contrast, male magazine readers are fed features on fitness, diet, work, and biohacking their way to Chris Evans's abs. The word "toxic," if ever used, predominantly refers to an unhealthy relationship with one's boss.

Renfrew acknowledges that the clean movement was primarily built on women. "If you light the fire under the asses of women about something they care about," she says, "they're going to fight tirelessly," whether it's Mothers Against Drunk Driving or child safety initiatives.

Companies also target moms because they still bear the brunt of decision-making in the family, upholding the legacy of the woman's domain. Branch Basics—a line of all-natural, nontoxic home cleaning products—showcases a smiling woman washing her hands with her child in a pristine white kitchen, alongside the caption CREATE A HEALTHY HOME: EVERY-THING YOU NEED TO REPLACE DOZENS OF TOXIC CLEANING PRODUCTS. The Honest Company, which primarily focuses on moms, promises customers can "rest easy" knowing their products are made without "health-compromising chemicals."[11] The brand's campaigns and social media posts show mothers happily cuddling their children, including founder Jessica Alba. The actress turned entrepreneur claims there are "a lot of toxic chemicals in everyday products" and especially in baby products. With her line of products, however, moms don't have to choose between "what works and what's good for you."[12]

In a way, not much has changed since the 1930s. Back then, as the American historian Roland Marchand writes, advertisers believed women possessed a "greater emotionality" with "inarticulate longings."[13] Manipulating women's emotions continued for decades to come, as the feminist writer Betty Friedan expounded on in 1963's *The Feminine Mystique*. And the tactics continue today. Precautionary consumption plays on women's vulnerability and demands our vigilance. Made fearful of "hazardous" ingredients, our intense risk aversion manifests into a bible on what we can and cannot consume. Some items are forbidden to us, hence we scout for a kosher "clean" symbol ensuring we're on the right path.

Shopping becomes a layer of protection, but at a cost. Personal purity mandates drain time and resources—a limited commodity in an already hectic existence. Women still do more laundry, grocery shopping, and household cleaning than their male partners, regardless of any recent discourse on gender equality. Now they need to do it even better and *safer*, with noxious chemicals peering over their hunched shoulders. Adding to their sense of urgency, their children's lives could presumably be in peril; cancer and chronic conditions loom on the periphery.

In time, women might come to blame themselves should they fail to buy their way to healthy freedom. Dafna, a marketing consultant and mother of three young children in New Jersey, considers her home "clean." She buys strictly nontoxic cleaners, consumes only organic produce, and counts seven natural deodorants on her nightstand. Plastic bottles are banned, as is most processed food. "I'm basically the CDC of our household," Dafna explains. Naturally, she was shocked when her eight-year-old daughter showed signs of early puberty, including breast development. Her pediatrician's tests confirmed follicle growth on her daughter's ovaries.

The discovery sent Dafna into a tailspin that caused her to fault her diligence, believing if she'd just *tried harder* and completely banished all synthetic chemicals and GMOs, her daughter wouldn't be in such a predicament. She joined parenting groups and read health sites that stressed the need to eradicate anything that didn't grow straight out of the ground.

"It's so easy to lose yourself in these forums, you don't know which way is up," Dafna recalls of the avalanche of information. In detoxing her home, the worried mom threw out any items that she believed could be contributing to her child's unwelcome development. Dairy was replaced with almond milk (much to her husband's dismay), and the perfumes were shelved away. "Could I have protected her better?" she asks with a strained voice. "I *thought* I was doing a good job."

The hectic mom likens herself to a smartphone running twenty apps at once—likely to crash—versus her husband, running just one. "It's not that my needs come last," she sighs, "it's that they don't come at all." Dafna doesn't blame her spouse: he doesn't encounter even a tenth of the information thrown her way. In frustration, she framed a quote—Michelle Obama's response to Sheryl Sandberg's *Lean In* philosophy: "That shit doesn't work all the time."

Dafna is not alone in her frustrations. It's neither cheap nor easy to carry the safety burden. For those unable to afford the expense of clean products, questionable chemicals will simply have to do. Lacking the disposable income to assemble a pure bathroom counter, most women continue to worry about ingredients as the media warns they'll jeopardize their future health. Meanwhile, it's not like women can opt out of the entire system: our labor market demands a certain level of hygiene and beauty. Women need to smell nice, look good, and be "presentable" not only to get a job but to keep it. A female professional cannot simply forgo consumption; she might feel as if she cannot stop dyeing her hair (with products made from ammonia and peroxide) unless she's willing to be subjected to ageism.

Although "clean" is a relatively new concept, it has hijacked women's anxieties, not only about beauty but about food, household cleaners, and even over-the-counter medicine. Suddenly we're all terrified of chemicals. Justifiably? Perhaps. Or not.

"The Real Thing":
A Return to the Natural Order

"Clean" isn't the only buzzword taking over your local Sephora. "Natural beauty" exploded in popularity alongside it, propelling luxury brands like Tata Harper into an industry worth billions. The naturals market is defined by products made from naturally derived ingredients stemming from plants and minerals, presumably free of synthetic chemicals. Think botanical ingredients that are usually in a fruit salad but somehow end up in your facial toner.

The appeal of nature is obvious, if not nostalgic. Nature worship has deep roots in American culture. (The naturalist John Muir, for instance, wrote that "nothing truly wild is unclean.")[14] By the more religious, nature is regarded as God's handiwork; therefore, the closer we get to it, the closer we are to godliness. In nature, we feel stripped down, minimal, and pure. We're clean in the most fundamental sense. And maybe that's a logical desire in a society in which we're divorced from nature and tether ourselves to tech in our artificial environments (like our cubicle offices).

We long for that which we feel missing, and what we're missing is minimalism. Everything feels overdone, overstimulating, and overwhelming. Less—as Marie Kondo tells us—is more.

A return to the natural order of things can presumably undo modern brutality, all the man-made "toxins" polluting our space and our world. More to the point, it signifies an awakening to the unhealthy environment around us. We want remedies and products to reflect our values: local, small, or handcrafted alternatives. The farmer's ideal. We long for days of yore, romanticizing village life when we personally knew the pig that ended up on our dinner plate.

Roughly 75 percent of millennial women say "natural" ingredients are an important factor in their purchases.[15] Consumers are drawn to naturals because they're "the real thing," believing that their bodies intuitively reject synthetic chemicals. They appreciate the authenticity of ingredients that have been "crafted" by nature, extracted from the beautifully evolved plants of the wild. Some women from ethnic communities use herbal remedies to reconnect to their cultural heritage, a link to a long maternal history. Likewise, people are attracted to the foreign, exotic, and ancient—centuries-old cures assumed to contain wisdom.

Corporate behemoths have flocked to this natural flame, eager to cash in. Clorox bought Burt's Bees, Colgate-Palmolive acquired Tom's of Maine, Unilever scooped up Schmidt's Naturals. Retailers built up entire "natural" and "organic" sections. Chemicals are out, "natural" is in—even in fashion. By late 2020, Gwyneth Paltrow could be found walking around her Brentwood neighborhood in a $100 white sweatshirt adorned with a single word: NATURAL.

All of this marketing does make you wonder: What even constitutes "natural"?

The Natural Fallacy

In 2019, the natural skin care brand Herbivore Botanicals advertised their $44 jars of Pink Cloud, a moisturizing cream reportedly made without harsh chemicals. "Everything we make is natural, chemical-free, non-toxic and entirely good for you," reads their website. The pretty, minimalist jars, inspired by the soft pink clouds of a Hawaiian sunset, quickly sold out. *Allure* posted a story to announce when it was restocked.

Alas, some who had scooped them up in time opened their jars of coveted loot only to encounter clumpy, funky-smelling goo. Their promised clouds of moisture? The texture of yogurt. A portion of Herbivore's naturally formulated products turned out to be moldy, and a recall was issued at Sephora.[16] As it happens, some "natural" beauty preservatives don't always work as well as their traditional "chemical" competitors. "Natural" preservative substitutes, if ineffective, can allow more contaminants—bacterial spores, yeast, and others—resulting in something more akin to a third-grade science experiment.

Herbivore wasn't the only company to experience this problem. The FDA increasingly recalls beauty products over bacterial contamination resulting from less effective preservation. And since "natural beauty" took off, dermatologists have reported an increase in patients reporting itchy red rashes, bumps, swollen areas, and other allergic reactions.[17] Such products often contain high concentrations of botanical extracts that can also be skin irritants. Not to mention that many "natural" ingredients are far less effective when it comes to results-driven skin care (aimed at wrinkle reduction, moisturizing, acne treatment, and other remediation) and lack the same rigorous level of clinical research. That means people are potentially paying a premium for inferior ingredients that not only underdeliver but (in rare cases) might irritate them.

But isn't natural supposed to be better than chemical?

Personal care products are all, technically, made of chemicals. The term "chemical-free" perpetuates science illiteracy because *everything* is composed of chemical compounds. Just because a company arbitrarily labels a product "natural," doesn't mean it isn't chemical. As one irritated Twitter user once tweeted at me when I wrote a story on the popularity of "natural" fragrances, "natural essential oils are complex chemical mixtures."

"[Beauty products] are all processed in some way," explains Perry Roma-nowski, a cosmetic scientist and formulator who delves into these com-plicated issues on his podcast *The Beauty Brains*. "You cannot go out into nature and pull a bottle of shampoo off a bush. There are no lipstick trees." A chemical is a chemical is a chemical; only its source and synthesis differ. But corporations love misusing the term "natural" as a way to distinguish their products, as if their concoctions are yanked right out of a garden.

The narrative surrounding chemicals in beauty products reminds me of a famous 1983 April Fools' Day prank. The *Durand Express*, a Mich-igan weekly newspaper, reported that dihydrogen monoxide—"a chemi-cal known to cause death" if inhaled—was discovered in the city's water lines.[18] How terrifying! After paragraphs alerting readers to the chemical danger, the joke was later revealed: dihydrogen monoxide is simply the chemical name for water, literally H_2O. The lesson? Everything sounds scarier if you identify it by its chemical terminology.

There might be less confusion if the use of the label "natural" to market products was clearly defined and regulated somehow. But although there have been efforts to establish a standard for the term "natural," uniform definitions simply don't exist. Any brand can slap "natural" on a label regardless of the ingredient list. These distinctions are often false adver-tising, offering consumers nothing more than a pricey placebo and a way to satisfy conscientious shoppers despite negligible botanical content.

"Natural," by definition, means existing in or caused by nature. Any-thing beyond that is conjecture. In fact, many natural substances (e.g., arsenic, asbestos, mercury) are more toxic than man-made ones. Even the seemingly most benign of naturally derived products can be harmful if used in the wrong way. This includes "natural" remedies like essential oils, which can act as irritants and allergens—or worse. Our illogical deference to Earth's bounty has become so widespread that researchers had to give it a name: the "appeal to nature fallacy," which occurs when we automat-ically assume something is better just because it's natural, and likewise, worse if it's not.

When I interviewed scientists to get their perspective on the natural product press releases flooding my inbox, I learned that the issue is not about synthetic versus natural, but whether the ingredient is safe and effective for use in the way intended. But *why*, I pressed, do brands continue to push a skewed beauty narrative? Why incorporate incorrect terminology?

Because it works. Over 90 percent of consumers believe natural beauty ingredients are better for them, according to a survey.[19] "If that kind of marketing wasn't effective with the people that are buying cosmetics, they would do other things," says Romanowski.

This is Branding 101. To create a need for a product, one must differentiate it from its competitors, as Douglas Atkin explains in *The Culting of Brands: Turn Your Customers Into True Believers*. One must create a mythology that marks a clear distinction and flatters the shopper through shared values.[20] Much as Apple fans buy in to the notion that their hardware purchase makes them "think different" than humdrum Microsoft drones, natural products make consumers feel good, educated. You know something others don't, and your face wash reiterates your inherent authenticity and environmental concern. Only "normals" buy in to the mainstream system. But not you: You know what's up. You are not satisfied with the status quo. *You care.*

Brands and influencers capitalize on legitimate yearnings. But they sometimes take it up a notch, assigning to nature fantastical traits and inherent virtue. They lean in to near-religious associations to sell nature as "purer" and "safer" (often without scientific backing) or to claim unsubstantiated superiority. Nature becomes something to worship. In some cases, you could easily substitute the word "God" and the copy would read like any devotional dogma. "Get rid of all of those harsh chemicals and come over to greet Mother Nature. She always has your back," reads an ad for the skin care brand Allure of Nature. Fiddler's Greens tinctures, composed of extra virgin olive oil and cannabis, are described as "just Mother Nature giving us exactly what we need."

Nature now possesses all the wisdom once afforded a bearded man up in the clouds. Trust that nature has a plan, brands state, while ignoring the earthquakes, tsunamis, pandemics, famines, and poisonous mushrooms plaguing this troubled earth. Nature, as science shows, does not signify goodness: nature is brutal, relying on survival of the fittest. And yet it's exalted as a higher power we can put faith in or that can transport us to a more wholesome era.

Shoppers gravitate toward this trend because of how cleverly it's been marketed. "Natural" is mentioned alongside words such as "pure," "authentic," "good," "real," "honest," "fresh," "wholesome," "worry-free," "gentle," and "safe." Compare that to demonized synthetic chemicals, which are regularly called "fake," "unnatural," "harsh," "toxic," "harmful," and "man-made." Juxtaposing chemical versus natural creates a narrative that these two categories are at odds with each other when in reality that's a false dichotomy.

"Household CDC" Dafna admits that highly publicized product safety scandals drove her to natural products. "In this fake world, you want fewer steps away from the source," she explains. "It feels a little more innocent, less consumerist." Having children also sparked a greater interest in what she describes as instinctual, innate womanhood. "You want to be in touch with nature."

But when Dafna finally visited a pediatric endocrinologist for her daughter's puberty spurt, she was advised to refrain from using lavender oil, which some studies have suggested may be a factor in premature breast development. Dafna was aghast. She used lavender oil every evening at bath time and rubbed it on her daughter's feet because wellness websites suggested it as a "safe" alternative to most drugstore moisturizers. "For eight years, I've been buying all organic, natural, beautiful organic shit to protect my kids, and then this. How fucked is that?" seethes Dafna. "You can't win." This is not to say one can identify what caused her daughter's early puberty. Studies have found associations with stress and obesity, among other potential factors (not to mention the randomness of genetic or hereditary traits). The point is that natural ingredients can potentially harbor the same concerns as "chemical" alternatives.

So why are we being told "alternatives" are always better?

A Clean Beauty Revolution or Marketing Confusion?

When I started writing this book, I called a cosmetic scientist who told me the clean beauty "movement," for all its promises of revolutionary change, is decidedly murky and chock-full of pseudoscience. His claims felt a bit inflated. So I called another. Same thing. Then another. Again, the same hesitance. By the fourth call, I began to accept what they were saying.

It's all marketing, they said.

Several additional calls later, here's what I learned about clean beauty. For one thing, it's complex. There's no simple answer here. But what is clear is that the science, as it stands now, is not being communicated to the consumer.

How so? For one, ingredients' presumed effects are often exaggerated, especially in cases in which topical use of an ingredient is equated with ingesting it. (You aren't eating your skin cream, right?) In addition, it's also common to cite studies conducted on animals exposed to high doses of the ingredient under question, significantly higher than the amounts any human encounters. These studies' findings therefore aren't immediately applicable to humans, who are much larger and have far different biology.* And if you think that something harmful to an animal is automatically problematic for us, then perhaps you also think we should stop eating chocolate because it's toxic for dogs.

In general, most ingredients in question are often used in amounts that are considered safe by toxicologists. Ingredients are studied for how much can be used, and cumulative exposure is accounted for. Toxicologists often repeat "The dose makes the poison," which means that at a high enough level, even water can be toxic. The result depends on how an

---

* However, toxicologists can establish safety for humans based on animal studies. The safe dose for humans based on animal toxicity studies is determined by its own science-based process.

ingredient is *used*. Focus shouldn't be placed on the potential dangers, but on the actual exposure, much as you shouldn't equate a splash of water to a tsunami. Water is not inherently dangerous, but it can be in the form of a fifty-foot wave.

"Toxicologists distinguish hazard from risk, wherein risk is the likelihood that a hazard will occur," explains the toxicologist Jay Gooch. "The fear game that is played is one where you simply mention the hazards that sound the scariest."

For example, lead is a natural element that can get into cosmetics, including lipsticks, at very low levels from a variety of sources. Beautycounter warns that lead poses health risks such as neurological effects, thyroid dysfunction, and reproductive toxicity in exposed adults. In response, the brand puts forth their own lipstick formulation, attempting their best to reach "non-detectable" heavy metal standards.[21]

But the level of lead in most conventional lipsticks is so minuscule and the exposure is so inconsequential that it can't be measured in routine blood testing, explains Perry Romanowski. "You could chew lipstick every single day for a year and you're not going to get lead poisoning."

We're not being given the full picture. "With a lot of ingredients that have been used for many years, there's still no strong link between these ingredients and any long-term health effects," says Michelle Wong, a cosmetic scientist who runs the popular website Lab Muffin Beauty Science. Contradicting the popular myth that "60 percent of skincare ingredients get into the bloodstream," Wong explains that the skin is a very tough barrier, with very few ingredients possessing the right properties to penetrate it in significant quantities, which is why most drugs are administered orally. For the overwhelming majority of molecules to get through the skin, you generally need some sort of penetration enhancer, because the skin's job is to keep the environment out. (I guess that's why we don't fear jumping into a chlorine pool.) Skincare formulations are crafted to stay within the first few layers of the skin. Beauty products are actually quite low on the list of potential hazards in comparison to something like air pollution or drinking water.

"The beauty industry is largely male, and they've largely ignored women's concerns about these [ingredients]," says Wong. "And because they haven't been addressed effectively, it's made it really easy for pseudoscience to take hold and get ingrained into our consciousness."

Often reporters believe in clean beauty's exaggerated claims because they are, like many unsubstantiated theories, based on real, existent anxieties. "The problem is that we humans, as a whole, have an inclination to believe negative information," explains the cosmetic chemist and formulator Esther Olu, who runs an Instagram account called The Melanin Chemist to combat misinformation in the beauty industry. We're more inclined to prick up our ears when faced with terrifying tidbits than we are when presented with science. Humans are built that way, evolutionarily hardwired to focus on threats.

Olu, along with Romanowski and others, is part of an emerging class of science experts producing content through podcasts, Instagram, TikTok, and YouTube to share a more nuanced take on the beauty industry. Cosmetic formulators and scientists were once quite content to work on their craft and leave beauty writing to underpaid twenty-six-year-old magazine writers. But as the clean beauty campaign ballooned, they became motivated to peek out from the lab and address false information and oversimplified arguments. Remember, it's not toxicologists running the beauty industry. It's marketers. And even dermatologists cited in articles might be incorrect because they do not necessarily specialize in toxicology and might not grasp the complexities of formulation as an experienced cosmetic chemist would.

In speaking to these cosmetic science experts, you pick up on hints of annoyance and weariness, of having to explain basic fundamentals for the hundredth time. They sound a lot like public health experts in 2021. *Tired.*

The Prickly Parabens Debate

One topic that can reliably get these scientists fired up is parabens.

Parabens are preservatives used to prevent the growth of bacteria and mold in everything from shampoo to shaving cream to mascara. They are probably the most rigorously tested ingredients in beauty. But some researchers hold that parabens may mimic natural hormone function, harm fertility, or increase the risk of cancer, and therefore have no place in personal care. The EWG cites animal studies in which certain parabens impacted female reproductive development and human studies that show a potential association with negative effects.[22]

But a blanket targeting of parabens is like saying *all* animals are dangerous. Which ones and at what level of exposure? Toxicologists I interviewed say the most commonly used parabens at their usage levels are *not* dangerous. The FDA, whose scientists continue to review any new paraben studies, states there is no proof that parabens' cosmetic use has an effect on human health.

Some critics mention the fact that parabens are found in urine, which doesn't sound great. But that doesn't necessarily prove harm: our bodies are meant to expel parabens from our systems. Not that parabens should even be assumed to be the devil. Parabens are derived from para-hydroxybenzoic acid (PHBA). Hydroxybenzoic acids naturally occur in some fruits and vegetables. The ones that show up in your skin care are synthetic versions of that.

The dispute over parabens is a complicated issue that took off after a highly contested 2004 study published in the *Journal of Applied Toxicology* discovered parabens in breast cancer tissue. However, in this study, the tissue was taken from samples of just twenty patients and not from a control group (that is, the researchers didn't test healthy breast tissue).[23] And, as critics have pointed out, "they didn't know if any of the people who donated tumor tissue used paraben-containing products."[24] The study did not demonstrate that parabens cause breast cancer, according to scientists I interviewed.

Some researchers challenge toxicologists on these matters, stressing that several studies suggest certain chemicals can be harmful at low doses. This is especially true of endocrine disruptors, since our hormone systems are activated at very low doses. Subsequent studies have suggested a possible link between parabens' estrogenic properties and breast cancer development.[25]

Heather Patisaul, the associate dean for research at North Carolina State University's Department of Biological Sciences, is a neuroendocrinologist who studies endocrine disruptors and says that they might be more subtle. "There can be this more insidious harm, like one could lose their fertility or could become obese," she explains. "It opened up this complicated dialogue about [if we are] harming ourselves in a way that's harder to see and evaluate than 'Oh, I just had a major stroke because I got massive exposure to a pesticide.'"

Discovering exactly what is going on is difficult because the impact is rarely immediate. "We know that the incidences of many diseases are going up and up too fast to not have an environmental cause, but it's incredibly challenging to establish cause and effect," explains Patisaul. It could be, she argues, that there are significant mixture effects. "What if it's parabens + phthalates = higher breast cancer risk? Or parabens + high sun exposure = higher skin cancer risk? . . . Those questions are rarely asked, let alone tested."

Perry Romanowski agrees that some chemicals can be harmful at low doses, but reiterates that cosmetic ingredients are tested for safety at low dose levels. As for potential harm, he asks, where is the proof? "Lots of things could be true," notes Romanowski. "Eating pizza could result in infertility. Exposure to soybean oil could cause birth defects. It's simple to dream up potential problems . . . These things have been studied. There just isn't any evidence to support the claim that cosmetic ingredients are causing 'insidious harm.'"

So we're always stuck with these questions: What do we do when the information is seemingly inconclusive? It's a complicated field of science, and one that, like all areas of health science, continues to evolve and incorporate new information. Experts call for more scientific research.

It's especially complicated when a host of other factors might play in. Take deodorants, many of which contain parabens. Because breast cancer is found near the armpit, deodorant is often blamed. But both the National Cancer Institute[26] (the federal government's principal agency for cancer research) and Susan G. Komen[27] (the world's largest breast cancer organization) state there isn't sufficient evidence to support this claim. And why blame the parabens when there are more likely candidates? The American Cancer Society notes, "Although parabens have weak estrogen-like properties, the estrogens that are made in the body are hundreds to many thousands of times stronger. So, natural estrogens (or those taken as hormone replacement) are much more likely to play a role in breast cancer development."[28]

One reason breast cancers grow not far from the armpit is that tissue is denser in that region and dense breast tissue is linked to an increased risk for breast cancer, suggests the University of Pennsylvania Health System. Denser tissue is also more difficult for doctors to detect via mammo-grams.[29] "So far, studies have not shown any direct link between parabens and any health problems, including breast cancer. Many other compounds in the environment mimic naturally produced estrogen," concludes the American Cancer Society.[30]

Isolating one culprit is extremely difficult because we are exposed to so many chemicals in our environment. Finding the smoking gun is nearly impossible because of the large number of chemicals we encounter each day in the air, the soil, and our frizz-free hair conditioner. For that reason, medical researchers (a conservative bunch) err on the side of caution in presuming culprits. Correlation does not equal causation. But that answer isn't definitive enough for some consumers.

A final note on parabens: the entire purpose of putting parabens in products is to avoid the growth of funky bacteria and fungus. So some-times there's a weighing of risks. And we shouldn't always err on the side of nature, because nature isn't necessarily safer. In fact, parabens have been far more tested in comparison to newer, more "natural" substitutes which have less data. Parabens have thousands of studies assessing their safety. They also remain one of the least allergenic preservatives.[31] That might be because "natural" preservatives, which aren't as effective, need to be used in *higher* concentrations. "The reason that parabens are so difficult to replace is because there's no other preservative that works that good and is that safe," says Romanowski.

But ultimately, even when the body of evidence heavily leans in a particular direction, it's a tough call for the average consumer. One might think there is no concrete causal evidence, but who's to say they won't find it down the line?

Even if we concede there's a debate, the inconclusiveness doesn't stop companies from exaggerating probable harm. Some brands tout a refusal of fourteen hundred ingredients already banned by the European Union, in seemingly stark contrast to the United States, "which has banned or restricted only thirty [ingredients]."[32] These numbers give the impression that the oversight process is an indiscriminate free-for-all. But the majority of those fourteen hundred "questionable" ingredients—like rocket fuel—never end up in beauty products, so restricting them is unnecessary. Just as banning Legos from food production is pointless.

Some clean brands love to say the United States hasn't passed a major federal law governing the cosmetics industry since 1938, implying that regulators have sat on their laurels for eighty years. This accusation is disingenuous. The framework is the same, but the FDA regularly updates regulations. Potential issues can and sometimes do slip through, and the FDA could certainly do more. But claiming that nothing is regulated is an exaggeration.† "It's just taking little points out of context and then confusing the marketplace," says the science communicator

---

† The FDA has the ability to require a company to recall or halt sales of any product deemed unsafe. It's also illegal to knowingly sell an unsafe product.

and formulation chemist Jen Novakovich, founder of the podcast and blog *The Eco Well*.

Most conglomerates and well-known brands, such as L'Oréal and Unilever, are obligated to take safety very seriously. Plenty of toxicologists point to their Scrooge McDuck–size budgets to research ingredient efficacy and safety. Big brands, especially in our highly litigious society, generally (though certainly not always) try to ensure safety because the consequences of not doing so can be very costly. If they face a class action lawsuit, they know they need to substantiate safety, and if they can't, they will have to pay out millions, if not billions, of dollars. This is why many also push for cosmetic regulation bills—because they already abide by many of the requirements proposed for legislation.[33]

What about all those lawsuits? If it's all just pseudoscience, how are lawsuits being won against big companies? On this front, the wellness shopper's concern is understandable. Product fiascos have left us wary of major manufacturers. But there's not always a simple answer—even for incidents that seem like a done deal. Thousands of women sued Johnson & Johnson, claiming the company's talc baby powder caused ovarian cancer due to naturally occurring asbestos contamination. Johnson & Johnson was ordered to pay over hundreds of millions of dollars, while other juries have ruled in favor of the pharmaceutical giant.

Johnson & Johnson denies their product was liable, and indeed some scientists say there's no conclusive evidence to suggest a causal link between talc and cancer development. A few experts I spoke to accused law firms of aggressively recruiting clients for class action lawsuits. But then other scientists defend women's claims. Studies are mixed, with some suggesting moderate risk and others unable to establish causality. In 2020, a study of a quarter million women was unable to find "a statistically significant association" between talc-based powders and ovarian cancer.[34] It's an ongoing scientific debate, one with worried consumers caught in the middle.

What does seem clear, however, is that J&J failed to disclose asbestos contamination to regulators and consumers, even if it was trace amounts. Ultimately J&J pulled the baby powder from U.S. store shelves, discontinuing a product that—harmful or harmless—was now too tainted by all the negative publicity. The company's lack of transparency fueled suspicion that they now admit simply cannot be overcome. Perhaps there's a lesson in that lack of transparency.

Everyone should have some skepticism toward any industry, so I'm not advocating trusting big brands en masse. Rather the point is to recognize that the activists in the clean beauty industry are *also* selling something—and profiting on anti-conglomerate sentiment. Any investigation into the beauty industry needs to be one that looks into the corners of the clean one as much as the mainstream one. Slapping a "free from" label on a bottle doesn't absolve a company of scrutiny. Just look at Jessica Alba's The Honest Company, which has recalled products and been hit with lawsuits, including one that charged it falsely mislabeled forty-one personal care products as "natural." (The company settled the class action lawsuit in 2017.)

Another industry-wide issue: many of these clean and independent brands outsource their manufacturing. They're not in full control. The Honest Company's baby wipes, which were voluntarily recalled over mold concerns, were made in China.[35] "[Some companies] don't have the type of oversight over their production and quality that a company like Procter & Gamble does," says Kelly Dobos, a cosmetic chemist and a member of the American Chemical Society's expert panel. Although conglomerates also make mistakes, "bigger companies have the resources to investigate, to be extremely thorough, and to handle a recall situation."

It's a lot to consider, but it's obvious that it would be helpful to take fear and hysteria out of the equation. Granted, science does change based on new information, but all we can do is act on what the current evidence shows.

The beauty industry, as it stands, isn't explaining the available evidence. Instead, wellness marketing perpetuates chemophobia—an outsized fear of synthetic chemicals or "chemical exposure." Though many of us are quick to parrot popular catchphrases like "trust science," a substantial portion of us are not well equipped in science basics, evaluating evidence, or critical thinking—thereby making us susceptible to pseudoscience. All the more so when we're taking advice from "experts" who aren't necessarily experts in the field they're weighing in on (or worse, dermatologists failing to disclose they're being paid by a brand). In fact, one 2021 study published in the *Journal of Experimental Social Psychology* found that people who are pro-science were more likely to believe and share misinformation when presented with articles and arguments packed with supposedly scientific lingo.[36] The bottom line: we're easily duped by academic language, seduced by the mirage of science. If it sounds like Bill Nye, we're sold.

Yet for all the debate surrounding clean beauty, Beautycounter did succeed in opening the floodgates of transparency. Before this movement, says Renfrew, the beauty industry had been built on secrets, which surely didn't help with industry mistrust. Now consumers demand to know the ingredient list and take a strong interest in what they buy.‡

Conglomerates and institutions could certainly do more to better test heavily debated ingredients and fund more research. But to do better, we need to take an honest look at what the current challenges are in our marketplace and not just make stuff up, which would only prevent real change, says *The Eco Well*'s Novakovich. "Consumers have to be given the right information," she says, reiterating that current regulations aren't perfect by any stretch. "Otherwise, we're misdirecting the energy."

The Environmental Working Group, which has been nicknamed "Environmental Worry Group" for relying on inflammatory, fearmongering language, isn't necessarily helping. The organization's methods for assessing risks are not uniformly shared by all experts, making it "beloved

---

‡ An ingredient label, however, does not inform you of a product's safety because it lacks specifics on dosing, production processes, potential contamination, and much more.

by activists but detested by scientists," according to the American Council on Science and Health. Critics say the organization peddles "scientific half-truths and outright fabrications."[37] In one survey of nearly one thousand members from the Society of Toxicology (an association of professional toxicologists), nearly 80 percent believed that the EWG overstated the health risks of chemicals.[38] Some scientists I interviewed have accused the EWG of depending on obscure, flawed, or dated studies with minuscule sample sizes—cherry-picking those that support their theories—and misinterpreting data to their liking.

The EWG cannot even be described as an impartial party, as it has a lobbying arm and receives heavy financial backing from the organic food industry, corporate brands, and "clean" beauty, including Beautycounter. The EWG also participates in affiliate programs (like Amazon's) and sells a certification label to make money off the very same products it recommends.§ If you go through their tax forms, you'll find folks like Michelle Pfeiffer, founder of the "clean and transparent" fragrance brand Henry Rose, who paid the EWG for ingredient guidance.

The EWG instills fear, then pushes certified products that will make it all go away. "So many people forget how much money they've made by doing the certification programs for brands," says Olu.

• • •

When clean beauty companies say they opt for "safe" ingredients, they imply that the competition doesn't. But toxicologists reiterate that the personal care aisle is not oozing slime, and that the body of evidence should be communicated to the consumer. Marketing cannot claim your face wash is out to harm you without being able to back the claim up. This is no longer even limited to small clean brands. Even conglomerates have pivoted to get in on the trend of the day because that's what the consumer responds to. They just give in to what's fashionable—exploiting doubt, fear, and guilt—regardless

---

§ An EWG representative noted that many nonprofits receive corporate support and sponsorships.

of the science. It's why you'll see CoverGirl promoting its "sulfate free" clean pressed powder even though sulfates wouldn't make their way into such a product. I'm surprised it isn't also labeled "fat-free" or "cage-free."

Still, with ingredients' impacts being debated, more research is required; perhaps that's what we should be lobbying for, considering beauty doesn't receive as much research or funding as other sectors. Although one thing is certain: we are worshipping a golden calf of misinformation. Novakovich and others would love to see the word "clean" removed from the beauty lexicon altogether because it perpetuates so much undue apprehension around safe products. The term reinforces the idea that if someone experienced bad effects or poor health, it's because they didn't buy the right products. It's fueling a culture of self-blame. "*That's* toxic," she says.

Don't get me wrong: I still buy Beautycounter (specifically their lightweight cleansing oil that dissolves makeup faster than any other cleanser I've tried). But I don't buy it out of fear, as though it's some magical amulet protecting me from chemical demons. I buy it because it *works*. And I like it. Maybe we can return to a space where we enjoy our products without fueling unsubstantiated assumptions. As the back of my Beautycounter cleansing oil informs me, "beauty should be good for you." Agreed. Perhaps that should apply to our psychological health as well?

The teachings of clean and natural beauty can cause bigger problems. Instilling an irrational fear of "chemicals" and claiming that nature reigns supreme—in other words, science illiteracy—can change the way we think about a whole lot of other stuff beyond lipstick. Some women take those simplistic lessons and apply them elsewhere. Because confusion or distrust over what's inside a package isn't just an issue with beauty. This concern reaches far beyond our bathrooms and extends to so many of the products we depend on. More and more women are asking, What's in my food? What's in my medicine? What's in my vaccine? *What's in everything?*

Chapter 4

Gym as Church

On the screen before you, a darkened stage is awash in purple neon lights. At the center of a circular podium sits a woman decked in a purple sports bra and leggings set. She is beautiful. She is hard-bodied. And she draws thousands of viewers on any given weekend.

Welcome to Sundays with Love, hosted by the Peloton fitness instructor Ally Love. This streaming stationary cycling class can gather seventy thousand viewers—what Love sometimes calls a "movement." A movement mostly, that is, of customers who put down anywhere from $1,745 to $2,495 for Peloton's connected bike.

Our fitness instructor begins with her eyes closed and hands in a casual prayer position. As the beat of an R & B tune kicks in, Love opens her eyes and stares directly into the camera. Extending her toned arms, she invites you—the audience—to join her. We are here, she explains, for a thought-provoking and spiritually grounding experience. "It's a celebration of life," Love offers.[1] In the background, the faint R & B song grows louder. It's Samm Henshaw's "Church," an apt title for this morning's work: "Mama said we in the church / You best believe this ain't no hotel."

"Today's virtue is honesty," Love proclaims. Honesty is supposedly the foundation of all other worthwhile virtues, and today we will hone this craft. Love then strengthens her voice to the uptempo beat: "Twenty-five to forty on resistance!" she shouts as you fiddle with your resistance control. "Welcome to your three-and-a-half-minute warmup."

Love pedals forward on her stationary bike, a makeshift pulpit. Bobbing up and down, her gold necklaces motion left and right like ping-pong balls. Five minutes in, she is ready to share more of her wisdom: What's the reason people are dishonest? Why do they shun this virtue? They fear embarrassment, want to avoid awkward situations, or simply hope to evade punishment. If you feel like you've committed any of these transgressions, it's okay, Love empathizes, pausing for effect: "Add one or two on resistance if you've done it."

You could call Love the patron saint of modern workouts. Incorporating religious lingo and pop psychology, her classes are motivational sweat sessions dripping with nondenominational faith. Sundays with Love begins with a mini-sermon centered on a chosen "virtue," like determination, honor, or courage, which Love peppers with moving personal anecdotes. This high priestess on handlebars might technically instruct clients in physical movement, but her real goal is to elevate the stationary bike into a soaring Pegasus of self-reflection with our fellow man. (Peloton integrates live rides with a digital social experience where users can "see" and compete with other members.)

Ally Love wants you to feel spiritually fulfilled. But also totally ripped.

Love has ascended to celebrity status with this creation. Peloton even sells a Sundays with Love capsule fashion collection, including $88 purple branded leggings that "inspire you to push into each week with passion and purpose." In just a few years, the energetic model/dancer has amassed nearly eight hundred and fifty thousand Instagram followers and snagged coverage in publications such as the *New York Times*, *BuzzFeed*, *People*, *Vogue*, and dozens more outlets. Fans dress up as Love on Halloween, complete with branded tank top and highlighted wig.

Peloton describes her class as "creating a sensation of deep connection with yourself" and declares that Love offers herself "to be used as a vessel."[2] Even the class artwork evokes the idea of a prophetic leader: Love is photographed with her arm outstretched and purple auras emanating from her bike pedestal, like Jesus at a disco. That is if Jesus, like Love, had an advertising deal with Adidas. (For all those who demean the humanities in college education, Love's success demonstrates otherwise. She seemingly got her money's worth from her theology program at Fordham University.)

Love is instantly likable, even inspirational. She offers up a dramatic origin story rooted in pain, perseverance, and ultimately independence. At the age of nine, Love was hit by a car as she walked away from an ice cream man. The horrific accident broke her hip and left femur. Love lay in a hospital bed for a week; the staff weren't sure she would make it due to massive blood loss.[3] She came out on the other side but to devastating news. Doctors informed her she would never be a runner, nor could she expect to ever be athletic. She was told to expect arthritis by the time she was fifteen.

Just a year after her accident, however, Love pushed the boundaries of her mortal body to overcome medical expectations. "I was able to defy those odds and decided that I really wanted to move my body," Love proclaimed decades later.[4]

People adore Love. Nearly all the Peloton fans I interviewed for this book detail how she impacted them. "Peloton saved my life . . . I feel like myself again," declared Danielle, a working mom of two who overcame postpartum anxiety. During a time when the elementary school health educator had stopped showering and cried every day, Peloton came to the rescue: the combination of motivational "life lessons" and hard-hitting exercise proved stronger than her antidepressants (which she's since ditched). Each morning, Danielle logs on to Peloton's streaming fitness classes where she is surrounded by happy strangers joining her in this mass ritual.

Danielle finds she has sustained energy throughout the day, more hope for the future, and even more patience for her children. "I don't go to church, but I can imagine that's sort of what church would feel like."

Today, Peloton has more than 6 million members, surpassing the population of Ireland.[5] Peloton grew to be a market leader for several reasons, one being that it was far more convenient for overwhelmed Americans (especially parents) who struggled to commute to and from physical studios. Walking upstairs to the guest room turned home gym trumped driving to a boutique gym.

But we already had NordicTrack and many home fitness options, so what catapulted Peloton to upper-middle-class stardom? What did it offer that other brands didn't?

An intoxicating blend of community and motivational interactive content.

Peloton promises far more than cardiovascular stamina; it promises all kinds of things that have nothing to do with cycling—by way of stirring language. So to call Peloton a "church" on a bike or their classes "mass" would not be a stretch. In fact, the similarity is intentional.

In 2017, the Peloton founder and CEO, John Foley, gave a presentation at a tech industry event. In describing the need for his 140-pound exercise hardware, Foley said there's been a dramatic slide in people's association with organized religion, but "that is not to say that people do not still want that guidance and ritual and identification and community and music and ceremony and spirituality and reflection—that stuff that happened on Sunday morning at church or in your synagogue."

Foley went on to say that people want fitness *and they want something else*, before pausing for dramatic effect. The heralded solution? "Enter instructor-led group fitness classes. Replete with the candles on the altar and somebody talking to you from a pulpit for 45 minutes." He goes so far as to liken a Star of David or a crucifix draped around one's neck to a branded fitness tank top. "That's your identity. That's your community. That's your religion."[6]

It's not that far-fetched an idea. Going to a gym can be sacred depending on the meaning one gives it. Purpose, ritual, fellowship, discipline, and prayer all make their way onto a fitness bike. As the sociologist Wade Clark Roof once observed, religion is socially produced and is constantly being reproduced. Faith is always being creatively tinkered with and interpreted to fit people's heritage, environment, and cultural norms.* And the most successful faiths adapt to the demands of the day.[7]

The ultimate Peloton mission is "to better ourselves, inspire each other, and unite the world through fitness."[8] By this account, Peloton is something to *believe in*. If not talk of virtues, Peloton instructors share uplifting one-liners reminiscent of elementary classroom posters: "Anybody can give up, but you're not just anybody," or "Don't do what you can do, do what you should do." The body is something to conquer, to mold into something greater. Much like the concept of original sin, our bodies—as is—are weak, imperfect, and keeping us back. But with perseverance and labor, we can transcend the pitiful state we're in; we can change our destiny.

While Peloton's digital platform might be the new Vatican, it wasn't the first to market sweat-dripping faith. When it comes to mixing spirituality and group fitness, no brand is more on the nose than the upscale fitness studio SoulCycle. Though it may have forfeited its papacy to Peloton, its ascent explains a lot of current fitness trends growing stronger by the day. SoulCycle walked so that Peloton could run (or rather bike) to fitness domination.

Over the years, I've gone to SoulCycle more than a dozen times, and each time, I was amazed at how enjoyable it was. Class never felt like work. It felt like being taken on an interactive amusement park ride with a bunch of ecstatic women way too enthusiastic for morning exercise.

SoulCycle lived up to a term thrown around too easily these days: cult

---

* In 2020, I wrote a *New York Times* piece about how organized religion was turning to wellness to woo back audiences. Churches, synagogues, and mosques have begun implementing cardio classes, hikes, and even forest-bathing prayer programs.

brand. Fans built their work schedules around classes. Women rose before the sun for their favorite instructors. It even governed real estate choices. "I can never live anywhere where there's not a SoulCycle," one follower noted in a report on nonreligious communities studied by Harvard Divinity School students.[9] It went beyond being just a boutique fitness studio. It induced religious fervor.

So what exactly was in the sugar-free Kool-Aid?

Evangelists on a Transcendent Bike

Julie Rice was *over it.*

Her seemingly perfect Malibu life wasn't cutting it anymore, even though it looked like a Hollywood success story. For ten years Rice served as a talent manager to A-list stars at a well-known management company. Jennifer Lopez was a firm client, as was Will Smith. She took on Ellen Pompeo and Justin Long before you knew who they were, and you know who they are now largely because of her.[10] Rice knew everyone, was well respected, and negotiated deals with a lot of zeros behind the dollar sign.

But Rice was missing something. She flashed forward and saw a future full of long days with uninspired meetings surrounding the whims of demanding clients. She saw herself more like a prisoner with golden handcuffs than as a power player on a golden path. Rice didn't even want to stay in Los Angeles. She wanted to return to her native New York, "to keep it real."[11]

When she thought about her next pursuit, Rice kept thinking about the one thing she loved about Los Angeles—the city's active lifestyle. Like many Angelenos, Rice treasured weekends spent hiking with friends, reveling in the majestic mountains while chatting away. Or, if she wasn't climbing the canyons, she was engrossed in a local running club where camaraderie trumped speed. Her social life didn't revolve around drinking cocktails so much as it did around burning calories.[12]

When Rice moved to Manhattan, there was nothing quite like the social activities that filled her L.A. weekends. Acclimating to the concrete jungle, Rice joined big-box gyms, but they failed to provide the intimacy or awe readily built into California fitness culture. The instructors at a New York cardio class yelled at her to work harder, which wasn't exactly emotionally supportive. Going to work out felt like "part of the grind."[13] She missed the sense of connection. It was a real void.

So Rice turned to one pastime that New York has on lock: venting. She complained to her cycling class instructor that nothing felt quite right. She wanted to be dazzled, not bullied—or worse, ignored—by her gym's staff. The cycling instructor set her up on a friend date with another client who had expressed similar gripes. That's how Julie Rice met Elizabeth Cutler, her business soulmate.

Like Rice, Cutler came from an outdoorsy social culture—in Colorado. She too missed the bonding moments that came with hiking with friends. Without her mountains, Cutler had no social fitness outlet. She missed the ritual.

Cutler and Rice found themselves imagining their perfect gym over lunch at the members-only club Soho House. It would be an uplifting fitness "experience" staffed by life-changing instructors who nurtured a supportive community. The clients should connect, not compete. The studio should be a center for empowerment, with exercise treated like a theater production and fashioned as a "lifestyle." And unlike the membership model, they wanted a pay-per-class system to ensure that people had a reason to come back—the classes would have to be *that good*. So good that a brand wouldn't need to spend much on marketing; their users would automatically spread the word to their friends, co-workers, and family. And if their friends couldn't get in, they wanted them to feel only the most visceral Manhattan reaction: FOMO.

They wouldn't create clients. They would create *evangelists*.

"It was like we had the same exact idea, and we were just completing each other's sentences," says Rice of their fateful first meeting. "When I left lunch that day, before I even got in my cab, my cell phone rang and it was Elizabeth. She said to me, 'I'm going to look for real estate, and you look at towels. I'll call you on Thursday.'"[14]

Sure enough, by that Thursday, Rice's new best friend had found a 1,200-square-foot former dance studio on the Upper West Side ("which we found on Craigslist!" Rice proudly recalled years later).[15] It was perfect. Rice, who had a five-month-old baby at the time, went all in: she quit her job, locked away her credit cards, put her family on a $400 weekly budget, and signed the lease.

The very first SoulCycle opened several months later. The boutique studio offered an "inspirational, meditative fitness experience" in the course of a forty-five-minute indoor cycling class. Rice hit the pavement, traversing Manhattan with a baby stroller as she begged people to let her post flyers in their storefronts. If she saw someone open a door to an apartment building, she'd stick her foot in before it closed and then flyer-bomb the mailroom. It was, as she called it, guerrilla-style marketing.[16]

Within a year, SoulCycle sign-ups were crashing the server as New Yorkers rushed to snag a seat.[17] The studio's popularity was due in large part to how the brand trained its employees in hospitality. Instructors were hired full time and paid above market rate so that they could take the time to invest in their students—learning their names, sharing favorite songs, and chatting with them before class. "People felt seen . . . like they mattered," said Rice.[18]

Within a few years, what started as a need for social exercise turned into one of the hottest and most exclusive boutique fitness studios. Soul-Cycle earned a celebrity following and acquired the kind of status usually reserved for luxury fashion labels. How? By formulating a transcendent collective experience that women couldn't resist.

Boutique Piety for Mystic Sweat

At seven in the morning, a group of stationary cyclists furiously pedal to the uptempo electro-beat of a Britney Spears remix. The song is "Till the World Ends," an uncanny title given that the cyclists are there to find something akin to salvation. "How you do anything is how you do every-thing," calls the energetic class leader, readjusting her headset. "Hell yeah!" responds a member from somewhere in the back of the room.

Lights are dimmed to near blackout, save for a few grapefruit-scented candles in the corners of the intimate SoulCycle studio. You're cocooned in the darkness—a muted support system that lets you, the individual, shine. Working individually but in the reassuring presence of others, members can focus on themselves. There's an element of freedom despite being squished together like sardines, a closeness purposely manufactured. Rice, who along with Cutler stepped down after selling SoulCycle to Equinox in 2016, explained:

> When people were done complaining about "Can you believe they're going to charge $27[†] and I'm going to have to sit that close to somebody?" what actually happened was, the lights were dark, and people could all feel the music at the same time, and you could almost feel somebody breathing next to you. Your foot was on the same beat as their foot was on, and all of a sudden it became connected, and it became tribal, and it was dark, and there were candles. The music was amazing and an instructor is telling you that you could be more than you thought you could be . . . There's something about a moving meditation with other people that are rooting for you, that are holding space for you, that aren't there to compete with you, that are there to elevate you so that they can be elevated as well.[19]

Heavily contributing to this altered state is the combination of music with movement, similar to the way EDM concerts inspire euphoric emo-tions. Such strong emotions can spark a spiritual connection to something outside ourselves; we submit ourselves to see the world as something good,

---

† Note: It's now approximately $36.

beautiful, and powerful. And when we're deeply entrenched in something, like when we're wildly dancing at a party, the absorbing activity puts us into a near-trance-like "flow" state.[20] We shut off that nagging voice in our head (with all its to-do lists) and redirect our focus to repetitive rhythmic motions. Hence the term "losing yourself" in an activity: when you're so absorbed in pedaling, there's no room for intruding, ruminating thoughts.

The self, as you're accustomed to it, melts away. A "we" takes over. And suddenly you feel nothing but love and connection to your fellow rider. You look around the room and think, "we're all getting through this ride together."

Pedaling in unison takes on a powerful force, even in its digital equivalent, Peloton. But according to researchers at Oxford University, it is exercise's mood-enhancing endorphins and serotonin (nature's uppers) that might be responsible for some of those feel-good bonding emotions. In experiments where strangers were brought to row together, they discovered that moderately intense group exercise creates more meaningful social benefits than lower-intensity exercise. "It may be that experiencing exercise-induced natural highs with others leads to a sort of 'social high' that facilitates group bonding, friendship, and cooperative behaviour," wrote the study's co-author.[21]

Of course, much of SoulCycle's success also lies in its talent. (Before there were Peloton influencers snagging brand endorsement deals, there were SoulCycle star instructors, often known only by their first name, like Oprah.) The brand does not hire the average fitness instructor. It recruits charismatic *performers*. Dancers, cheerleaders, actors, models, Broadway veterans, and professional athletes audition in what Rice once called *"American Idol* on a bike." The company scouts for charismatic showpeople oozing star presence—the same kind of people who can lead a congregation. Fitness pastors, you could say. SoulCycle promotes talent as the main attraction, some of whom reportedly earn up to $1,500 per class. And they make sure to live up to the hype.

Instructors say they "strengthen faith muscles," supplying a kind of emotional catharsis for those in need of healing. As one teacher explained,

"I get them to a point where they are so tired that emotionally they are so much more vulnerable. They no longer rely on their physical strength; they have to go deeper. That is when the experience becomes more than a workout."[22] Instructors motivate, but they also exhibit a slice of vulnerability to connect with congregants. "Sorry I'm late, my four-year-old was sick," one instructor told a class. "If you thought I looked too young to have a kid, I also have a six-year-old, a ten-year-old, and a divorce."[23]

Plenty of SoulCycle instructors develop strong ties with repeat customers, who at times rely on them during moments of crisis—a divorce, a breakup, Barneys closing. Fans report that they'll text their fitness mentor when they're going through a rough patch or stop them after class to seek counsel on sensitive matters. This attachment is not unlike the dependence on self-help books, which some researchers say fill in the gaps once filled by organized religion or closer-knit female communities.

"It is possible that the emphasis placed on friendship in women's lives has diminished as we have entered the paid labor market in greater and greater numbers, as the division of labor has become more specialized, and as families have become smaller and more isolated," writes the sociologist Wendy Simonds in *Women and Self-Help Culture*. "All these trends may have helped to professionalize the giving and receiving of advice, at least among the rich and middle class."[24] What was once a mainstay of female friendships—of telling someone to dump their dumb boyfriend—has now been outsourced to "professionals" as a commodified service. One's psychologist or Peloton instructor has replaced a once ordinary exchange because we're all too darn busy or far away to be there for one another.

Fitness brands may have created new ministers, but people need more than just a priest. They need a congregation. People need people. And with those people, they need to *feel* something. SoulCycle emphasizes "community" as much as it does its impressive talent, and Peloton advertises working out "together" in your living room. As the beloved indoor cycling brand posted on Facebook in 2020, "Sun up to sundown, you'll never ride alone."

So exercise classes are group therapy and High Holiday services and country club social time all rolled into one. They are, as the sixties "seekers" sought, an experiential spirituality. Whereas once mankind shook at Sinai to bombastic commandments or participated in gleeful revelry with faith healers, now we get a spiritual boost from group cardio. There are now even wellness festivals where ten thousand or more people (80 percent of them college-educated women) join in mass yoga like a Zen revival tent.[25] Women are expressing a need for intense tribal gatherings. And Beyoncé goes on tour only so often.

Flashback: The Original Group Fitness Fad (with a Nude Twist)

The April 1937 issue of *Life* magazine was keen to investigate a new "body culture" taking the Western world by storm: a peculiar new fitness fad that had groups of women doing leg circles and spine twists in a classroom setting—and completely in the nude. Not only were they stark naked, but they were performing a medley of slow-moving exercises in between two mirrors.[26] Double the view.

Called the Mensendieck system, it was a set of functional exercise movements to strengthen muscles as well as improve posture. Its creator was Dr. Bess Mensendieck, one of the first female physicians (European-trained but American by nationality). She inspired a generation of women to gracefully move their bodies. She also exalted nudity, believing it "fundamental in enhancing body consciousness."[27]

In 1905, Dr. Mensendieck published the first of several books centered on gentle movements, with picture tutorials on how to properly iron or reach for an item on a shelf. (Since Dr. Mensendieck's exercise manuals featured photos of demonstrations in the nude, they initially were deemed too risqué to be sold in the United States.) Some exercises were in direct response to what she saw as society's increasingly negative effect on women's health—modern constrictions such as fashionable narrow shoes and corsets so tight they resulted in fainting.[28] The body required full physical freedom, she preached. These ideas stemmed from Victorian dress reform, an attempt to make fashion less suffocating and more comfortable. In place of constricting undergarments, Dr. Mensendieck advocated "nature's corset": exercises to strengthen abdominal muscles and align the spine.

Over the next two decades, Dr. Mensendieck would open schools across Europe, and eventually her teachings spread to New York.[29] Her gymnastic training became a worldwide hit, with a reported two hundred thousand students enrolled in her programs. Two-thirds of them were women. By 1937, Yale University was teaching her revolutionary theory. Elite private academies incorporated the nude classes, although teen girls were permitted to wear underwear if they had "the curse."[30] Hollywood took to the Mensendieck system too, with devotees reportedly including screen sirens like Ingrid Bergman and Greta Garbo.

On the one hand, fitness was still a relatively new idea: tending to one's own body was a foreign concept to those who were raised to care solely for others. Throughout history, women weren't afforded the same opportunities as men to build strength. Now they were encouraged to work on their own physical well-being. And to do so with other women.

On the other hand, Dr. Mensendieck's teachings—which mostly catered to upper-class women—overemphasized beauty and grace, flat-out equating appearance with health and virtue. Maintaining an attractive body, by her logic, cemented one's social standing. "Sculptors tell me they are in despair over the lack of models with perfectly proportioned bodies," she told the *New York*

Times in 1924. "I go to the opera or a bal masqué [masquerade ball]. I am ashamed of my sex when I see the backs and arms and torsos revealed by décolleté evening gowns."[31]

Exercise fads come and go. The Mensendieck system is rarely heard of today. Although, some historians believe she had an influence on Joe Pilates, who created one of the most popular exercise routines of all time; Pilates is now taught in group classes everywhere.

Craving Connection: Wellness Fills the Void

By now we're all aware many Americans are lonely, isolated, and increasingly detached from meaningful socialization. There is no shortage of literature on this. The seminal book *Bowling Alone* by Robert Putnam flagged the crumbling dissolution of robust social infrastructures. We've heard that loneliness is rumored to be as damaging to health as smoking fifteen cigarettes a day. We've read headlines on millennials who struggle to find friends and hear about new moms grasping for advice on message boards. And we've come across startling social media groups, like a 300,000-member-strong Reddit group titled NeedAFriend.

More telling: thousands join virtual and silent co-working groups, where they keep a muted collective Zoom on in the background just so they can feel the presence of others. That's how bad it is. That's how *real* it is.

Today, a vastly different landscape confronts the lone American from a century prior, thereby shattering communal bonds and in effect, their identity. If in decades past, we automatically inherited fraternity through our large families, walkable neighborhoods, and religious institutions . . . in the twenty-first century, we cobble together a hodgepodge of friends here and there and stay in touch via frantic text exchanges. Meaningful social activities have been replaced by paid services that rob us of the chance to connect: quick Amazon book deliveries stand in for local libraries while Grubhub replaces communal home-cooked meals. Consumed with convenience, career success, and independence, we never stopped to ponder whether all these advancements hampered our social health.

Tech is another double-edged sword. Many Americans feel isolated despite "friends" at their fingertips, just a text away. If anything, recent research finds that heavy social media dependency—those who mainly use it as a substitute for real, in-person connection—increases loneliness. One reason is because so much of online postings are situated around performance, status, and showing off what's going superbly well. It's a toxically positive exaggeration of real life. When everyone is posting only the highlight reel on Instagram, that might just make you feel only lonelier: *Does everyone have an amazing life but me?*

Loneliness adds stress, accelerates physiological aging, and increases rates of depression. But interestingly, strong bonds are a female superpower. Research suggests women, more than men, engage in something called the "tend-and-befriend" phenomenon. When shit hits the fan, they are better able to handle stress because they're more inclined to seek social support (versus the "fight or flight" response to a threat). Reaching out to others releases oxytocin, the "love hormone" that facilitates bonding and reinforces commitment to those in your group.[32]

Prioritizing support isn't that easy, though. Would people prefer to have friends over for dinner and get to know their neighbors? Absolutely. But working Americans are so pressed for time that they barely have the opportunity to cook a meal for themselves, let alone for the Joneses next door. On weekends, when they presumably do have time, they're exhausted, preferring just to veg out on the couch watching Netflix. Facing an ever-growing list of errands and pressures, they simply can't be bothered to socialize as much as they'd like. If they don't belong to a built-in community with scheduled events, like, say, a church, that means they'll need to make plans. And who has the patience to make plans?

That's where boutique fitness studios come in. Like church—which has long been a communal gathering place—you don't need to orchestrate brunch plans or figure out friends' availability: people are just there. There is a set time. It's a social hour programmed into your life. And so, it becomes part of your routine, *a habit*. And if you give fitness a sense of purpose, as many women do, it evolves into a ritual—one that brings meaning, if not a sense of belonging. It's why I hear so many women call their local studio their "tribe."

Turns out that despite all the loneliness, connection continues among women, albeit in altered forms and by virtue of new wellness enterprises. Maybe they're not chatting in the church pews or baking cookies together for the sisterhood, but they are creating new and useful models. Ones where they can ask: Why not reach and connect with someone while also toning that butt?

The wellness industry has succeeded in convincing consumers they can master their life—and solving the problem of isolation was no exception. Over the last two decades, boutique fitness studios marketed their intimate social settings, spurring rapid expansion over the last decade. Some studios host book clubs, holiday parties, even weekend retreats. These gym societies draw millennials with the allure of meeting new people. Instructors ask participants to high-five their neighbors and to hang out at post-class happy hours. Planet Fitness throws pizza parties where members socialize over a free slice and bodybuilding tips.

In a 2019 survey of two thousand Americans conducted by *Vox* and Morning Consult, respondents were asked what kinds of social or ritualistic activities regularly provide "purpose, community, or identity." More than book clubs, bar outings, recreational sports, or political meetups, people named . . . exercise classes. They hit the gym once a week or more.[33] In Los Angeles, you might find the young, toned, and athletic hitting up trendy gyms like CrossFit or Barry's Bootcamp. Type A Manhattanites join early-morning running clubs that meet in both sweltering and freezing temperatures. The Midwest sees rapid growth of Females in Action (FiA), a free and peer-led workout program for women in which each workout finishes with a prayer or secular intention.

Boutique gyms wax poetic on how their enterprise provides "family" and "connection." Promises sound like, "At SoulCycle, we are a pack—we look out for each other." As with any group dynamic, participants' reason for banding together sets the motivation: the why is just as important as the who. A shared passion or experience is the point. And naturally, no one wants to be merely with people; they want to be with their own perceived kind. This can be distinguished by race, class status, interest, or psychographics. No matter who these spaces cater to, they attempt to gather the scattered, anchoring them in a familiar place—a twenty-first-century Cheers.

Some say the communal benefits outweigh the primary health draw. A small Brown University study suggests that with instructor-led mindfulness programs, the social factor is potentially "more significant than the type or amount of meditation practiced."[34] The "with whom" may just trump the "how" because face-to-face contact has been shown to lessen anxiety, stress, and depression.[35] In interviewing more than a hundred participants, researchers found they frequently spoke about their relationships with fellow participants and the class instructor, notably "the expression of feelings and the installation of hope."

Others might question whether building your communal identity around the ability to perform push-ups rings hollow. They turn their nose up in favor of political movements, traditional religion, or more intellectual pursuits, believing them superior modes of communal power. But if the ultimate need is to connect, then whatever gets the job done is worthwhile. And if you are concerned with your health, then why wouldn't you seek out like-minded parishioners?

What Kind of "Community"?

Questions I've long had while peering into these newly established wellness spaces: How much of a community *is* it? What kinds of bonds are we forming? Perhaps things aren't as bad as they seem with this whole "loneliness epidemic."

From a macro view, wellness acts as a social signifier. When individuals see others carrying a yoga mat, it's a clear signal: *I'm one of you. We share the same interests.* So often I see women strike up a conversation with someone spotted in yoga leggings, sparking discussions on products or practices. It's a common language. That's one type of belonging.

Then there's the belonging to a specific gym. Boutique studios can truly act as a tight-knit clan, where members check in with one another and rally around a member going through chemotherapy. I've heard several remarkable stories about the close bonds forged within CrossFit gyms, a chain well known for welcoming people of all backgrounds and sizes. It all depends on the space or the leadership, which sets the tone for community engagement. Is there a sense of obligation to one another? Is there room to socialize? It also comes down to what you put into it. If you loiter around the water cooler, you have a better chance of making new friends.

The same goes for digital groups. There are over a hundred Peloton Facebook groups for fans to unite over a shared identity, hobby, or goal, some boasting hundreds of thousands of members. There's Peloton Riders for Christ, Working Moms of Peloton, Peloton Military & Veterans, and instructor fan groups that feel like rock star fan clubs. For the LGBTQ community, Peloton can feel like the church they were never quite welcome at. When instructors mouth Lady Gaga lyrics such as "I'm beautiful in my way, 'cause God makes no mistakes," they can feel seen in a way that feels nearly therapeutic, a radical acceptance in a society that doesn't always extend it. One superstar instructor told *Vogue* he helped students come out to their parents.[36]

Even the seemingly casual networks can foster real support and substantial dialogue. It's not uncommon to see issues of self-worth, feminism, and the meaning of a good life pop up on fitness platforms. Members boost up those in need of emotional assistance, like a new mom sharing her body image issues. Far beyond cardio tips and oatmeal recipes, these spaces become beacons of help for those in need.

One member of the Peloton Law Moms group—a group of mostly

young and middle-aged lawyers—told me that if someone posts about needing a job, another member will call in a favor or offer a referral. Another time, a member shared that her child was in the hospital, prompting Law Moms members to order flowers, food, and gifts straight to her daughter's ward. Maybe they weren't there in person, but their virtual support proved they were united by more than just $1,895 exercise equipment. "It's not superficial," this member assured me.

While sociologists debate the quality of virtual interactions, others hold that the structure of a community is changing. After the pandemic, we are not returning to a world where everyone counts on Sunday service or social clubs for socialization. So the question becomes: With this new reality, how can we make it the best it can be?

Critics worry that people only socialize with their own kind in these communities. Peloton's core demographic, for example, is college-educated, has a household income of over $100,000, and skews female. As Americans gravitate to smaller, single-purpose groups (like the Peloton Law Moms Facebook group), they retreat from a more diverse pool of people. We naturally tend to silo ourselves off into groups where others look like us, act like us, and think like us. As Putnam wrote, if once upon a time we came face-to-face with our disagreeable neighbors, now we opt for groups "purpose built to represent our narrower selves."[37]

That said, I also hear from plenty of Peloton riders who learn about different groups of people through fitness classes. Diverse instructors share their personal experiences of discrimination with their audiences. Gay instructors recount how they have struggled in a society that wasn't always hospitable to them. This is where, specifically, digital connection brings together people from all walks of life.

Maria Doerfler, an assistant professor at Yale University's Department of Religious Studies, is skeptical of digital fitness communities. Without suggesting that every person who purchases a Peloton or works for the brand is of a certain mold, there is a very strong overlap and strong homogeneity.

"It's a very curated sort of diversity—exactly the level of diversity that is tolerable for the lowest common denominator of consumers," Doerfler told me. "If that's the extent of your encounter with persons of different ethnic background than yourself, persons of different sexual orientation, of different gender identity, I think you're being sold a bill of goods."

Now, not everyone is looking to their gym to be their diversity outlet—or their community. In most cases, gym connections are loose and casual. Some just enjoy seeing the same faces every week, like their own little buff Sesame Street. I attended a cardio fitness studio two to three times a week for nearly three years. And though I adored my instructors, I bet none could tell you anything about me save for the fact that I love working out to Prince and hate doing burpees.

People might dismiss these "loose affiliations," but the pandemic proved how being barred from those acquaintances felt like a real loss. People spoke of how surprised they were that they missed schmoozing with the yoga studio receptionist or joking around with their fellow gym members. They often wondered what happened to that one guy they would high-five after class. Were they best friends? No. But it did mean *something*. We need both loose and strong connections, and the former might just even turn into the latter if you cultivate them.

But here's another question I have: While these gyms act like religion, feel like religion, and nearly market themselves as religion, should we expect them to deliver like religion?

Spiritual Leaders in What, Precisely?

Gym members might consider instructors their surrogate pastors, but the majority of fitness instructors are as trained in chaplaincy as Gwyneth is in gynecology. They're trained in showmanship. In SoulCycle's case, talent undergoes an *eight-week* training program where they learn cycling, DJ skills, and "how to be spiritual and emotional leaders."[38] Fitness instructors aren't necessarily equipped to handle a client's issues with divorce, trauma, or loss. They might not know how to navigate suicidal tendencies or spot dangerous downward spirals. They are potentially being put in positions that they're not ready for.

Fitness instructors also tend, inevitably, to be much more mobile than their pastoral counterparts, who are often stationed for life with a congregation. The result can be devastating for their flock. As one member lamented on Twitter, "my regular SoulCycle Instructor is moving to Southern California and I don't even know what to do." And vice versa: in the early months of the pandemic, SoulCycle furloughed or cut a percentage of their staff without severance.[39] One former instructor felt it was at odds with the company's preached ideals: "A brand that talks about honesty, transparency, community and supporting each other all seems to all be a big myth," wrote one former instructor of being let go with no severance, and by his account, no explanation.‡

Now, of course SoulCycle, like all companies, had to protect its finances during the pandemic's economic upheaval. But just like companies promoting social justice causes without practicing it in their hallways, SoulCycle's "community" evangelizing came to bite them in the firm ass.

In 2020, numerous reports found that not only did the company transgress its "family" ethos by unceremoniously dumping staff, but that top management turned a blind eye to inappropriate behavior. By boosting fitness stars to prophet proportions, SoulCycle inadvertently created untouchable gods. Clients and former employees accused top-performing instructors of sexist, racist, and bullying behavior. A *Vox* investigation unearthed a note that hung in an office, penned by a top instructor

---

‡ A SoulCycle rep offered the following statement: "Like many organizations at the start of the pandemic, we furloughed a percentage of our employees and maintained benefits coverage. Whether someone impacted by a position elimination received severance was based on our severance eligibility criteria at that time. If not severance eligible, impacted employees received benefits continuation for three months or a stipend to cover benefits continuation for three months."

trainer: "If someone asks you if you are back on cocaine or if you have an eating disorder, you know you've hit your goal weight."[40] One popular instructor allegedly fat-shamed front-desk staff. Other instructors were accused of diva-like antics like hurling objects at fellow employees, berating staffers if they got a green-juice order wrong, or sexually harassing non-talent staff.[41]

But SoulCycle reportedly did nothing.[§] Why? Because, as former corporate employees attest, the instructors were just too valuable to the brand. They brought in too much money.

Gym-goers seem to forget one important point—at the end of the day, *these are businesses*; their goal is profit. Unless you're the Murdochs, "family" bonds do not report to shareholders. For although SoulCycle's IPO filing claims the brand intends to "help people connect with their true and best selves," it also states a very definitive goal: make gobs of money, as evidenced by plentiful income stats like "expanded total revenue from $36.2 million in 2012 to $112.0 million in 2014, representing a CAGR of 76 percent."

On one hand, SoulCycle claims its "mission is to bring Soul to the people." On the other, it proudly touts an intentionally exclusionary reservation system that "has created a frenzied experience . . . when approximately 30 percent of our weekly rides are selected within 15 minutes." Some classes had waitlists of over 400 people. In a 2010 *New York Times* report, one besotted member compared snagging a seat in a top instructor's class to getting a reservation at Momofuku,[42] which was then among *GQ*'s top five hardest restaurant reservations to score.

You also have to ask what a "family" entails when it relies on very

---

[§] In December 2020, SoulCycle responded with a statement, noting, "When we receive complaints or allegations within our community related to behavior that does not align to our values, we take those very seriously and have internal processes in place to both investigate and address them, as needed."

specific criteria. If your community membership is dependent on a level of physical ability or financial status, you're out of luck should either fall by the wayside. (A *Business Insider* investigative report alleged that one instructor booted a pregnant woman from her reserved front row seat to make way for a thinner rider.)[43] Here is where wellness spaces lack the infrastructure of more established institutions; a religious congregation, for example, spans multiple touchpoints versus one particular (ableist or financially dependent) touchpoint. And while organized religion also relies on money—as anyone who has paid a hefty temple membership fee can attest—it's usually better equipped to help those who have fallen on hard times.

Do you really think SoulCycle would let someone attend for free if they lost their job?

This is not a spirituality intended for the masses. Scarcity—or more like *exclusivity*—is the point.

Boutique studios are meant to be small, exclusive, and special to keep the Planet Fitness masses out. One former fan wrote that attending a Soul-Cycle session felt "more like going to a debutante ball than going to the gym."[44]

That too can backfire. When people become so crazed about booking a class or securing a front-row seat because fitness is their new sense of purpose, they'll resort to bad behavior. They'll pay off the front desk (in money or in "personal favors") and harass employees to secure what they believe they must have. Building such a cult brand can also lead to elitism and fanaticism. You run the risk of replicating everything that soiled certain sects of organized religion: bribery, arrogance, and abuse of power. You run the risk of *bad* religion.

In the early years, the media found the SoulCycle fandom rather amusing. As one member described "groupies" to the *New York Times:* "If [the instructor] said they could go to the pharmacy with her, they would be thrilled . . . Anything to be close to her."[45] But some clients became obsessed with fitness instructors to the point of treating them to holiday vacations, cash bonuses, and fancy meals. Several went so far as to romantically pursue them.

SoulCycle contributed to the idolatrous excesses: "Our riders should want to be you or fuck you," was one master instructor's advice to trainees.[46] It worked: Some women bullied other riders they believed to be competing for a beloved instructor's attention. Jealousy ran amok, with women vying like *Bachelorette* contestants for a chance to chat up their teacher after class. Some even verbally assaulted fellow riders whom they deemed unworthy of the front row. "I watched grown women cry," an ex-employee told *Vox*. One popular instructor sent nude photos of himself to riders, which were then shared among other riders. "That became problematic because people's spouses were complaining, and then it caused a lot of infighting with riders as well," a former employee told *Business Insider*.

Others had their confidence shot if they weren't invited to drinks after class or freaked out if the instructor didn't acknowledge them in class. There's an account of one woman, like some sort of unsanitary mafia, sneaking a used tampon into a fellow rider's purse as punishment for riding on the podium with a star instructor. Call it tribalism, pettiness, or desperation—but a wellness community can devolve into something not unlike a (very expensive) religious cult.

Tampon-bombing is the rare occurrence, the offbeat turned fitness apocrypha. Despite a fall in popularity, die-hard SoulCycle customers will continue to go, enjoying a calorie-burning catharsis (or more likely just buy a Peloton instead). As the spiritual landscape continues to expand beyond organized religion, we start to see that faith isn't disappearing, it's evolving. New players will find ways to reimagine what women sorely feel they're missing. At the same time, we need to accept that selling something bigger, more "meaningful," is just how business is done these days. Every brand shooting for cult status knows it needs to stand for something larger than itself.

But what happens when you buy in to the gospel and are left holding the bag?

Testing Deconstructed Faith in
Troubled Waters

In early 2020, my father passed away. He had been sick for several years, but his death occurred suddenly. Or at least it *felt* sudden. Even those who anticipate a passing feel gobsmacked by having their loved ones taken away. There is no real way to "prepare" for such an event. It unmoors and devastates and shocks no matter the warning signs.

My father was my hero. Gentle, curious, and soft-spoken, he was a physician and academic heavyweight who devoted his life to the sciences and Judaic history. He was remarkably down-to-earth, preferring to discuss science fiction novels or recount impressive football strategy moves. On Sabbath afternoons, when we refrained from watching TV or driving anywhere, we'd play games of chess to pass the time. Then, as soon as the Sabbath ended, we'd jump into the car to head to the movies. After that, we'd go out for ice cream or frozen yogurt, and he'd insist on either a waffle cone or a root beer float.

My dad was earnest and nerdy, in all the best ways. He quoted *Star Wars* as much as he did the physicist Richard Feynman. When I was twelve, my father gave me a copy of *"Surely You're Joking, Mr. Feynman!,"* filled to the brim with witty and brilliant observations. One that has stayed with me is "The first principle is that you must not fool yourself—and you are the easiest person to fool."[47]

After his death, I was devastated. Insomnia returned, as did the anxiety. But I did find solace in joining my family in abiding by Jewish rituals that seemed bizarre on paper but made sense in practice. As soon as the nursing staff announced my father's departure, we tore a piece of our garments—signifying the tear in one's heart—which we then wore throughout the week. We kept shiva, the structured seven-day mourning period in which friends and community members console the immediate family during waking hours. It's nearly all day, every day, for an entire week. Shiva also has its own laws: our family covered up mirrors and abstained from cosmetics, serving as a break from caring about how we looked.

On the last day of shiva, it's customary for observers to walk around the block, marking the end of intense mourning and the need to move on—to reengage with society. These were powerful, helpful traditions.

When I returned from my parents' home, I felt adrift. Basic household tasks and routine errands felt overwhelming. Talking to friends about standard fare—politics, new restaurants, celebrity gossip—infuriated me. I was out of sorts. The first week back, friends visited to express their condolences, and it was all appreciated, but my mourning didn't subside after seven days. I'll say I'm not sure our society is well equipped to handle lingering grief. We seem to expect everyone to buck up and mourn a loss all too quickly, to be back in the office by Monday.

Self-care went only so far. To be honest, I needed consoling. I needed support. I needed a way to express and make sense of my grief. Mainstays like The Class or SoulCycle were unappealing because I didn't want generalized pep talks for what was a very specific, sensitive process. There wasn't anything they could offer at that moment, not in terms of rituals nor counseling. It was outside their purview.

Of course, none of my fitness instructors were going to show up with a casserole. Nor was there any program in place to support milestones or crises. Unlike religion, gyms have not had centuries to perfect communal outreach and manage difficult life transitions. Although I instinctively knew it was ridiculous to even suppose your local gym could help in such times, I started to wonder: What was I investing in? Not just the gyms, but everything? In centering career success, a toned body, and nonstop consumption, what was I getting in return?

Surprisingly, the strongest support came from what I had veered from the most in years prior: my synagogue. Though I wasn't a member and generally showed up only on holidays, the community came out in full force: The staff sent an email out to all the other members. The rabbi invited me to participate in rituals that acknowledged the passage of time, such as saying the kaddish, a communal mourner's prayer, week after week with others who had also lost loved ones. Community members asked me to share memories of my father, then invited me to group meals. They showed continued support far beyond what I had anticipated.

Obviously, thriving humanist churches and grief support groups exist. I am in no way suggesting religion has a monopoly on ritualistic activities and community. Not in the slightest. But my gym as a grief outlet felt absurd: *I'm not working on my body during a crisis*. It was the first crack in the armor of my otherwise complete devotion to my wellness regime.

I wasn't necessarily committing to going to synagogue every day moving forward or chucking my gym memberships. But I began contemplating the energy I devoted to my "healthy" lifestyle, which absorbed more and more time, energy, and money. I enjoyed working out and eating well, and would continue to do so, but doubts were creeping in about what exactly I was consuming in those Sunday morning workouts. Despite the quasi-liturgical platitudes in classes, I couldn't help but shake the feeling that this was all still an exercise in perfecting the physique and not too much else, thereby confirming that what mattered most was . . . my body.

I had bought in to my gym's gospel of community. It served a purpose, but it hadn't turned out to be what I wanted or needed when I reached the spiritual milestone of parental loss. The promise of gym as church had led me somewhere though. It led me to this book. Now more than ever, I felt the need to investigate why I was so preoccupied with these elements of my life—and how much of what I was being sold was true, and how much was simply what I wanted to hear or believe.

Chapter 5

A Plea to Be Heard

A smorgasbord for the curious, a blur of theater and wellness, the Goop conference could just as easily have been called the Alternative Health Convention. Six hundred well-groomed women paid between $500 to $1,500 for a full day of healthy eating, toxin-free pampering, and guilt-free Gwyneth gawking. Inside a Century City warehouse that resembled a luxury jet hangar, guests learned the importance of gut bacteria, how our minds manifest sickness in the body, and the use of poisonous frog venom as a healing agent. They sipped "brain-boosting" Bulletproof coffee as IVs dripped vitamin B_{12} into their bloodstreams. The younger ones analyzed their futures with a crystal-wielding shaman. Others had their "auras read."

Goop founder Gwyneth Paltrow brought along her celebrity pals. They were, as she attested, friends she "constantly" swapped healers' phone numbers with: the actress Cameron Diaz, the designer Nicole Richie, and the supermodel Miranda Kerr. The latter was eager to share her most recent discovery: leech therapy, in which creepy crawlers suck on one's face and the collected blood is then smeared back on the skin. "Health is wealth," Kerr told the crowd.

To be fair, not all Goop fans take Paltrow seriously. To them, she and her lifestyle site are more entertainment than a solid news source. For them, knowing that some of the health information Goop promotes raises more than a few questions is part of the fun; part of "the journey," as Gwyneth might say.[1] They welcome the $135 coffee enema kit and vaginal steaming (reportedly to "cleanse" the uterus) with Pilates-toned open arms.

In some ways, Goop isn't all that different from the traveling salesmen of the nineteenth century, who turned medical road shows into popular venues of entertainment. Brandishing magical elixirs and opium-laced concoctions, the salesmen knew the psychology of persuasion; they recognized a gap that could easily be filled with tonics, a bit of empathy, and mesmerizing onstage antics.[2] And the audience had no issues with that. Plenty knew the Rattlesnake King straddled the line between health and sensationalism. To them, seeing the snake oil show was their version of dinner and movie. Santa Monica's finest aren't any different: they take their colonics with a dash of skepticism.

The conference alternated from informational and empowering to kooky and downright pseudoscientific—but above all, it was highly entertaining. Women reclined on chaise longues in the branded outdoor picnic area, making friends and swapping notes on meditation practices and sneaker styles. While I got an "organic manicure" (a manicure with "nontoxic" nail polish), I spoke to a woman in her late twenties who had spent the last hour taking in the parade of fashion.

"Aren't they all just wearing yoga leggings?" I asked.

"Yes," she responded, "but the *best* yoga leggings."

Naturally, the longest lines led to the checkout counters in a scene that can best be described as self-improvement Black Friday. Goop fans might have been eager to learn about the latest health fad, but their consumerist tendencies drive the site's ad and product revenue. Starting at 9:30 a.m., participants crowded numerous indoor shops, each one dedicated to a different sector, such as athleisure, beauty, and home. And of course, all the panelists hawked their own books and supplement lines. No wonder the company is believed to be valued at over $250 million.

But Paltrow remains the biggest attraction. Inside, as participants crowded into their auditorium seats, the founder took the stage, her designer paisley dress brushing the floor. "Why do we all not feel well?" she asked the audience. "And what can we do about it?" A good question, and one the actress turned leader purports to solve, one diet cleanse at a time.

Looking around the hall crammed with Louis Vuitton handbags, I did not doubt that the audience had access to doctors and specialists, if not some of the finest health care in the country. No one there *looked* sick. No one acted sick. A Black beauty stylist working at a touch-up station—one of only a handful of women of color in the room—remarked, "They look fine to me."

And yet they were there, spending hundreds if not thousands of dollars on health advice from an actress who had no medical credentials. No schooling. And certainly no mainstream acceptance. The very same actress who, when confronted by the late-night TV host Jimmy Kimmel about Goop's more bizarre suggestions, admitted, "I don't know what the fuck we talk about!" As long as Paltrow provides hand holding, Goop fans don't question an adult woman who once declared she was on an eight-day goat-milk cleanse—a diet that medical experts have concluded offers no benefits save for "more flatulence."

So, if it isn't mainstream acceptance or the backing of scientific studies, what *has* become so very seductive about Goop? How has Paltrow been able to so effectively crawl into her patrons' ears?

Part of the answer lies in the fast-growing field of alternative health. Goop is part of a larger and flourishing ecosystem: 30 percent of Americans now use alternative medicine, with women more accepting of it.[3] Some turn to alternative treatments as a complementary add-on, though many fully adopt them instead of Western medicine. Women, or more accurately, *dissatisfied* women lead this movement.

Women are stepping outside their doctor's office, searching for something. And Gwyneth's fattened golden goose is happy to lay vaginal jade eggs for them. But what precisely is inspiring this mass conversion?

Dismissed and Disillusioned: A Frustrating Patient Experience

The crisis of faith in modern medicine starts long before someone buys a ticket to the Goop show.

The inefficient and, at times, mind-bogglingly frustrating patient experience starts with sorting premiums, deductibles, hidden fees, and a maze of coverage limitations. (And that's for those fortunate enough to even have medical insurance.) In the U.S., the consumer faces a cat-and-mouse chase of referrals and sign-offs to see specialists or get approval for a treatment. Long wait times and onerous paperwork can make a simple procedure seem like applying for a mortgage. Who has the time? Amidst work, parenting, household chores, and little to no time off, medical appointments only add to an already hectic schedule.

And it doesn't end with just nabbing an appointment. So many times, I've gone in for a routine checkup, then weeks later received separate surprise bills for blood work, lab testing, etc. In my thirties, medical bills have been sent to collection agencies not because I didn't have the money, but because *I couldn't keep track* of all the various individual bills.

Then there are the experiences that leave women's faith in the system badly shaken.

Jacquelyn Clemmons from Baltimore, Maryland, is one such woman. In 2003, the friendly and no-nonsense Queens, New York, native was two months into her first pregnancy when she visited a local doctor for help with a persistent yeast infection. Her mother was a physician, so she had full confidence in the doctor's capabilities—what she called "a healthy respect" for the experts. But the appointment proved less than assuring. The doctor and personnel spent only a few minutes chatting with Clemmons, then quickly penned a prescription. "They didn't touch me, they didn't really look at me," Clemmons told me. "They kind of sat at their desk and then wrote the script. I felt dismissed."

Clemmons says she looked up the medicine prescribed, Metronidazole, only to discover it was linked to an increased risk of miscarriage, which she was not made aware of.

The questionable treatment didn't end there. While pregnant with her second child, she experienced severe abdominal pain and back-to-back contractions and sought hospital treatment. The staff assumed Clemmons was overreacting because she didn't seem like she was "in enough pain." They sent her home.

Clemmons returned, demanding attention. This time she came with a plan. Clemmons turned to her partner and said, "I'm going to have to fake it because they're not believing me. So don't look at me crazy." She then proceeded to scream and wail at full volume. The Oscar-worthy performance did the trick. Staff discovered Clemmons was dehydrated and experiencing preterm labor, thereby endangering her unborn child. Afterward, Clemmons was placed on three months of bed rest.

As Clemmons recounts, pulling theatrics "is nutty to do on any day, but when you're experiencing contractions and you just want to be comfortable, it's even crazier."

Then came the third pregnancy. Clemmons said she was subjected to a forceful cervix check and dealt with an anesthesiologist who attempted to administer an epidural while half the lights were out. Terrified and angry, her perception of medical care shifted. She explains, "I felt like I could no longer just safely walk into a doctor's office, trust what they're telling me, and walk out without harm being done to myself or my child." Clemmons soon found herself asking "a million questions about everything, and not taking anyone else's word about anything that I needed." She decided to independently seek solutions, including natural remedies or changes in diet to alleviate ailments. "From then on, I was just going to do my own due diligence," she says. "If it was something that I could do, I was going to do it before I decided to involve a doctor."

These experiences inspired Clemmons to become a doula. She founded her practice, De La Luz Wellness, to be an advocate and pillar of support for women who also felt disregarded by medical personnel. Incorporating wellness modalities such as traditional herbal medicine, Reiki energy treatments, breath work, and relaxation techniques, Clemmons mostly serves Black and Indigenous women who come to her with the same goal: "I don't want to die."* These women distrust hospitals, and that alone is enough to make them opt for an at-home birth. "They get very tense and very afraid because they've had other hospital traumas and they don't want that reaction to come up subconsciously while they're giving birth," explains Clemmons. "There's this tension that builds, you automatically go on the fence. You walk in there already knowing you're going to face a fight."

Clemmons tallied multiple transgressions before throwing in the towel, but sometimes all it takes is one bad experience to taint one's entire view. Whether it was a physician, therapist, or health expert, if someone hurt or dismissed you at your *most vulnerable time*—which is generally when we interact with medical providers—you will need to get over that experience. Some might need to break away for a while. But others, especially when it pertains to trauma, might vow never to return.

Clemmons is Black, part of a segment of the American population that has historically not experienced the same level of "care" as other patients. (More on this later.) Surely wealthy white women aren't in the same boat. Affluent individuals presumably live a far different existence, for which the adage "see your doctor early and often" still holds considerable weight. Blessed with health insurance and access to top docs, they must have a better go at the whole medical appointment game. *Right?*

Unquestionably, wealth helps. *A lot.*

But wealth doesn't necessarily protect you from everything. Having

---

* In the United States, Black and American Indian women are two to three times more likely to die from pregnancy-related causes than white women, according to the CDC.

legitimate concerns dismissed by a physician is a problem that cuts across race and income.

In 2019, the actress Selma Blair appeared on *Good Morning America* to share what had been a silent struggle: an agony-inducing medical experience that spanned years. At just forty-six years old, thin and clutching a cane, the *Legally Blonde* star leaned on host Robin Roberts as they walked on the balcony of her Cape Cod–style L.A. home. Sitting down indoors, Roberts asked her a simple question: "How are you doing?"

Blair, sporting a chic blond bob, shocked viewers with her answer. It wasn't what she said, but how she answered. Through broken and stuttering speech, Blair struggled to respond. Nobody had known that the Hollywood star had become so sick. She persevered through the interview, which covered years of attempting to convince doctors that something was wrong with her body. Blair said she was besieged with pain and bizarre symptoms like blurred vision, extreme exhaustion, and numbness in her leg. Sometimes she had trouble walking, experiencing a sense of vertigo. She started falling.

The single mother would become so fatigued that she'd need to pull over and take a nap while driving her son to school. She'd truly feared how she was going to get by from day to day while taking care of her child. "I was ashamed, and I was doing the best I could, and I was a great mother, but it was killing me," she explained.[4] Thinking she might have Parkinson's disease, Blair reached out to actor Michael J. Fox, who was diagnosed with the neurodegenerative disorder in 1991. "I said, 'I don't know who to tell, but I am dropping things. I'm doing strange things.'"

Doctors didn't take her seriously. "Single mother, you're exhausted, financial burden, blah, blah, blah," she recalled. They blamed it on postpartum depression or a hormonal imbalance. One said she was simply being "dramatic."[5] None of these doctors offered further significant testing, even as symptoms worsened. The unrelenting strain became so unbearable that Blair turned to self-medicating the old-fashioned way. "I was drinking. I was in pain," she told Roberts. "I wasn't always drinking, but there were times when I couldn't take it."[6]

Finally, after years of pleading with doctors, Blair's condition was ultimately diagnosed as an aggressive form of multiple sclerosis—a chronic autoimmune disease that affects the nervous system. When Blair received the diagnosis, she cried. They weren't tears of sadness, but of relief at finally being acknowledged. She thought, *Oh, good, I'll be able to do something.*

The actress's story struck a nerve with women across the country, many of whom showered the frail star with gratitude on social media and offered their own medical mishaps and battles with chronic conditions. "My symptoms were chalked up to stress," wrote one woman in solidarity. "[My doctor] said I was having a panic attack!" shared another. Like Blair, they described doctors who denied their pain and brushed off medical inquiries. They felt they had to prove their case. Doubling over in agony, they were told to "suck it up" or simply accept that "this is part of being a woman." Others were told to go see a psychotherapist, implying that their pain was purely psychological. Some were offered the most patronizing advice of all: "Just have a glass of wine."

It would seem that average American women and Hollywood celebrities are united by their medical experiences. (Stars: they're gaslit just like us!) It's quite telling that Real Housewife Yolanda Hadid titled her memoir about Lyme Disease with a simple request: *Believe Me.*

When some women describe a medical condition, their doctors tell them they're exaggerating or overreacting. If they dare express emotion (as opposed to the more stoic male stereotype), it is used against them as evidence of the "hysterical woman." Although if they are *too* stoic, doctors will still not believe them; a lose-lose scenario if there ever was one. Worse, practitioners dismiss symptoms as a by-product of the patients' own failings: Higher-weight individuals report being told it's their own fault. Even younger patients face prejudice, as doctors just can't believe a twentysomething-year-old could have a serious health condition. In one chronic pain treatment survey of twenty-four hundred women, 90 percent said they felt the healthcare system discriminated against female patients.[7]

The list of dismissed or misdiagnosed chronic conditions runs as long as a CVS receipt. Women suffering from fibromyalgia—a chronic condition that causes fatigue, pain, and tenderness in the body—usually see several doctors before they receive a proper diagnosis. Same for vulvodynia, a chronic burning and soreness in the vulva that affects roughly 16 percent of women at some point during their lifetime. Of those who seek treatment, 60 percent consult three or more doctors, many of whom can't provide a diagnosis. The condition is often misdiagnosed.[8] Some vulvodynia patients deal with constant pain across months and even years, at times so severe that they cannot sit, let alone have sex or use tampons.

Endometriosis is another chronic condition that often gets ignored. It occurs when tissue that generally lines the inside of the uterus develops outside it, and can be marked by intense pain in the lower back and pelvis, nausea, fatigue, cramping, and infertility. Those living with endometriosis have been shown to have a 52 percent greater risk of heart attack (in comparison to women without the condition).[9] The painful disorder affects an estimated 190 million worldwide—one in ten reproductive-aged women. These women are often handed birth control (which manages some symptoms) and sent on their way.

Samantha Bee, host of the TBS talk show *Full Frontal,* best immortalized the issue in the public eye when she likened endometriosis flareups in the body to the horror slasher flick *Saw.* Bee asked the audience to imagine all their furniture thrown onto their front lawn, only for the police to say, "That's life. Wanna take the pill?" She further declared, "One in ten women suffer from endometriosis and it's just one of the many painful, debilitating lady diseases that get treated with birth control and a shrug."[10]

And it's not just male doctors—women experience subpar treatment from both genders. One study found that emergency room doctors were less likely to prescribe painkillers to women for acute abdominal pain.[11] And statistically, women received far less aggressive treatment for heart disease than men, even though heart disease is the leading cause of death for women in the United States. This cardiology gender gap is called "Yentl syndrome," a reference to Barbra Streisand's iconic role as an aspiring Talmud student who disguises herself as a boy to enter a yeshiva. In medicine, this term connotes underdiagnosis and undertreatment, implying that women's symptoms need to be more like men's to receive adequate care.

Meanwhile, male patients undergoing coronary artery bypass graft surgery receive more opioids and pain medication than female patients. Women, however, are given *more sedatives*.[12]

Disillusioned and fed up with a system they feel doesn't believe them, a growing number of women have taken it upon themselves to course correct their own medical care.

But the problem of not being heard starts with a medical structure that disinvests in meaningful physician-patient relationships even as it invests in bureaucracy and speed. For many women, traditional Western medicine seems built to make a buck, not to significantly care for their needs.

Just Tired of It All:
Hurried and Impersonal Care

Fortunately, not every woman has a horror story or a traumatic history with medicine. But too many harbor a general dissatisfaction that opens the window for more alluring competitors to breeze in.[†] And this has a massive impact because they're the stakeholders: women serve as the "chief medical officer" in their households, accounting for 80 percent of health-care decisions for their families.

When I have gone in for a routine checkup, the experience has often been less than inspiring. Modern gynecology is best described as awkward. Convention forces me and so many women to strip down and don

---

[†] Women generally interact more with the medical industry than men, and starting from a younger age (gynecology, etc.). As such, they might accrue more complaints.

an embarrassing, paper-thin cloth gown, all while shivering like a hairless cat, and lie on a clinical examination table. The physician asks perhaps one question before crudely inserting tools, making patients feel more like a lab specimen than a human. Little is done to make us feel safe, comfortable, or welcomed. A quarter of women who skip their yearly OB-GYN appointments give this simple reason: they hate going.[13]

Let's put it this way: I have seen at least six gynecologists over the last twenty years and cannot remember most of their names. But I know the names, hobbies, and favorite musical artists of nearly all of my hairstylists.

Maybe that's a problem.

Surprisingly, the only time I found medical personnel willing to take the time to get to know me was at the NBC News onsite medical station, the inspiration for Chris Parnell's Dr. Spaceman on the TV comedy *30 Rock*. But that was likely because the staff were as lonely as the Maytag repairman—no one was ever there, since most NBC employees didn't want their employer knowing their private medical issues. (As a Loehmann's shopper, I valued a good deal and convenience over privacy.) I almost felt I was doing them a favor. Nurses would invite me to take a nap if I had a headache, listen to my fear of bedbugs, and ask how I was managing stress. I'd swing by to thank them following a recovery, and they'd offer me a hug along with free Tylenol packets for my purse.

But that's not the norm. The current clinic model produces a hurried appointment, leaving little time for a well-intentioned doctor to meaningfully engage with the patient—a system that can be demoralizing for both parties. A 2018 study in conjunction with the Mayo Clinic monitored conversations in doctors' offices, only to find that most patients were afforded eleven seconds to explain the reason for their visit before being interrupted.[14] The average length of a primary care office visit runs 17.4 minutes.[15] The system incentivizes productivity; some doctors are paid according to how many patients they see, not by the quality of health outcomes. Physicians see an average of twenty patients per day.[16]

With all too often lackluster impersonal care, diminishing allegiance to the medical system is understandable. A study by Harvard confirmed that although the United States spends nearly twice as much as other countries on health care, it has poorer health outcomes.

And that's just the general population. Minorities are more likely to face discriminatory healthcare practices, which feeds into a general apprehension of medicine.

One study published in the *American Journal of Public Health* found that among Black patients, physicians were more likely to dominate conversations. Patients feel less involved in decision making and then less receptive to the doctors' guidance.[17] Results from a 2017 survey conducted by NPR, the Robert Wood Johnson Foundation, and the Harvard T.H. Chan School of Public Health showed that a third of Black patients felt discriminated against at a doctor's office or health clinic, while nearly a quarter avoided medical care all together lest they suffer the same treatment.[18]

In 2017, ProPublica and NPR jointly collected over 200 stories from Black mothers, and "the feeling of being devalued and disrespected by medical providers was a constant theme."[19] Likewise, some women I've spoken to insist they were pressured into hurried and unnecessary cesarean sections to limit a lengthy labor or to accommodate a doctor's shift.

"I am not a person who believes Western medicine is totally unuseful, and I'm also not going to say that traditional medicine or alternative healing is unnecessary. There's a balance," clarifies Clemmons, who longs for the days when family doctors took the time to know individuals. "There is a level of connection, compassion, and tailor-fit care [missing from institutionalized medical care]. Someone has to take time to ask you questions, discuss your background and body composition . . . It's so personal and so detailed. And I think that's what is attracting women to wellness."

Many doctors are equally unsatisfied with how care is currently managed. Do they want to rush clients out the door? Do they want to spend precious time dealing with multiple insurance companies? They didn't break their backs throughout medical school and exhausting residencies to treat humans like factory inventory. Neither do they want to star in their own version of *The Office*, filling out piles of administrative paperwork. As the physician Dr. Danielle Ofri writes in *What Doctors Feel*, doctors spend over 60 percent of their time documenting ailments, reviewing records, and communicating with staff. "For physicians, this 'indirect care' is perceived as time they are spending on patients' cases, but for patients, this indirect care is invisible. Patients are aware only of the time they actually see their doctor, and it feels like almost nothing . . . the patients, rightly, feel shortchanged."[20]

It's not necessarily the doctors. It's the system. Too many physicians are overwhelmed—working long, stressful hours—and beholden to the current healthcare model. Some research suggests patients feel more satisfied and better adhere to treatment compliance when cared for by empathetic doctors, but for that to happen, we need a system that lets doctors flourish. Instead, 47 percent of physicians report burnout, which naturally affects their patience, empathy, and quality of care.[21]

Of course, doctors also have their own legitimate gripes about patients, including the frustration that comes with doling out guidance that's ignored: *stop smoking, exercise, eat your vegetables* . . . When patients repeatedly refuse to take responsibility for their health, doctors—who are human too—can feel as if they're living in their own *Groundhog Day* in which their empathy is constantly tested.

Still, some patients take issue with the outcome of such visits, which often end with a prescription. Although most symptoms—say, a cough or rash—will mend themselves in time, doctors and patients succumb to the "do something" psychology in which a specific remedy must be provided at the end of a consultation.[22] Nearly half of the U.S. population took a prescription drug in the last month.

Once lost, it's tricky to regain trust, especially in an age of ever-proliferating information. Constant access to the Internet pushes people to believe they can self-diagnose, while conflicting media reports erode faith in one consistently reliable source of medical information. Much of the general public is likely to encounter misleading information on social media because sensationalized headlines perform better. They're *juicier*. False stories prey on emotions like fear, disgust, or shock, and people are more likely to share what moves them—for example, an emotional anecdote.

In 2019, a bipartisan network of scientists examined the one hundred most popular health articles of the previous year; specifically, those with the highest number of social media engagement. Of the top ten shared articles, they found that three-quarters were either misleading or included some false information. Only three were considered "highly credible." Some lacked context on the issue, exaggerated the harms of a potential threat, or overstated research findings. Others, it seemed, had a skewed agenda.[23]

With doubt seeping in at multiple points, U.S. women are looking to try something different. Many women have had less than stellar doctor appointments. Or perhaps they're convinced they alone can self-diagnose and treat an ailment, MacGyvering their way to better health. The question is: What is the alternative?

Roaming to Alternative Health Pastures

In 2018, the journalist Sarah Graham founded *Hysterical Women*, a blog documenting personal accounts of biases in women's health care from the UK, the United States, and Canada. Female patients write in with complaints covering the spectrum: reproductive health, chronic illnesses, and disabilities. Graham found the consensus to be *Hysterical until proven otherwise*. According to testimonials, doctors accused patients of seeking attention, imagining symptoms, or attempting to acquire drugs. Often, women were reluctant to push back or challenge a doctor's authority because they were raised to trust and obey them. Some reported they were taken more seriously only when a male partner accompanied them to an appointment, like some sort of medical chaperone.

Plenty didn't get what they needed. So they pursued alternative self-care methods, including acupuncture, marijuana, and dietary changes—

not necessarily as cures, but as complementary treatments to minimize symptoms. Many joined patient advocacy groups or online communities to share knowledge and to find peer support. "People are looking for alternatives outside of medicine, even if that's just about sort of managing day-to-day life," Graham told me, noting a prevailing sense of desperation. "There is definitely a sense of people being willing to try just about anything."

I meet women all the time who want nothing to do with Western medicine, which they call "sick care" rather than health care. They believe the system isn't all that invested in solving "root causes" (a trope used to slam doctors; mainstream medicine addresses both causes and symptoms, though there's certainly room for improvement). The system doesn't incentivize preventive medicine, they'll say, so it's no wonder people are unable to stave off chronic illness.

Alternative health is presented as a proactive approach—trying to prevent ailments in the first place, as opposed to traditional Western medicine's reactive approach. Wellness advocates promise partnership over "patientship," heralding ways to fine-tune the machine so it doesn't break down as often, which is why seemingly fit and healthy women attend a Goop conference. That's the point; they want to stay healthy. Or more like: *what they believe* is healthy. And they'll work damn hard—or spend lavishly—pursuing it.

Western medicine's approach is simply too myopic, these women say. Hospitals and physicians are ideal for acute problems like heart attacks or broken bones, while alternative medicine is preferable for chronic conditions. Eastern medicine or "natural" remedies appeal to those who say they want more personalized, less potentially harsh methods. They only need to turn on their TV to see how prescription painkillers like opioids have harmed millions of Americans.

More and more often, women are asking, What else is out there? Is there some other way besides pharmaceuticals? And how can I manage symptoms on my own?

Take Naomi, a marketing executive and mom of two preschoolers in

Brooklyn, New York. She was diagnosed with rheumatoid arthritis and ulcerative colitis, an inflammatory bowel disease. Pharmaceuticals prescribed by her gastroenterologist failed to manage the symptoms; Naomi was besieged by fatigue, rectal bleeding, and abdominal cramps.

Naomi decided to visit a holistic doctor, who told her three things acted like "shards of glass" in her digestive system: gluten, dairy, and sugar. He told Naomi she must never consume them again. "That diet was the first thing that ever really helped my symptoms," she recalls. When Naomi went back to her gastroenterologist for a routine colonoscopy, she mentioned her newfound strategy only to receive a heavy dose of skepticism. The doctor stated it wouldn't work, even though it seemingly was working. "I said, 'I have stomach issues all the time. How can you look me in the face and actually tell me that the things I'm [eating] are not affecting the pain that I'm feeling?'"

In the following years, Naomi began researching alternative methods of self-care, becoming more and more entrenched in the wellness world. Now she pretty much avoids traditional Western medicine, save for surgical needs. Her health regimen incorporates whole, gluten-free foods and fresh juices, which she says helped heal her gut. When she last got sick, she went straight to an energy healer. "You have to just take [your health] into your own hands," declares Naomi.

In self-preservation, the sick and vulnerable might avoid what let them down in the past, then invest their faith in promising cures. If they find the system isn't addressing their concerns, they'll find new sources to meet their needs.

Flashback: When Americans Succumbed to "Puke Doctors"

Samuel Thomson faced the court, a sea of serious faces stretched along the wooden pews. It was winter 1809 in Massachusetts. The mood was solemn, the cold air filled with tension. Among those in attendance were Thomson's lawyers and an array of witnesses who at one point had been his patients. Thomson knew the press would turn the court case into a media circus, as this was no slight accusation. Thomson was on trial for murder.[24]

Thomson was famous for his botanical treatments and purging techniques, which he sold to licensed administrators across the country. He believed that sickness stemmed from an internal temperature imbalance, that all an ailing body needed was a restoration of heat and a release of toxins in the stomach and bowels. To that end, he employed steam baths, oral purgatives, and enemas laced with cayenne pepper. His licensed operators were soon dubbed the "puke doctors."

Thomson had prescribed one patient the emetic herb *Lobelia inflata*, also known as Indian tobacco. The patient was forced to puke daily, to the point that he lay in perpetual sweat. He died within one week. At one point, Thomson's lawyer dangled Indian tobacco in front of the courtroom. The lawyer then abruptly swallowed it whole, drawing gasps from the audience. He claimed he felt just fine and in fact could easily consume three times the amount without ill effects. The press ate it up like a page-turning thriller.[25]

Thomson was ultimately acquitted, but that didn't satisfy him. He saw the trial as the product of a power-hungry, corrupt medical establishment attempting to quash alternative medicine. At that time, who had access to information—and how it was wielded—was shifting. The "anti-establishment" President Andrew Jackson, who campaigned on a populist platform, celebrated the average citizen who relied on nothing more than grit and intuitive wisdom. The idea of rugged self-reliance permeated more than just D.C. politics; it became a siren song for the Everyman to revolt against what was seen as a two-tiered system of health care, making do with herbal remedies while access to doctors was reserved for the privileged few. Playing up a common perceived enemy, as always, bolstered support and galvanized communities. Medicine—both access and quality—became fuel for class conflict.

For Thomson, it was also personal. As a young man, he bore witness to the rudimentary medical care administered to his mother, who suffered from the measles. By prescribing mercury and opium, the doctors "galloped her out of the world in about nine weeks," he reported.[26]

By the 1830s, the Thomsonians had grown into a sizable movement, and botanic physicians came to be seen as on par with medical doctors. The ordinary people applying this new democratic approach sometimes obtained better results than those who were bled by doctors. Reportedly, 2 million Americans—more than a tenth of the population—adopted the Thomsonian system, which stressed a key motto: "To make every man his own physician."

Thomson wasn't alone in taking on the medical establishment. Americans soon embraced a hodgepodge of alternative healthcare methods, everything from magnetic healing to homeopathy. For better or worse, medical care was no longer concentrated in the hands of a select few.

Give Me Your Tired, Your Sick, Your Dissatisfied Masses

Those who flock to Paltrow's altar take comfort in believing that the Oscar winner (or more likely, her team of employees) is playing lab rat for them, although it's unclear whether any of these rituals in any way make her, per the mission, healthier. But that doesn't matter, for Goop provides a seductive fantasy of health and beauty. There's a strain in American culture that leads us to believe we can have or do anything as long as we put in enough effort. We live by the prevailing creed of personal control over one's environment—the very same creed that propelled man to the moon. Our go-getter mentality, bred by a Puritan work ethic and a belief in American exceptionalism, made us hard workers but also big dreamers. This unique mix finds its way into our leaders, our markets, and our health landscape. High expectations coupled with rugged individualism push health seekers to greener, more holistic pastures.

Goop also lends women a much-needed ear. It caters to a population longing to hear three simple but powerful words: *I believe you*. After years of feeling minimized and discredited, women gravitate toward those who validate their pain, who take them seriously.

Gwyneth Paltrow embraces this disillusioned group, filling a vacuum in which no empathetic or aspirational brand captured the market. Goop publishes pieces on Lyme disease, fibromyalgia, and other chronic conditions. Paltrow and her publication share alternative treatments, such as biomagnetic therapy (to balance the body's pH levels) or bee venom (which involves live bee stings to supposedly treat inflammation). For patients whose doctors offer nothing more than a shrug, these kinds of alternatives feel like manna from heaven. Just buying her pricey wares makes them feel cared for and comforted.

That's because navigating a chronic condition isn't just extremely aggravating and painful. It's lonesome too. Many women describe how friends and family are quick to offer a helping hand at the start: casseroles, babysitting, pharmacy runs. But when they fail to improve—over weeks, months, even years—the attention wears thin. Meal delivery tapers off, the visits more seldom. It's not that people don't care, rather they just don't quite know how to react to someone who isn't getting better. We're not accustomed nor equipped to manage medical failure, even on a social level. (We Americans are far more comfortable with success stories; we want to hear of triumph, of overcoming the hurdles!) The long-suffering know there are only so many times they can reach out for help before they're considered a "burden" or labeled *that* person who is "still" sick. In this regard, digital patient communities and websites provide crucial emotional support.

Even those with minor chronic ailments seek solutions and support. With that mindset, Goop launched its most ambitious product—a collection of supplements to address women's everyday health issues. The cleverly named Why Am I So Effing Tired? pill to "help re-balance an overtaxed system" was created because Paltrow found herself feeling sleepy all the time. She joins a big club: fatigue is the most common complaint for 10 to 20 percent of primary care visits.[27]

The pills, $90 for a monthly pack, were also designed for people suffering from "adrenal fatigue," a theory suggesting that overworked adrenal glands might not produce enough cortisol. Western medicine doesn't officially recognize this malady (which is not to be confused with myalgic encephalomyelitis, also known as ME/CFS or chronic fatigue syndrome). The Mayo Clinic describes adrenal fatigue as a lay term given to a collection of nonspecific symptoms, like body aches, fatigue, and nervousness, but one without an accepted medical diagnosis. Goop's Dr. Alejandro Junger, in comparison, likens it to an "epidemic."[28]

Adrenal fatigue is a new, invented term for feeling tired or stressed. It's possible that one's adrenal function is shot, but it's generally not a primary problem with one's adrenal gland, doctors I interviewed tell me. But as soon as it was *suggested*, consumers were convinced they had it. Before hearing the term, they might have assumed feeling sleepy sometimes was just a marker of modern life. Now they were self-diagnosing and buying Goop vitamins in bulk. It then becomes socially contagious, with friends suddenly discussing the "condition." And this is where Goop and unproven remedies can become potentially harmful. Some buyers might be ignoring actual symptoms with actual solutions. Their sleepiness could be the result of real medical conditions, including immune disorders, a thyroid condition, or depression.

Goop's supplement line sold $100,000 worth of product on its first day. (Even though you can buy the supplements' equivalents for half the price at your local GNC.) If women feel more understood by Gwyneth Paltrow than their own doctor, there's a problem with medicine.

Many of Goop's quasimedical suggestions lack solid scientific evidence. Moreover, their health advice always seems to converge to one end point: Buy more stuff. And not just any stuff, *expensive* stuff. At their conference, I noticed a $42 "transformational" flower essence oil—also called "vibrational" medicine—to combat a wide assortment of ailments: social anxiety, self-consciousness, self-criticism, and the "tendency to isolate." (What, it doesn't also cure my Netflix addiction? Align my bowel movements to my horoscope?) Is this science? Probably not. Is it great salesmanship? Definitely.

This hasn't gone unnoticed. In 2018, Goop agreed to pay $145,000 in civil penalties after an investigation by a task force of prosecutors from ten California counties claimed its product advertisements lacked reliable scientific evidence. Consumers who bought their jade vaginal egg, marketed for "hormonal balance," were entitled to a full refund. A year earlier, the advertising watchdog group Truth in Advertising filed a complaint with two California district attorneys against Goop after it found more than fifty instances in which Goop claimed it could treat, cure, prevent, or reduce the risk of developing a number of ailments.[29]

Goop was on a roll at that time. Their signature perfume claimed its collection of ingredients "improves memory," "treats colds," and "works as an antibiotic." Then there were Goop's $120 wearable energy healing stickers, which generated as much media scrutiny as Ben Affleck's back tattoo. These stickers reportedly "rebalance the energy frequency in our bodies" and were said to be made of the same conductive carbon material NASA used in space suits to monitor an astronaut's vitals. Not only did NASA deny the existence of the material, but a former NASA chief scientist went so far as to respond, "Wow. What a load of BS this is."[30]

Goop products and content now often include a convenient disclaimer: "This article is not, nor is it intended to be, a substitute for professional medical advice, diagnosis, or treatment, and should never be relied upon for specific medical advice."

Goop as a company does not shy away from controversy and has defended its practices. The brand said it anticipates questions surrounding its content but takes issue with attacks on its methods, reframing them as an attack on women's empowerment (and thereby appealing to consumers' feminist leanings). "We always welcome conversation. That's at the core of what we're trying to do," read an open letter Goop published in 2017. "Being dismissive—of discourse, of questions from patients, of practices that women might find empowering or healing, of daring to poke at a long-held belief—seems like the most dangerous practice of all."

Goop's strategy is to put edgy wellness ideas out into the world and let readers make up their minds about them. In a way, the company absolves itself of any responsibility because their role is to simply introduce new ideas—not to ensure their efficacy. It's a brilliant business model—the possibilities are endless.

While there is a glimmer of logic to Goop's openness to new treatments, the issue is that many of their products are not put through any kind of rigorous medical evaluation process. And without an approval process that involves rigorous testing and standards, their claims of benefits are just that: claims, not medical advice.

But Goop is not the whole of alternative medicine, and it would be unjust to presume as much. There are plenty of other players in town who don't resort to steam-cleaning their private parts. So, one might ask, what about all the other alternative healers and clinics exploring new treatments? What if they know something mainstream medicine doesn't?

The Gray Zone: The Space Between Medicine and "Something Else"

When it comes to poorly understood or chronic conditions, a gray area does exist between evidence-based medicine and unorthodox treatments. I tread lightly here—appreciating mainstream medicine while fully accepting its current limitations—because physicians have yet to truly figure out some of these debilitating conditions that leave women in agony.

Many conditions go undiagnosed or misdiagnosed, especially ailments that don't show up on blood tests.[31] That does not invalidate mainstream medicine, rather it reminds us that medical mysteries still exist. Also, it doesn't necessarily follow that alternative practitioners *do* have the answers. Some alternative medicine practices have little, mixed, or no scientific backing. Homeopathy, for example, is based on the philosophy of "like cures like"—that a condition can be treated with an ultra-diluted ingredient that has similar symptom effects. So an allergy remedy, by this logic, might contain onion because it too causes irritated eyes and a runny nose. This "similar" symptom concept goes against basic scientific principles. Besides, ingredients are generally so diluted that it'd be hard to label them an active ingredient. Homeopaths argue that dilution increases potency, while scientists counter that they're diluted to the point of being negligible.

Homeopathy (which is often conflated with herbal remedies) hasn't been proven to significantly affect specific diseases or symptoms even after thousands of papers.[32] In this regard, we need to separate interventions that have been *disproven* from interventions that are *unproven*.[33]

As for patients, their suffering should be taken seriously. While people can certainly convince themselves of symptoms or illnesses, we should not be quick to assume "it's all your head."

Doctors I interviewed say we aren't always equipped to deal with complex chronic conditions, particularly those that lack clear causes and treatments. Part of this has to do with how we think about medicine. We generally think of acute infectious diseases, in which there's this *one thing* that causes a disease, and if you take an antibiotic it all goes away. That's the gold standard: a simple cause-effect-treatment paradigm. "That is actually the exception, not the rule," explains Dr. Adam Gaffney, a critical care physician and assistant professor at Harvard Medical School. "A lot of our symptoms have not one cause, but a multitude of causes."

Many chronic conditions need more than one intervention, and conditions can manifest very differently in each individual. This is especially true for some contested chronic illnesses—those that some doctors debate are even real. ME/CFS, for example, is marked by extreme fatigue and severe body aches over a long period of time. It's a brutal condition that can leave some patients with dizziness and intense brain fog and others unable to get out of bed. Uniform cookie-cutter treatments just won't cut it.

What you hear from women with chronic conditions, many of them living with agonizing pain and fed up with what little medicine has to offer, is defeat: *Doctors aren't going to save me. It's up to me.*

It might be up to them because doctors generally abide by the philosophy "First, do no harm." That mentality can translate to "do nothing" if they don't have treatments they believe are guaranteed to work when it comes to patients with a certain constellation of symptoms. There are always trade-offs with any intervention, so doctors balance risk versus benefit. But if someone is desperate, they might be willing to take more risk—provided there's *some* scientific plausibility to the treatment in question. Given what we know about the human body, chemistry, and biology, does this intervention make sense?[34] Their best bet is to find a doctor who fits their threshold of risk-taking if they are open to experimenting with treatments that have less evidence behind them. Ideally, that doctor could interpret the available data and safely see what works for them.[35]

Those doctors exist but are rare. Inevitably, this puts desperate patients in a sleuth-like position where they search for under-the-radar therapies within patient support communities. Throughout my research, I have spoken to women who experiment with (and swear by) unconventional treatments few Western doctors would endorse: water cures, laser therapy, mold avoidance, mixing of pharmaceuticals, and the like. Some will be money-sucking bunk, some will nary move the needle, and some might actually help. A portion might be dangerous (certain interventions carry real risk of harm). But patients will say the best they can hope for is to lean on that which has the most data—or, more likely, anecdotal success stories—to manage symptoms.

Anecdotes are a fine place to begin the process, but personal tales of recovery are subject to all kinds of biases and misleading contributing factors. Anecdotal "data" is not reliable. Thousands of people who attest to something can very well be wrong. (Exhibit A: flat-earthers.) At first glance, it may look like a strong grouping of evidence, but because the data was collected in a nonscientific way, it can leave out pivotal information.

Anecdotes are powerful and potentially misleading. Too often, especially in alternative medicine, we only hear the success stories. We rarely hear about the person who depended on energy healing, then got sicker, and ultimately died. They're not here to warn us. *Dead men tell no tales.*[36]

It's also at times difficult to measure the efficacy of any one treatment. This goes for both mainstream and alternative medicine. Generally, common medical conditions improve on their own, whether or not a patient took something, so intervention is hard to judge. It's very easy to assume causation when it's in fact correlation or placebo. If you take an herbal supplement at the height of a flu and then you start feeling better the next day, you might think it was the pill's doing. In reality, it was just the passage of time; in the normal course of things you were going to improve regardless.

Likewise, when patients go for an energy healing appointment, it might be the calming spa environment that relieves pain and stress or reduces tension headaches. It could be the act of something touching you or even the practitioner's personal attention and reassurance. In one study, participants who received a sham acupuncture (placebo) treatment said they experienced a 43 percent reduction of headache frequency.[37] Some might also believe a treatment works because they've invested time and money, in the same way I'm "certain" my pricey Estée Lauder serum dissolves wrinkles.

For these reasons, alternative medicine flourishes: people believe whatever they're taking or doing is what's aiding their recovery.

But alternative medicine isn't completely harmless, much in the same way mainstream medicine isn't. One element in mainstream medicine's favor is that—when practiced correctly—doctors evaluate the best body of evidence and weigh it against risks before recommending a particular intervention. Not always so with its competitors: "Sometimes alternative medicine gets a bit of a pass in the risk assessment department because it's seen as being 'natural,'" explains Jonathan Jarry, a biological scientist and science communicator with the McGill Office for Science and Society. "So it's seen as having only potential benefits and no real risks."

But there are risks: of side effects, physical harm, and just wasted time or money. There are cases of people who got liver damage from Chinese herbal medicine. On rare occasions, acupuncture has resulted in a punctured lung.[38]

Of course, most alternative remedies are not actively dangerous. But here's another issue: they potentially replace actual science-backed interventions and rob consumers of real therapeutic opportunities. It's sort of like how believing in flying carpets is harmless, but if you're stranded on a desert island and you wave off a rescue boat to wait for Aladdin's mode of transport, you've got a problem.

Alternative medicine can induce a rejection of traditional medicine, potentially leading down a slippery slope of conspiracy thinking or overconfidence in alternative methods. A 2018 observational study published in the medical journal *JAMA Oncology* found that cancer patients who depended on complementary medicine (herbs, vitamins, homeopathy, and other alternative therapies) were more likely to refuse conventional cancer treatment such as chemotherapy or surgery and therefore had a twofold higher risk of dying than those who never sought complementary care.[39]

Once you start questioning medicine, researchers warn, you might just take it too far. Steve Jobs shunned what might have been timely and lifesaving cancer surgery in lieu of alternative therapies and a strict vegetable diet. (Jobs had a rare form of pancreatic cancer, a neuroendocrine tumor, which is less lethal than the more common forms of pancreatic cancer.) He died at age fifty-six. His biographer, Walter Isaacson, reported that he later regretted his rejection of orthodox medical treatment.[40]

There are those opting for a more hybrid approach when it comes to medical innovation. Dr. Lucinda Bateman is the founder and medical director of the Bateman Horne Center, a medical center devoted to ME/

CFS and fibromyalgia. She was inspired to dedicate her career to these conditions after her older sister became sick with ME/CFS. Dr. Bateman has gathered other doctors and specialists to come up with expert recommendations that could be used in the absence of a large evidence base.

As a physician, Dr. Bateman readily admits it's "heresy" to criticize the high standards of evidence-based medicine, but "the concept that everything has to be evidence-based before it can be taught is a problem because when you have something new that you're discovering, it takes a while to build an evidence base." COVID-19, for example, helped us understand we can't wait to initiate care. Yes, double-blind, randomized, controlled trials are ideal, but when a crisis hits, we don't always have that luxury. "In order to have more rapid progress, we've had to let down our standards in the United States about what constitutes good evidence."

While Dr. Bateman recommends working with a physician, she fully understands that that isn't always a possibility. To that end, she advises: Buyer beware. "There's lots of good education online, but don't go hook, line and sinker, especially after someone is making a lot of money from selling products," she says, singling out supplements, for one. "As soon as people are earning their living by selling these [pills and products], then all credibility goes out the window as far as I'm concerned."

The Alternative MD Will See You Now

Mainstream doctors don't have all the answers, but it doesn't follow that then *anything* goes. All science is evolving, though there are stark differences between pseudoscience and that which is supported by evidence.

The commercialized wellness space can lend itself to predatory practices by those who seek to profit from the needs of the struggling. Uncredentialed influencers assert themselves as legitimate substitutes. They push pricey placebos masquerading as supplements, sham "detox" diets, and unsubstantiated IV vitamin injections. If you were to believe the marketing hype on cannabidiol (also known as CBD), you'd think the cannabis extract could cure cancer *and* solve the Middle East conflict; while CBD shows promise, cure-all claims are supported by little conclusive evidence and lack sufficient clinical trials. The Federal Trade Commission has pursued companies like HempMe CBD—which sells oils, creams, and gummies—for what they say were misleading claims regarding AIDS, autism, bipolar disease, cancer, depression, epilepsy, and seizures.[41]

It can be hard to judge "other" treatments when the marketing, branding, and presentation are just so good. A great example is the hot new trend of an alternative medicine MD or a functional medicine practitioner.

These are primary care doctors trained in a variety of alternative medicine modalities. Functional medicine says it treats the patient "as a whole" using herbal remedies, acupuncture, and other unorthodox methods along with lifestyle changes, but it doesn't necessarily shun pharmaceuticals if necessary. "The best of both worlds" is how it's described: bridging wellness and medicine. These practitioners are available for lengthy, in-depth appointments at sleek new clinics that feel more like fancy spas. Patients are welcomed into a beautiful space boasting lots of natural light, potted plants, stocked kombucha, and a comfy hotelesque lounge.

Upper-middle-class women in their thirties and forties, many dealing with chronic conditions, flock to these coastal clinics. Some clients likely saw functional medicine billboards sprouting up around L.A., preaching "You deserve a better doctor." These are women, as one clinic founder told me, who just can't get a doctor to "investigate" their medical issues. Here they will not be rushed out in seventeen minutes. They get more like a full hour.

These alternative clinics are attractive because they advocate preventive lifestyle habits that no one would argue with: eat more vegetables, exercise, get proper sleep. In many cases, they do help people by holding them accountable to these modifications. But they sometimes add on treatments with little or any rigorous evidence, such as detoxes and hefty supplement regimens. It's a mixed bag: a bunch of great recommendations combined with what sometimes amounts to pricey pseudoscience and unnecessary lab tests.

What's wrong with endless rounds of fancy-sounding tests? Well, it insinuates that conventional doctors are keeping essential information from you ("Why doesn't my doctor check XYZ?") while encouraging a preoccupation with details that might not lead to anything worthwhile, especially since some functional medicine tests are considered bogus by mainstream medicine.

Science communicators liken overtesting to conspiracy thinkers who fixate on teensy details as if they're holy grails. Too often, these details prove to be nothing more than red herrings. Unnecessary lab tests without a specific reason aren't recommended because the more tests you order, the more likely you are to get a false positive result *because tests aren't perfect*[42] (as anyone who has taken a COVID-19 test knows). The likelihood of an "abnormality" is high. This results in heightened anxiety, then more pricey tests, and then more supplements.

Many functional medicine clinics lambaste conventional doctors' relationship with pharmaceuticals even though they often follow the same format with supplements.

Part of this fixation with testing lies at the intersection of the quantified-self movement and the "do something" medical mentality. Dr. David Scales, a sociologist, physician, and assistant professor of medicine at Weill Cornell Medical College, also observes a psychological component: "[Wellness seekers] tend to be uncertainty avoidant people. There is the thought that more data is better, more data is going to provide more certainty." Usually these are people who believe the worst thing possible would be to "miss" something, without realizing that overdiagnosis (and overmedicating) pose their own risks.

Regardless, functional medicine's messaging is effective because it positions alternative care as empowering and anti-authoritarian even if it too can be plagued by exploitative practices. Or, more simply, this messaging and marketing is a heck of a lot better than that of mainstream medicine. Functional medicine clinics look like spas, and they understand women's pain points. They know exactly what we want to hear: that we are unique and therefore require tailor-made treatment, that Western doctors aren't listening to us, and that medical care can be enjoyable.[43]

It's hard to understate how much women want a better relationship with their physician—the primary reason they go to these clinics. Patients want more time to talk. They want doctors to help them retool their lifestyle and better emphasize preventive medicine. Many women are not getting this from traditional medicine. If we only look at treatments strictly from a medical perspective and not a psychological one, medicine will continue to lose patients. The experience *does* matter.

• • •

The hard left turn to alternative health has been galvanized by the dissatisfaction women have experienced in their doctor's offices. None of this, however, should undermine an appreciation for medicine and great strides in scientific discoveries. Antibiotics, vaccines, and proven medical methods ensure that most of us reach an age well beyond what any of our ancestors ever dreamed possible. No one should throw the baby out with the rose quartz–filtered bathwater.

And yet a gender bias continues to plague a portion of female patients dealing with a laundry list of mistreatments at the hands of an imperfect system that can ignore, trivialize, or misdiagnose ailments—and then follow with inadequate treatment.

But this phenomenon almost doesn't make sense. Why would those who take the Hippocratic oath purposely ignore women's calls for help? Surely they don't intend to hurt their patients who come to them in tears and desperation.

Undeniably, some harbor discriminatory tendencies, but in light of such a large volume of complaints, a bigger story must be behind it. There's an explanation for why physicians shrug their shoulders and rattle off perfunctory prescriptions. And it goes way back: back to when women were purposely excluded from the halls of medicine solely because of their sex.

Chapter 6

Can't Treat What You Don't Know

Since she first got her period at thirteen years old, Noémie Elhadad, had had constant pain in her legs. It was sometimes so painful she had trouble walking. Then other debilitating symptoms popped up: agonizing pelvic pain, chronic inflammation, and exhaustion. At times it got so bad that she ended up in the hospital only to be told "there's nothing wrong with you."

Doctors eventually diagnosed Elhadad with endometriosis. While validating, the diagnosis didn't do much of anything. "I knew I wasn't making it up, but that was it," Elhadad told me on a call. She underwent various hormone treatments, including being put on artificial menopause, with little success. "There's a lot of uncertainty and a lot of frustration because most treatments don't work," she explained. As Elhadad got older, her health took a nosedive. She was forced to take several leaves of absence from work. In total, she endured seven surgeries.

Elhadad ultimately became a computer scientist and an associate professor of biomedical informatics at Columbia University. Her personal experience inspired her to take action, specifically with what she knows best—data. She realized that what endometriosis needed more than anything was . . .

research. "When I started looking into endometriosis, there was no good quality information in these large data sets and it didn't fit at all what I was experiencing as a patient," Elhadad explained. "I started talking to a lot of support groups and I realized that I'm not the outlier here. *The data is the outlier.* And I knew from my research in other diseases that if you don't have an accurate representation of disease, you're doomed. You're not going to be able to identify what treatments work or what or who is at risk."

In 2016, Elhadad founded the Citizen Endo project, which aggregates female patients' experiences through "the power of crowds." She launched an endometriosis monitoring app called Phendo for women to self-document day-to-day symptoms and treatments, which it couples with existing patient health records. This crowdsourcing platform builds a stronger data set so researchers can better understand how different subpopulations precisely experience the condition.

It's an innovative approach. Already, the research project has collected data from 2 million endometriosis patients—making it the largest collection of endometriosis patient clinical data to date. The hope is that the collected and analyzed data will produce better self-management treatments. "We're using AI to learn what works specifically for you and what doesn't, to the point where I can build a tool that would say, given how you feel right now, it would be best to go for a walk for half an hour rather than rest, for instance," said Elhadad.

Elhadad isn't alone in her mission: she's part of a growing group of women servicing their peers. But the Citizen Endo project also hints at a fundamental piece of the puzzle in the growth of the wellness market, a growth that's often led by women. And that explanation lies in exactly the problem that Elhadad confronted: not just the present-day but the historical failure to develop effective treatment solutions for women.

Keep Out of Medicine: No Girls Allowed

Many issues we experience today have their origins in decisions made long before we agreed that both men and women deserve equal rights. The effort to keep women out of the official practice of medicine extends back to the Middle Ages, when women paid with their lives to administer care. Female healers were labeled as witches, seducers, and heretics for tending to their sisters. "No one does more harm to the Catholic Church than midwives," reads the definitive witch-hunter guide, *Malleus Maleficarum*. Published by Catholic clergymen in 1486, the manual served as the ultimate expression of distrust of females.

As the clergy saw it, the only reasonable way to account for women healers was as testaments of malicious magic. Their herbal concoctions and childbirth techniques became proof of consorting with the devil (as if Satan were, of all things, a doula). A high percentage of women who practiced what we would call medicine were accused and subsequently burned for "practicing witchcraft," though undeniably because they circumvented (and threatened) the Church's authority. Fueled by religious dogma, those in charge successfully pushed women out of care, thereby restricting their role in society.[1]

For centuries, women were sidelined out of medicine until it turned into an elite, male-dominated industry. And once medical schools required college education as a prerequisite for admittance, minorities and lower-income groups also faced exclusion. Maya Dusenbery writes in *Doing Harm: The Truth About How Bad Medicine and Lazy Science Leave Women Dismissed, Misdiagnosed, and Sick*, "The regular doctors had finally gained a legal monopoly over the practice of medicine, and in the process created a profession that was overwhelmingly white, male, and wealthy."[2]

This medical reorganization resulted in a massive loss of valuable health information, tools, and remedies that had been passed from generation to generation. For centuries, midwives and village elders oversaw childbirth; now, this task was outsourced to male doctors. The normal transmission of knowledge about sex or the female body by word of mouth stopped flowing. By the end of the nineteenth century, doctors discovered that 25 percent of young women were unprepared for their first menstruation.[3]

Sometimes doctors did attempt to learn more, but not always in the most ethical ways. *How* many of these doctors perfected their surgical techniques was often just as sinister as how frivolously doctors treated female bodies. Dr. James Marion Sims (1813–1883), considered the father of modern gynecology, practiced ovary operations on enslaved Black women. These women were not anesthetized and were sometimes operated on numerous times.

Medical misogyny no longer involves flaming torches and barbaric research practices. More women are becoming doctors, as they now constitute half of medical school students and more than a third of the U.S. physician workforce.[4] But while women increasingly joined the fold, structural sexism has hummed along through the modern era.

Problems in the Pipeline:
The Gender Health Gap

Here's one of the biggest issues in medicine we still feel today: Females were largely excluded as subjects from clinical research up until a few decades ago, leaving wide gaps in heart disease prevention, cancer treatment, and drug research. More recently, women represented only 19 percent of HIV drug trials and 11 percent of cure trials despite constituting half of the world's cases.[5]

Before the nineties, many researchers scoffed at testing drugs on women because they believed fluctuating female hormones might obscure results or they were worried about reproductive effects. (And, well, it was just easier and cheaper to omit them.) Instead, the standing presumption was that male findings could represent findings for both sexes. Hence the male "norm."

But hormones, immune systems, responses to chemicals, and the stages experienced over a lifetime differ between the sexes, such as female menstruation, pregnancy, and menopause. Women experience conditions differently. They have, for example, a higher tendency to experience migraines, and their migraines are more painful and longer-lasting than those of their male peers.[6] Women also make up 80 percent of autoimmune disease patients.[7]

Women's bodies can and do respond differently to drugs, putting them in greater danger of side effects if they're underrepresented in research. Between 2004 and 2013, women experienced over 2 million drug-related adverse events, in comparison to 1.3 million for men.[8]

To give an example of how this plays out: For years the media reported strange incidents involving women who took the insomnia medication zolpidem (also known as Ambien). Women woke up to a chaotic kitchen with a bizarre hodgepodge of ingredients and pots in disarray. Mysterious packages began arriving—a fire extinguisher, fifteen boxes of decaffeinated tea, used wigs, T. rex erotica—the result of two a.m. online shopping splurges no one could recall. Some were sleepwalking, sleep eating, and even sleep driving in the middle of the night.

A former manager of mine had the scariest story of all. She wrote an email to her boss in the middle of the night signed "I love you!"

It turned out that women process zolpidem at a slower rate than men, so it lingers in their system longer. But without proper research on the biological differences between the sexes, women weren't aware of that effect. In 2013, the FDA finally announced that manufacturers must lower the recommended zolpidem dose for women by nearly *half*.

Speaking of gaps, remember how Samantha Bee said that women receive just birth control pills and a shrug to treat endometriosis? Well, now you may have a better idea why. Women's concerns are dismissed due not just to bias but to a literal lack of knowledge. There's a painful need for more inclusive research.

Granted, doctors aren't handing out hysterectomies like Halloween candy, as they did during the nineteenth-century hysteria craze, but we're sometimes still defaulting to catchall labels instead of thoroughly investigating conditions. Occasionally, doctors dismiss or tell women, "It's exhaustion" or "It's all in your head," because they truly do not know what to make of symptoms. They are sincerely baffled; your body is a Picasso to their realist minds. But at the same time, the issue is almost circular: women are also not progressing on issues because medicine doubles down on the hysteria myth, dismissing telltale signs instead of investigating them.

"Doctors sometimes aren't very good at just saying, 'I don't know. We don't have enough research on this,'" says Sarah Graham, founder of the women's health blog *Hysterical Women*. "For a lot of women, although it doesn't necessarily give you the answer you want, it would still be better than being sent away feeling like you're going mad."

Many endometriosis patients do indeed feel like they're going mad. Endometriosis is one of many underrecognized, underresearched, and underfunded chronic conditions affecting women. It's pretty nuts considering endometriosis is estimated to affect nearly 10 percent of American women of reproductive age—roughly 6 million women.

In 2020, the U.S. House of Representatives doubled funding for endometriosis research, which amounted to just $26 million per year. Kim Kardashian's home is worth more than double that. All in all, that comes out to about $4 per U.S. woman afflicted with endometriosis.

This relates to the flawed outcome: If half of the population isn't properly studied, how can we expect proper diagnoses, let alone effective treatment? Insufficient data influences how all doctors—both male and female—then treat patients.

It's also just counterproductive. Increasing women's health research initiatives would save money in the long run: not as many women would have to quit their jobs or seek as much medical attention. One study commissioned by Women's Health Access Matters—an advocacy organization that aims to increase funding for women's medical issues—ran economic simulations to analyze the potential impact of increasing research investment. Chloe E. Bird, a senior sociologist at the RAND Corporation who co-led the study, predicted a "shockingly high return" on investment.[9]

"What we don't know about these diseases with tremendous impacts on women's health is costing billions," says Bird. For example, doubling the $20 million the NIH spent on coronary artery disease research related to women's health in 2019 to $40 million would yield an ROI of 9,500 percent and add 12,000 years back to the workforce. Doubling the $6 million spent on research for rheumatoid arthritis in women would conservatively deliver an ROI of 174,000 percent, saving $180 million in healthcare costs and adding $10.5 billion to the economy over 30 years.

There has been significant progress: sex as a biological variable is now a key part of the NIH's policy on research. Women now make up nearly half of all participants in NIH-supported clinical trials.[10] Still, that does not yet make up for the years they were excluded from medical research. There are gaps in our knowledge that can be filled with studies that take decades, not a year or two.

"There is a lot more work to do," says Kathryn Schubert, the CEO and president of the Society for Women's Health Research (SWHR). The nonprofit advocates for better representation of women in clinical research at the federal level and within various industries (pharmaceuticals, medical devices, etc.). Schubert says more women have been included in clinical research, although subpopulations of women—more ethnically diverse women, as well as specific groups like pregnant and lactating populations—"have not necessarily been included as we would like."

Schubert understands women's frustration. She too is frustrated, pointing to a telling stat: since 2000, there have been seventy-eight drug trials on erectile dysfunction, compared to fifty on preterm birth.[11] "When we think about the population impact and the return on investment, it's a little lopsided," says Schubert. Why is there such an imbalance in investment? Probably because many of the stakeholders in health care have been and are men. "It's not just about elevating these voices of women, but also making sure that we're getting women into leadership roles and decision-making roles."

A 2019 report found that women make up 30 percent of C-suite teams and 13 percent of CEOs in healthcare leadership. On average, reaching CEO status in the healthcare field takes women three to five years longer than men.[12] That means we're losing out on those who can better advocate for women's health needs.

Silicon Valley can prove just as challenging when it comes to femtech, a term encompassing apps, software, diagnostics, and consumer tech focused on women's health. Femtech start-ups—predominantly founded and led by women—still struggle to secure large-scale institutional funding.[13] I've interviewed roughly two dozen femtech founders across categories— fertility, menopause, chronic conditions—who told me they experience bias in the tech industry despite rah-rah enthusiasm in media outlets.*

One sexual wellness start-up founder told me she would walk into a typical investor pitch meeting, which would be composed of thirty middle-aged men and maybe one woman. She would begin her pitch with "I'm here to talk about vaginas," only to face an uncomfortable, beet-red audience. She went so far as to describe it as "looks of horror." This founder was never able to get a VC or a fund to write a check until she hired a middle-aged man—basically the carbon copy of the easily shocked middle-aged investor—as her CFO. "Literally just having my CFO stand in the room next to me gave me instant credibility with this group," she said, adding that the CFO was indeed qualified and not just VC arm candy. "He looked like them. He talked like them. And that made them [think], 'Okay, this is actually a real business, a real opportunity.'"

If venture capitalists can't personally relate to a health issue, they're less inclined to take interest. This could be why start-ups like Hims— which started by selling erectile dysfunction and men's hair loss pills— snagged $100 million in funding just a year after launch. Meanwhile,

---

* Like any Silicon Valley sector, femtech has its fair share of bunk and overhyped products—not to mention, it's limited in its capability to fix systemic issues—but an increasing number of companies are attempting to address the gender research gap.

menopause start-up founders tell me they still struggle to be taken seriously. Representation influences research and funding, as numerous entrepreneurs in the space attest.

"I've heard the same story over and over of male investors who did not really understand the problem well enough to get excited about a company," says Halle Tecco, an investor and founder emeritus of Rock Health, a seed fund investing in digital health start-ups, who has since co-founded and successfully exited the fertility start-up Natalist.[14] "And the few women and doctors that there are [in this sector] are spread so thin because they're overwhelmed with the amount of opportunity."

Women's digital health had a "banner year" in 2018. The subsector collectively stood at $650 million in funding across dozens of companies. That might sound like a lot, but Juul raised the exact same amount in one funding round that very same year. Basically, just one company (an e-cigarette maker, no less) was able to raise as much as an entire category devoted to women's health solutions. It's apples to oranges, no doubt, but it gives an idea of the money flowing in Silicon Valley.

This divergence could be because reportedly only 13 percent of venture capitalists are women,[15] meaning far more femtech founders continue to encounter blushing audiences. Having women on board makes a sizable impact: women VCs invest in twice as many female-founded companies than their male counterparts.[16] (It would be safe to presume that most traditional investors aren't dying to learn about vaginas.)

And yet there's much consumer interest in this field: women are 75 percent more likely to use digital health tools—e.g., pregnancy-focused apps or health management trackers—than men.[17] So not only can health tech make a sizable difference in research and treating women's issues, but women *want* it.

Femtech founders tell me that investors often ask the same question of their company's goal: Why hasn't this been done before? It could be because women shied away from freely discussing intimate issues, thereby reinforcing its hidden status. That tendency is changing as more open discussions erode the stigmas. But maybe they also avoided discussing these issues because they knew no one wanted to hear about them.

A "Shattered" Trust: Scandals, Controversies, and Lawsuits

A lack of research is more detrimental than just the paltry solutions it leads to. It can cause real, lasting harm. Many women are wary of medical institutions as a result of horrific episodes in healthcare history that stemmed from rushed, undertested research.

In the last two decades, more than a hundred thousand lawsuits have been filed against the makers of transvaginal mesh (a netlike implant used to treat pelvic organ prolapse) and midurethral mesh sling (a narrow strip of mesh positioned under the urethra to treat stress urinary incontinence—the loss of bladder control when sneezing, laughing, and coughing).[†]

Marketed as an easy and safe solution for patients dealing with weakened vaginal walls, millions of transvaginal mesh implants have been administered worldwide since the nineties. But some doctors weren't properly trained in optimal insertion techniques or on what could go wrong, says Dr. Maude Carmel, an associate professor in the department of urology at the University of Texas Southwestern Medical Center.

While many women were successfully treated, it's been estimated that between 5 and 15 percent of mesh patients[18] suffered complications, including bleeding, infections, severe cramps, nerve damage, and organ injuries.[19] Poorly installed mesh resulted in erosion, making patients feel like the implant sliced into their vagina, bladder, urethra, and bowel. Suddenly these women couldn't walk or sit without debilitating pain. New brides stared at a lifetime of painful sex. Moms deserted their jobs due to chronic complications. One marathon runner found herself crawling to the bathroom.

[†] Mesh slings and transvaginal mesh use the same plastic material, polypropylene, but they differ in their applications, how they're anchored, and the way they are placed.

Consider Kath Sansom, whose friends called her "the Ritalin kid" for her inability to sit still. "Too much energy," they said. Super active in her forties, the photographer and journalist boxed twice a week, swam most days, and went mountain biking on weekends. Sansom had experienced a little bit of incontinence after having her second daughter, which was embarrassing but didn't truly inhibit her lifestyle.

In 2015, Sansom's surgeon said the condition was simple to fix. The physician sold her on an "amazing" procedure which took only twenty minutes and had a "really quick" recovery. "Perfect for a career woman like you," her doctor told her. She was training to cycle up Snowdon—the highest mountain in Wales—right before her mesh surgery.

But immediately following the procedure, Sansom experienced an extreme reaction to the foreign material and all-over pain in the lower half of her body. The plastic mesh pressed on nerves and muscles, instigating excruciating pain—a feeling like being cut with a cheese wire. Despite being promised seven days for recovery, the pain intensified as the weeks wore on, causing burning sensations in her groin. Sansom couldn't even walk up a flight of stairs. "It felt like someone had taken a baseball bat and smacked me down the back of my legs all the way down to the bottom of my feet," she recalls through tears. "I would lie in bed at night terrified because I couldn't think of living the rest of my life in this much pain."

Some patients learned that mesh removal isn't always so simple. Their doctors told them that revision surgery is complicated and runs the risk of further damage. As one patient described it, revision surgery is like "trying to remove gum from hair."[20] Thousands of patients never fully regained their health.

Sansom wasn't warned of these risks. Had she known, she would have never agreed to have it implanted. "None of us [patients gave] fully informed consent. If we had been told of all the risks, we would have run out of the room."

Sansom never cycled again, and her boxing days are long over. She can no longer take part in many of the high-octane activities that once gave her so much joy. In addition, she began to experience constant joint aches, making even light outings difficult to endure. The once carefree, energy-filled Sansom no longer exists.

That same year, Sansom launched Sling the Mesh, a digital community support group for women harmed by and recovering from mesh implants. Many of the nearly ten thousand members report chronic complications, and in a site survey, seven out of ten say their sex lives were destroyed. To clarify, they didn't lose their sex drive. Rather, they lost the ability to *have sex* due to intense burning sensations and pain. For some women, the mesh quite literally slices through their vaginal walls and cuts their partner. Of those, a percentage say their doctors show little sympathy, some telling women over fifty they're too old to be having sex anyway. "If it was men losing their sex lives on that scale, you can bet your bottom dollar that operation would have been stopped years ago," says Sansom. "Men would not stand that kind of a risk."

In 2016, the U.S. Food and Drug Administration reclassified surgical mesh products for the transvaginal repair of pelvic organ prolapse (POP) as "high risk" following reports of long-term complications.[21] Three years later, the FDA ordered manufacturers Boston Scientific and Coloplast to halt the distribution and sale of any remaining surgical mesh products for the transvaginal repair of POP, stating that they had "not demonstrated a reasonable assurance of safety and effectiveness for these devices."[22]

In 2021, Boston Scientific agreed to pay $188.7 million to settle claims that it deceptively marketed their transvaginal surgical mesh devices, although the company stated that the settlement was not an admission of misconduct.[23] Subsequent reports[24] alleged that implant manufacturers hustled their products without sufficient testing,[25] reinforcing suspicions that women had been essentially treated like guinea pigs.

How exactly did these products slip through in the United States without the potential complications being made more apparent? Well, medical device companies can simply prove their devices are substantially equivalent to ones already available on the market in a process known as the 510(k) pathway. "If you use that process to have a device approved, you don't need to provide any patient data," says Dr. Carmel. "This is how they got around it." (In 2019, the FDA announced the agency would enforce stricter standards on its medical device program to increase transparency.)[26]

The medical community is split over vaginal mesh in terms of what should and shouldn't be banned.‡ Pelvic surgery experts I interviewed said it isn't necessarily the transvaginal surgical mesh devices themselves that are problematic, rather their incorrect placement by surgeons. Many were not adequately informed about the risks involved. A surgeon could be just one centimeter off and accidentally hit a nerve.

Still, there are lessons learned from this controversy, including the need to adequately train doctors, to implement stricter regulations, and to listen to female patients.

But while changes are underway, there are still those picking up the pieces.

Today, Sansom relies on alternative therapies to manage lingering aftereffects. For example, her nose began dripping immediately after the procedure, and she believes the ongoing symptom is directly related.§ Sansom makes a homemade paste with turmeric, known for its anti-inflammatory properties, which she says stops nasal leakage within half an hour. Fellow sufferers say they use cannabis or alcohol to manage their daily pain. "I have no trust in [the medical establishment]," says Sansom, who mourns

---

‡ Doctors reiterate there is a big difference between the use of mesh for urinary stress incontinence, which is still in wide use, and for that of prolapse surgery, which has more complications.

§ It is unclear whether it is directly related, as urologists I interviewed expressed skepticism. However, Shlomo Raz, professor of urology and pelvic reconstruction at UCLA School of Medicine, told the *Washington Post* in 2019 that he had seen "lupus-type" complications such as a runny nose disappear when the mesh is removed.

participation in all the sports she'd previously based her life on. "All gone. Absolutely shattered."

Flashback: The Scientist Who Protected Women from One of the Biggest Drug Fiascos

Decades peppered by horrific medical fiascos have at times eroded public trust and enabled peddlers of alternative care. Many women have been left questioning the attention to safety and adequate research precautions. But women have also fought to protect consumers, and they serve as a testament to why their inclusion in medicine is vital.

In the late fifties, one such pharmaceutical tragedy across Europe involved a new drug to combat morning sickness: thalidomide. It was heavily marketed to pregnant women, or, more specifically, to their physicians.

But when taken during the first trimester of pregnancy, thalidomide could cause severe developmental abnormalities. More than ten thousand babies were born with limb malformations and other birth defects including blindness, deafness, and brain damage.[27] The drug, which was not sufficiently tested, was estimated to have also caused just as many miscarriages.[28]

When the drug tried to enter the U.S. market—months before its effects were widely known—a female FDA reviewer and scientist named Dr. Frances Oldham Kelsey demanded more testing. The drug manufacturer behind thalidomide, William S. Merrell Co., complained to Dr. Kelsey's supervisors—calling, sending letters, and even showing up in person to try to rush their application.[29] Dr. Kelsey remained resolute, demanding more research demonstrating the drug's safety and efficacy. "I held my ground," Dr. Kelsey reflected decades later. "I just wouldn't approve it."[30]

Thanks to Dr. Kelsey's steadfastness, thalidomide was never approved in the United States. An estimated 20,000 Americans—600 who were pregnant—did take the drug as part of clinical trials conducted by drugmakers; seventeen cases of congenital deformities were reported, but "that could have been thousands had the FDA not insisted on the evidence of safety required under the law (despite ongoing pressure from the drug's sponsor)."[31]

As *Life* magazine wrote in 1962, "A woman of fortitude and determination had proved that the wheels of progress should occasionally be slowed and examined."[32] That same year, President John F. Kennedy bestowed on Dr. Kelsey the President's Award for Distinguished Federal Civilian Service, the highest honor granted to a civilian in the United States.

The thalidomide crisis pushed Congress to sign legislation empowering the FDA to have more authority over drug testing. In addition, Dr. Kelsey helped compose guidelines that govern clinical trials and which are now used worldwide.

Funny enough, Dr. Kelsey got her professional start in pharmacology because she was mistaken for a man. Dr. Kelsey had applied to be a research assistant in the University of Chicago's pharmacology department. She was offered the position—without an interview—after the hiring manager read her name as "Francis," and assumed she was "Mr. Oldham." Dr. Kelsey, realizing the mistake, asked one of her professors at McGill University what she should do: "When a woman took a job in those days, she was made to feel as if she was depriving a man of the ability to support his wife and child," Dr. Kelsey told the *New York Times*. "But my professor said: 'Don't be stupid. Accept the job, sign your name and put "Miss" in brackets afterward.'"[33]

Insufficient medical knowledge, which leads to misdiagnosis and medical fiascos, is improving, in part due to more women entering medicine, health tech, and research.

Kathryn Schubert of SWHR is optimistic: she points to several wins at the policy level, including increased funding for the Office of Research on Women's Health (ORWH), which coordinates women's health research across the NIH. The National Institute for Child Health and Human Development (NICHD), which handles endometriosis research, discovered "pretty critical scientific breakthroughs" regarding the progression of the condition and treatment options "versus just looking at hysterectomy," says Schubert. "It's hard to see the wins because there is so much work that needs to be done, but it is happening."

Elhadad, meanwhile, has her sights set on more than just endometriosis. She plans to take the Citizen Endo model and apply it to other underrepresented women's health conditions, including polycystic ovary syndrome. She's also working on an organization dedicated to building a community for female-focused medical research. "We're making sure patient voices and women are actually heard."

That's in addition to plenty more research-focused start-ups and biotech companies uniquely focused on women's health. (Digital health start-ups serving women's needs raised $1.3 billion in 2021.)[34] Researchers, for example, are building "smart bras" that are basically heart monitors; they're using medical-grade fabric sensors and machine learning to gather heart health data because heart disease is the leading cause of death for women worldwide. Universities are mining the databases of period tracking apps such as Clue to better understand menstrual cycles' effects on pain, mood, and ovulation. Big ideas are in the pipeline, with plans to tackle everything from nonhormonal birth control to neuroimmune disorders.

Women are also talking more publicly about their health, which helps bring attention to the cause and assists in finding solutions. Postpartum depression is a great example of this: in earlier decades, women weren't necessarily telling friends or their clinicians about the phenomenon, so nobody knew it was an issue, let alone one deserving of research. "People are not always talking about what they're experiencing, and I think that sets us back," says Schubert. "We need to have these open, honest conversations."

Either way, some might feel the growth is not keeping pace with the dissatisfaction and issues inherent in an overburdened medical system. (Not that it's an easy feat: research studies are time-consuming and costly, racking up millions and taking years.) And within that vacuum, alternatives take root. Patients who become tired of trying to change a system that doesn't prioritize them take their business elsewhere. Sadly, desperate women are often mocked or criticized for self-treatment, and doctors roll their eyes at "Dr. WebMD." But these women turn right back around and demand: What other option did I have?

Chapter 7

Nutritionmania:
Why Are We Confused About What We Eat?

You wouldn't think the Kardashian sisters would be the yin and yang of wellness, the light to each other's dark, but let me share my favorite episode of *Keeping Up with the Kardashians*: In 2019, the reality TV stars Kim and Kourtney Kardashian fought over an issue that would have puzzled viewers a decade prior. It was so petty and so emotionally charged—and yet representative of a growing sentiment in American households.

In the back of their chauffeured Range Rover, the siblings argued over what to serve at their kindergarten-age daughters' joint birthday party. And it was getting heated. Name calling, raised voices, and insults ensued. The party theme was Candy Land, but older sister Kourtney—founder of the wellness lifestyle brand Poosh—refused to go along with it. She wanted none of the "nasty" and "gross" gumdrops or lollipops from the iconic board game. There would be no homage to Princess Frostine's Ice Palace, nor a nod to the bountiful Peppermint Forest. This candy-free Candy Land would present nutritious treats instead of sweets. Maybe even some salads.

Kim, who couldn't fathom carrots masquerading as licorice, called her health-conscious sister "insane."

"It's Candy Land, Kourtney," emphasized Kim. "It's not going to be healthy." The two went back and forth debating whether or not candy canes had to be, well, literal. An astonished Kim accused her sister of foisting a completely "sugar-free, gluten-free, party-free, fun-free zone" on two innocent six-year-olds. "My kids eat at home really, really healthy. And the one day they want a Candy Land birthday party, and you're saying they can't have sugar?!"[1]

Kourtney disagreed, accusing Kim of hurting the children. "You're dated, you're in the past," Kourtney lectured Kim, claiming food coloring "literally" gives people diseases. "Everyone is going to come to this party and everything is going to be disgusting chemicals?!" *How can you not feel guilty about that?* she asked. Unhealthy food, she added, wasn't what she "stood for."

The disagreement continued for several days, to the point where other family members needed to mediate between the two. And it was real: long-term show fans (such as myself) can tell whether a fight is manufactured or legitimate. In the latter, Kim quickly escalates a heated exchange into threats (or actual instances) of physical violence. At one point during "sugargate," Kim threatened to hit her sister in the face with a piñata.

After refusing to come to a consensus, the sisters decided to break with tradition and settled on separate parties. Though the cousins were inseparable best friends, they were subjected to their mothers' nutritional divide. Kourtney would serve sugar-free organic cotton candy, while Kim displayed mounds of gummy bears, chocolates, and marshmallows. Later, after the episode aired and viewers took sides on social media, Kourtney tweeted, "I am actually shocked that people are so unaware of how harmful certain foods can be."

Perhaps no better issue demonstrates the fading trust in Big Food than that of sugar, which has been dubbed the "new smoking," declared "addictive as cocaine," and gives new meaning to the danger invoked by the *Ghostbusters* Stay Puft Marshmallow Man.* There's no question that too much sugar is an issue in American diets. And as the number of children with obesity has increased tenfold,[3] some parents ponder: How do we best feed our families?

But fear of eating the wrong foods can quickly devolve into confusion, extremism—and judgment. In mommy circles, peers can pour the gasoline: Six out of ten mothers of young kids say they have been criticized about parenting, with over half of those complaints centered on diet and nutrition.[4] Even Reese Witherspoon "incurred the wrath of the food police" when she shared an Instagram photo of glazed cinnamon rolls for her son's breakfast.[5] "Child abuse right there," wrote one critic.

If choosy moms once chose Jif peanut butter, now they must choose only the *right* healthful products to cement their parental reputation.

Cutting out sugar isn't a fad diet, but it's just one of several popular food doctrines, along with vegan, dairy-free, gluten-free, or (Paltrow favorite) "clean" eating. The United States saw a 600 percent increase in veganism between 2014 to 2017,[6] and 30 percent of all Americans now avoid gluten,[7] though only a small percentage actually have Celiac disease or a gluten sensitivity. Cookbook sales grew 21 percent in 2018 partially because consumers were sold on the nutritional superiority of cooking at home versus going out (where presumably unwholesome food awaits).[8]

Anxiety over nutrition has inspired new food commandments, much like the ever-growing list of lifestyle laws dictating exercise and other practices. Food is no longer neutral territory; strict views have polarized our daily consumption. Within specific middle- and upper-middle-class communities, the message has gone from *Try your best* to *Do exactly this*. Talk with the average woman and you will notice a disturbing pattern

---

* While one could certainly have sugar cravings, nutrition experts I interviewed note that sugar is not literally addictive like drugs. In addition, a 2016 study led by University of Cambridge neuroscientists found "little evidence to support sugar addiction in humans."[2]

surrounding what is or isn't "healthy," what supplements you should take, how many meals to eat per day, the need for organic . . . Americans are, quite frankly, a nutritional mess.

"There's so much information about food being thrown at you, it's hard to know what to believe and what really works," writes bestselling author and blogger Vani Hari. "As a reader of this blog, you're on the right path. I'm showing you how to become the smartest consumers out there."[9]

Vani Hari, who goes by the moniker Food Babe, has built an entire empire lambasting ultra-processed food while waging war against Big Food. A charismatic brunette with an inviting smile, Hari is perfectly put together: slim, hair styled in loose waves, unfussy makeup, like one of those cool moms from a Nickelodeon show in designer skinny jeans and a moto jacket. But unlike a Nickelodeon mom, Hari will not offer you a Pillsbury cookie: in fact, this food safety champion won't invite you to enjoy much of any conventional snacks. To her, "refined sugar is the devil." She tells fans to avoid artificial dyes at birthday parties. She warned that Kellogg's waffles are a "disaster for children's immune system." She lobbied Starbucks to stop using Class IV caramel coloring in pumpkin spice lattes.

Her other big beef? That those pumpkin spice lattes contain "absolutely no real pumpkin."[10]

Hari is not a nutritionist, food scientist, or toxicologist, yet she became a leading health blogger, activist, and one of *Time* magazine's "Most Influential People on the Internet." The former management consultant was revered and feared for demonizing common ingredients found in *everything*: preservatives, additives, GMOs, and added sugars, all of which she says carry great health risks. In criticizing food companies, she goes hard: "Big Food is deliberately confusing us," she tweeted. "They don't want us to know how to eat right." There's not much love for regulatory oversight either, for that matter: "The FDA is asleep at the wheel and the Food Industry is in charge."

She's right about one thing: it's a bit odd just how confused we are about a basic biological function (though who is entirely to blame is a bit more complicated). At first glance it seems surprising. After all, weren't those laminated United States Department of Agriculture (USDA) food pyramids posted in every classroom—telling us to eat our vegetables and fruits like good healthy soldiers—the quintessential guides to healthful eating? What happened?

Piling on the Plate: Corporate Greed Further Confuses Matters

The iconic food pyramid has played the villain as much as the hero when it comes to clarifying eating recommendations. The nutrition guidelines reshuffled mandates on categories like fats and oils. A failure to define serving sizes or distinguish between types of fat, let alone between minimally processed grains and refined ones (not all carbs are created equal), opened the doors to mass confusion.[†]

Surprisingly, the pyramid was built on the architecture of a widely adopted (though contested) food theory. In the 1950s, a physiologist named Ancel Keys proposed that heart disease was linked to high-fat diets and high cholesterol levels. To prove it, he studied seven countries, including Greece, Italy, Japan, and Finland. Great travel destinations, no doubt, but the world is bigger than just a half dozen countries. Regardless, the infamous Seven Countries Study's findings prioritized carbohydrates, discouraged saturated fats, and oversimplified the issue of cholesterol. Eggs were out, cereal was in.

Despite conflicting evidence, it took off.[11] Research circles and the media—which were both looking for solutions to the heart disease epidemic—pushed the theory. The government then adopted it for their first dietary guidelines. In 1980, the USDA advised Americans to cut back on red meat, eggs, and dairy products and pile on carbohydrates like pasta, rice, bread, and cereal instead, among other recommendations. The position

---

† In 2011, the USDA introduced MyPlate, which emphasized a more holistic approach to nutrition.

was solidified into nutritional dogma, then rolled out across companies, schools, agencies, and the media, but not with the clearest communication. The guidelines were often misinterpreted.[12]

The established viewpoint claimed that if you reduced fat, you would automatically reduce calories because fat is higher in calories than carbohydrates. There was just one problem: once fats were removed from foods, the result was less appetizing. The only way to make the now textureless morsel tasty was to *add sugar*. Food manufacturers quickly swapped one ingredient for another and capitalized on the health lingo of the day. Suddenly grocery stores were filled with rebranded "low-fat" but sugar-packed snacks, granola bars, and yogurt. That led to what's been dubbed "the SnackWell effect," which refers to the psychological tendency to eat more of a food marketed as low-fat.

Based on this logic, Americans became fearful of butter and cheese but embraced "fat-free" muffins. From 1971 to 2000, American women increased their carbohydrate intake by nearly 25 percent, as fat became enemy number one.[13] What started as a fight against heart disease ended as a surrender to carb overconsumption.

The ongoing battle between sugar versus fat was further complicated by sugar lobbyists and biased researchers, who weren't very helpful at preventing this nutrition misunderstanding. In the 1960s, sugar producers paid Harvard scientists to discredit anti-sugar science and downplay its role in heart disease.[14] Instead, these researchers (whose pre-existing work, to be fair, already supported these findings) pointed the finger at fat. However, studies show both fat *and* sugar can contribute to heart disease.

Today, the average American consumes almost 150 pounds of total sugar in one year (the equivalent of six full cups a week). Of that, 66 pounds are added sugar.[15] Why? Because it's in everything. Sugar is in pasta sauce, bread, even salad dressing. It's virtually inescapable. While other factors contributed to our nutritional issues, it's fair to say that poorly constructed messaging surrounding the food pyramid ought to shoulder a portion of the blame.

Incorrect guidance wasn't the only thing leading Americans further astray from the nutritionally sound path. The situation was compounded by pressure placed on food companies to maximize profits, as Wall Street changed the way it evaluated corporations. Long, slow returns on investment gave way to the shareholder value model, forcing corporations to provide higher, more immediate returns on investment. Companies, under intense pressure, were forced to look for ways to sell more; growth became the focus. Gordon Gekko seized the dinner table.[‡]

Cheap and easily accessible highly processed food took off. Some ultra-processed-food manufacturers also followed what's been dubbed the "potato chip marketing equation," selling 90 percent of their products to 10 percent of their customers, many of whom were low-income. They decided that spending marketing dollars going after an existing customer and selling them on increased consumption was more lucrative than targeting new ones.[16] Essentially, they're persuading current clientele to buy not one bag of chips per month, but one bag of chips *per day*.

Lay's potato chips slogan "Bet you can't eat just one!" is therefore actually quite literal. You can't eat one not only because ad dollars ask you to eat more but also because the product is chemically engineered to be as delicious as possible. Food chemists craft ultra-processed foods to appeal to our biggest cravings—added sugar, salt, and fats—which light up our brains' reward centers like a Vegas slot machine, researchers suggest.[17]

As more food was produced and marketed, portion sizes got bigger. Calories in the food supply increased, and people started eating more. The

---

[‡] Many twentieth-century food trends have roots that go further back in American history, touching upon technological advancement and agricultural policies. Food historian Sarah Wassberg Johnson says that after WWII, food companies expanded on defense-funded nutrition and chemical research to increase their bottom lines. Then, in the seventies, new government policies allowed food corporations to cheaply purchase commodity crops like corn and soy, which incentivized using them as additives.

Big Gulp trumped the soda can. Fast-food chains rolled out supersized meals. Restaurants introduced all-you-can-eat buffets. And even standard foods were reworked. The average bagel went from three inches in diameter (140 calories) twenty years ago to six inches in diameter (350 calories) today.[18] "We used to eat less, end of story," Marion Nestle, a consumer advocate and the author of *Food Politics*, told me.

The industrial food revolution and fast-food dependency clearly affected eating habits. A modern American consumes more than 3,600 calories each day, a 24 percent increase from 1961, in part because highly processed foods and snacks make up to 60 percent of their diet.[19] Just 7 percent of American adults meet the daily recommendation for fiber (because fiber is found in foods like beans and lentils).[20]

Granted, not all processed food is bad for you. Processed foods lie within a spectrum. Some foods are lightly processed to prevent spoilage or boost mineral content, like canned vegetables, whereas others are ultra-processed and packed with sugars, salt, and additives. But the latter is usually far tastier and hence more popular.

It should be noted that the 1980 dietary guidelines advised minimizing added sugars, advice that Americans ignored.[21] In all fairness, how could nutritionists compete against Big Food's billion-dollar marketing budgets? Our childhoods are marked by McDonald's Happy Meals and Pop-Tarts advertised on television. We can't recall too many cartoon characters shilling for vegetables (except maybe the Green Giant, but he was drowned out by the party-loving Kool-Aid Man). Even today, more than 80 percent of food advertising—nearly $14 billion—promotes fast food, soda, energy drinks, chips, and candy.[22]

As enticing as it may be to squarely blame the original faulty science, our modern food environment—cheap, processed food available at every turn, from the gas station to ubiquitous food vending machines—does need to be considered. We never stood a chance. In time, we all started to realize it.

Growing Distrust of "Big Food":
The Personal Becomes Political

Awareness of issues with processed food took off in the sixties, when the growing natural food movement—think hippies, communes, and food co-ops—confronted the mainstream food industry for its greasy grip on consumers. Young baby boomers voiced their dissent through what they ate, wore, and believed. By revolutionizing their private life, the conscientious rebel would also transform "the system." Rejecting the mass-produced hamburger was, in its own way, a radicalized act. And so brown rice wasn't just brown rice—the sticky grain was an act of defiance.

Healthier eating produced a new kind of discernment that motivated reformers to rally against agribusiness *and* their parents' kitchen. And "unlike sporadic anti-war protests, dietary rightness could be lived 365 days a year, three times a day."[23]

It was more than just disgust at McDonald's beef patties. Food politics were part and parcel of a larger shift in societal attitudes toward mass industry. People were fearful of nuclear war, toxic waste, and environmental issues and saw many issues reflective of industrial failings. Corporate manufacturers proved they couldn't always prevent damaging ingredients from seeping into a hamburger. Tainted, contaminated, or misrepresented food sparked skepticism then and continues today.

Meanwhile, media exposés reinforced suspicions that government agencies aren't fully invested in nutrition but are smoking cigarettes in bed with food lobbyists. Reports confirmed the USDA is under constant pressure from meat and dairy groups.[24] The USDA is obligated to promote food commodities, thereby facing intense opposition whenever it wants to recommend a decrease in any food group in dietary guidelines. At a Senate hearing, former Illinois Republican senator Peter Fitzgerald characterized this blatant conflict of interest, "like putting the fox in charge of the hen house."[25]

Even the health associations and leading nutritionists no longer carry the weight they once did, in part due to their participation in paid endorsements or studies sponsored by bigwigs like Coca-Cola. In 1988, the American Heart Association (AHA) raised money for research efforts by selling a "heart-healthy" label to food companies eager to capitalize on better-for-you marketing. A product only needed to meet a specific requirement for levels of saturated fat, cholesterol, and sodium. By labeling single foods as "heart-healthy," it "distorted basic principles of good nutrition which depend on overall dietary patterns," writes Marion Nestle in *Food Politics*.[26] Many sugar-laden cereals boasted the AHA seal of approval. Shoppers scanned the grocery aisle and wondered, *How the hell is Trix healthful?*

Then there are the food scandals. Here is just a sample from recent global headlines: Chicken from some major fast-food chains might contain only 50 percent chicken DNA.[27] Mars recalled chocolate bars in fifty-five countries over "fears that customers could choke on pieces of plastic."[28] Consumer Reports found that 97 percent of chicken breasts sold in retail stores contained potentially harmful bacteria (often the result of fecal matter contamination).

Though rare, such debacles seep into the American psyche. In one 2020 survey of five hundred consumers, less than half said they trusted the overall food industry. Instead, 77 percent of respondents said cooking in their kitchens was the best course of action.[29] And when health-conscious consumers shop, they're pickier; almost half considered whether a product was processed before heading to the cash register, according to a Nielsen report.[30]

Women not only learned not to take the word of Big Food on what to eat, they started having nutrition meltdowns like never before, spinning a revolving door of restrictive food rules. Which led to even more confusion. When it comes to nutritional guidelines, harsh restrictions like Kourtney Kardashian's "healthy Candy Land" rule for her kids are extremely clear. But are all the restrictions deserved? Or accurate?

Flashback: Yearning for Nutritional Nirvana

In a Depression-era ad for Post Bran Flakes, a young girl named Sally is mercilessly mocked by schoolmates for her dismal report card. Turning to her mother, she finds little refuge. "Sally Lennox! I'm ashamed of this report card. What will your father say?" the mother lectures the child.

But not so fast, the reader learns. The mother is the villain here. The problem was not caused because young Sally didn't study. Instead, the selfish mother is to blame. For you see, it turns out the poor grades were the result of constipation . . . from not eating enough cereal. "Maybe you have a little girl like Sally," the ad reads, laying the guilt on thick, "and perhaps like Sally's mother, you have been unjust to her."[31]

Starting in the 1920s, national government campaigns coupled with women's magazine articles stressed a very specific nutrition mandate, reinforcing the idea that fortified foods (products with added nutrients) were "necessary" for a normal healthy life. Some brand campaigns relied on scare tactics, like Grape-Nuts cereal, which suggested that a cereal-poor diet puts children at risk of "unfortunate personality traits" like shyness and self-pity.[32] In time, nutrition was imbued with a sense of morality and elitism, claiming to ensure good nerves, composure, energy, beauty, and steadfastness. Health, essentially, secured one's future prospects.

This messaging reached deep into women's maternal core, causing utmost anxiety and thereby frantic obedience. No mother would refuse Grape-Nuts, lest her child turned into Eeyore.

Taking aim at children's success was a calculated action. Advertisers were "fascinated" by a growing competitive struggle— specifically, how it played out with parents dissatisfied with their own ambitions. Brands discovered that parents could be pushed to pass their anxieties and quashed aspirations onto their children. In effect, the next generation was coerced into actualizing their parents' disappearing dreams and pummeled into competitive one-upmanship.[33]

This collective guidance led to a nerve-racking quest for nutritional perfection in the fifties, equating a morning bowl of cereal to extra tutoring. Vitamins were synonymous with health, even though consumers knew very little about food chemistry. Women were told to put their faith in experts and nutrition gurus, for fear of gambling with the family's fragile health, as Catherine Price documents in her book *Vitamania*. "Americans of both genders embraced the notion that careful homemakers had a responsibility to ensure that their families—through food and, later, supplements—had enough of each," writes Price. "How much was enough, though? Nobody knew."[34]

Organic or Bust: How Concerned Should We Be About Produce?

While shoppers rack their brains over what to eat, many seem to be certain about one thing: they want their whole foods to be organic. Despite the extra cost and often reduced shelf life, in certain circles, organic is the new given. Sales of organic foods more than doubled between 1994 and 2014.[35] I too favored organic for several years. It sounded right. Why wouldn't I want the "healthier" option?

The problem is that organic is a description that seemingly confuses the consumer as much as it supposedly clarifies what should or shouldn't be on their dinner plate. Is organic the same as "natural"? Does it mean GMO-free? It turns out that 23 percent of consumers think "local" is synonymous with organic.[36] (It's not.)

Not to mention that the health benefits of organic are—and I know this might come as a shock—nowhere near as proven as most consumers would like to think.

Many women I've interviewed switched to pricier organic after reading the Environmental Working Group's "Dirty Dozen" list, a shopper's guide to produce that purportedly contains high levels of pesticide residue and therefore should be avoided. Every year, the EWG announces which misbehaving fruits and vegetables made the naughty list, prompting mainstream media outlets to publish which conventionally grown produce is "in" or "out." It's ubiquitous to the point where we don't even question it.

In 2021, the EWG warned that "imazalil, a fungicide that can change hormone levels and is classified by the Environmental Protection Agency as a likely human carcinogen, was detected on nearly 90 percent of citrus."[37] This was all very scary-sounding! Who wants evil chemicals lounging on their fruit?

The thing is, organic farms *also* use pesticides and fungicides to ward off pests and fungal disease. They're less discussed because they're "organic." Organic means derived more from natural substances than synthetic. But "natural," as we have learned, doesn't necessarily always mean better. Organic farms generally try to minimize pesticide use, and some of their pesticides are gentler than synthetic ones, but they can sometimes be less effective, leading organic farms to use much more of the organic pesticides in order to achieve the same results.

As for conventional pesticides, the science might not overwhelmingly support a reason to switch for *health* reasons. I'm focusing on the health benefits here, understanding full well that people choose organic produce for other substantial reasons, including animal welfare and planetary concerns.

Carl K. Winter is a toxicology expert and professor emeritus at the University of California, Davis, Department of Food Science and Technology who specializes in pesticides. He says researchers have consistent data demonstrating that the very tiny presence of pesticide residues on most conventional foods is far too low to constitute a health threat. Winter investigated the EWG's 2010 Dirty Dozen list, homing in on the specific exposure to the ten most frequently detected pesticides on each discouraged fruit and vegetable. His researchers concluded that typical exposures to chemicals on those particular foods were at "infinitesimal" levels. "For most pesticides, if we were to feed consumers ten thousand times more pesticides in their diet than they're getting, those levels *still* wouldn't be of health concern," explains Winter. "It's the amount of a chemical, not its presence or absence, that determines the potential for harm."

The EWG's imazalil claim—the one that warned about fungicide on citrus plotting against us? Their interpretation is partially based on extremely high doses.[38] A 150-pound adult could consume more than eight thousand conventionally grown nectarines *in one day* without any ill effects even if they contained the highest pesticide residue recorded by the USDA. Scientists criticize the EWG for scaring consumers with "deceptive" sensationalized warnings that distort the science.[39] Several scientists told me the same thing: the organization blows things out of proportion. Mind you, the EWG is not merely inflating the danger to the size of a birthday balloon; they're inflating it to the size of a Goodyear blimp.

Toxicologists I spoke to attack the EWG's Dirty Dozen for what they deem a dubious, arbitrary methodology that ignores the basic pillars of toxicology. The three principles of risk assessment—toxicity of the individual pesticides, consumption rates of these foods, and actual levels of pesticide residues detected on foods—don't seem to have been taken into consideration. The EWG (which, again, is partially funded by the organic industry, including Organic Valley, Stonyfield Farms, and more) readily states as much if you dig into their website: "The Shopper's Guide does not incorporate risk assessment into the calculations. All pesticides are weighted equally, and we do not factor in the levels deemed acceptable by the EPA."

Now, studies have found that organic produce does indeed have a lower presence of pesticide residue. That could be because organic farms use pesticides after exhausting nonchemical methods, including crop rotation, among other reasons. But does that mean it's much "safer" to consume than conventional veggies? Not necessarily. There's no doubt that most pesticides, both synthetic and organic, are potentially dangerous, especially for farm workers exposed to high doses in a work environment. The issue I'm discussing here, however, is whether the level of pesticide *residue* in regular produce—after it's been rinsed—should be of concern.

The FDA announced that nearly 99 percent of foods sampled and monitored in 2019 showed pesticide residue levels "well below" Environmental Protection Agency (EPA) safety standards, while 42 percent had no detectable residue levels at all. According to the FDA, results confirmed that residues "do not pose a concern for public health."[40] This is not to say that there isn't room for improvement in FDA regulations, just that experts agree it's inaccurate to label conventional produce as "unsafe."

Okay, but what about the nutrition factor? More than three-quarters of consumers who buy organic are "looking for healthier foods."[41]

There's not enough information to meaningfully conclude how organic foods benefit overall health. To start, observational studies following eating populations are quite difficult to decipher because, for example, if one cohort ate organic and were less likely to develop cancers, was it due to the food consumed? Organic eaters usually have access to better health care, exercise more, and suffer less stress than those without the means to afford such food. So how do you prove causation and not correlation?

Food consumption studies are also extremely difficult (and often fundamentally flawed) because they're short-term and not controlled: they're generally self-reported. Unless you keep thousands of people cooped up in a lab for years, it's hard to determine whether they're actually eating what they say they're eating. That is, if they can even remember what they ate.

We do have research, although scientists are mixed on the inconclusive evidence. A 2012 Stanford University meta-analysis study of 237 existing studies (basically, a study of studies) compared organic to non-organic counterparts, only to conclude that, overall, they "showed no evidence of differences in nutrition-related health outcomes."[42]

Other studies suggest higher levels of nutrients in certain organics.

A 2014 meta-analysis study based on 343 previously published studies[§] found that organic produce contains a 17 percent higher concentration of antioxidants than conventional crops.[43] Published in the *British Journal of Nutrition*, it was reportedly intended as a scientific reply to the 2012 Stanford study. But while antioxidants are associated with health benefits, they are not synonymous with it, especially since there's a wide range of antioxidants. As one of the lead researchers told the *New York Times*, "We are not making health claims based on this study, because we can't . . . [the study] doesn't tell you anything about how much of a health impact switching to organic food could have."[44]

The researchers also found that organically grown crops produced lower levels of proteins and fiber than conventional produce.

The question remains: Are there *significant* health differences between organic and conventional? There is a strong general consensus among nutritional science experts I spoke to: that consuming organic food has no considerable health benefit. Even the USDA pauses before staking a claim to benefits. The *Washington Post* asked Miles McEvoy, the former chief of the National Organic Program at the USDA, a very simple question: Are consumers right to think that organic food is safer and healthier? McEvoy was evasive, replying, "The question is not relevant."[45]

The organic industry is betting on consumers conflating farming standards with supposed health benefits. More specifically, they're counting on moms worried about properly feeding their children and made fearful of overhyped pesticide risk (more on that in chapter 12).[46] As far back as 2001, General Mills—having acquired organic lines such as Small Planet Foods—was quite forthcoming about their tactics. In a *New York Times*

[§] The 2014 study included studies that the 2012 Stanford study excluded. Critics argue that this does not necessarily mean that the 2014 one had more robust or more critical data, but rather that it potentially included weaker studies that didn't meet the Stanford team's criteria. The 2014 study also received partial funding from Sheepdrove Trust, which supports organic farming research, while the Stanford University study had no external funding from a farming group.

piece by Michael Pollan, General Mills marketing executive R. Brooks Gekler acknowledged that Small Planet Foods targets "health seekers" even though he doesn't know if organic is healthier. "At first, I thought the inability to make hard-hitting health claims—for organic—was a hurdle," Gekler offered. "But the reality is, all you have to say is 'organic'—you don't need to provide any more information."[47]

What Gekler meant is that brands don't need to actively mislead shoppers. At this point, consumers fill in the blanks with their assumptions all on their own.

We might assume certain things about organic because there's a lot baked (so to speak) into our views of food. When NPR ran a report on the Stanford study, they got so many complaints ("prompted a powerful reaction," is how they put it) that they had to run another segment just to address the backlash. In an attempt to calm down listeners, they interviewed NPR's social science correspondent Shankar Vedantam, who is also the host and creator of the *Hidden Brain* podcast. He said something that applies to many of the things we buy or do: strong emotional values are tied up with organic food. It has come to represent so many other things—anti-industrialization, good parenting, nature, spirituality—that might not have anything to do with these studies' findings.[48] "There are these tensions between what we want organic to be at a psychological level, and what it actually does at a practical level," says Vedantam. "And the science is very good at telling us at the practical level what's going on. But sometimes, that could feel like the science is attacking our values."[49]

Normal nectarines aren't keeping nutritionists up at night (at least the ones I spoke to). What does worry them is far more practical: organic's scare tactics could make people more fearful of consuming conventional produce and may lead them to consume less produce overall. Indeed, here's what sometimes happens with some lower-income shoppers: nervous and confused[50] about pesticides—and too cash-strapped to afford organic— they end up skipping the produce aisle altogether. A small 2016 study of five hundred low-income shoppers' habits indicated that some planned to consume fewer fruits and vegetables after being alerted of pesticide residue concerns such as the crudely named Dirty Dozen.[51][¶] As the *Washington Post* speculated, the EWG "may be doing more harm than good."[52]

Because of our current nutrition discourse, those without the means or time to devote to an all-encompassing clean/organic/"superfood" lifestyle believe healthy living remains unattainable. This is especially true for those who do not have access to fresh organic food, or the time to prepare it.[**] The price of organic food varies from 5 to 100 percent more expensive, though on average, it hovers around 47 percent pricier than conventional alternatives, according to a Consumer Reports study. (Granted, organic produce is becoming more affordable and on rare occasions, it's actually cheaper than conventional produce.)

In one Facebook group for natural parenting, a moderator asked moms who eat 90 to 100 percent organic to share how much they spend each week. Quite a few were forthcoming about the challenges of trying to live their best Goop life:

"Ugh, I want to eat like that but I just cannot afford it!"

"I want to do better for my family food-wise, but geez, the prices are crazy!"

"We don't buy all organic because of this . . . We can't afford it. So we do half and half. The kids' stuff is mostly organic and then we eat the cheap gonna-give-you-heart-disease stuff."

[¶] The 2016 study did receive partial funding from the Alliance for Food and Farming, a nonprofit which represents both organic and conventional farmers. Though the AFF states it was uninvolved in the study nor made aware of the study findings until after the paper was peer reviewed, some could still interpret the findings as inevitably benefitting their members.

[**] Sylvia Klinger, a registered dietitian and the founder of Hispanic Food Communications, has witnessed decreased consumption of conventional fruits and vegetables within lower-income Hispanic communities. "I see the fear," she told me, noting that they can't afford organic alternatives. "We forget that almost half of the U.S. population is financially struggling."

"It's almost like supermarket shaming," says Winter of the two-tiered class of produce shopping. "We've got enough stress in our lives right now. We don't need to invent additional ways." Already, lower-income individuals consume fewer vegetables than higher-income groups.[53] Given that 90 percent of Americans fail to eat the recommended intake of produce, the food toxicologist shares only one piece of advice: "Just eat your fruits and vegetables if you're really concerned about health and don't worry so much about whether they're organic or conventional."

Health is obviously not the sole reason consumers choose organic produce. Organic can also taste better or fresher to some people. And taste is not to be discounted; for certain individuals, more delicious produce inspires them to eat more of it. Consumers are also influenced by production values, zeroing in on farmworker safety or environmental reasons. (The latter are also debated.)[54] These are legitimate, important concerns that aren't raised half as much as the health claims.

Although, if you're buying organic from Whole Foods—owned by Amazon, which generates millions of pounds of plastic waste per year—to "help the environment" . . . you might want to reconsider your patronage.[55] You're probably better off buying from regional producers (whether their food is organic or not).

Answering the question, *What produce should we buy?* is complicated. You're measuring a host of issues spanning environmental, financial, nutritional, and farmworker safety that go well beyond the conventional versus organic binary. I am in no way advocating against organic or suggesting it doesn't have merit. I am simply questioning a marketing-led narrative that has been so ingrained in our culture even though the science is more complex than advertised. Should we be made fearful about consuming "toxic," i.e., regular, produce when the evidence suggests otherwise?

Meanwhile, you'll notice that conventional produce is increasingly resorting to its own marketing tactics. It's why you might spot an apple with a sticker reading, "100% fresh!" or "All natural," hoping to compete against organic's seductive branding.[††] We've turned our supermarkets into a scream-ing match of flashy good-for-you labels. Everyone is pressuring us into nutri-tional choices. There's a lot of conflicting information out there—information from what should be trusted sources that just continues to proliferate.

Wait, What's Healthy Today?

Sifting through breaking news from nutritional researchers can prove just as challenging as navigating food labels. From a young age, Americans witness an ever-changing nutritional landscape that treats food like some sort of Whac-A-Mole game. One day avocados have too much fat, the next they're the crown jewel of any worthy millenial's toast. Red wine might be heart-healthy, but maybe it just correlates to a Mediterranean diet. Depending on the weather, red meat is a good source of protein or will usher in a cancer apocalypse.

This dietary nitpicking inspired the parody publication *The Onion* to opine, "Eggs Good for You This Week" but they "may be unhealthy again as soon as next Monday."

Having worked as a producer at NBC News for seven years, I can assure you that no one in the newsroom is afforded the time to sit back and consider what all this information cumulatively does to the audi-ence. Many news organizations suffer from a lack of resources and staff-ing, forcing journalists to hammer out pieces at breakneck speed. Junior reporters grab viral items from social media or newswire offerings based on attention-grabbing headlines or top audience interests. I vividly recall laughing when some provocative food study would come across a news-wire service vehemently contradicting a previous one. "Those perform well," an editor would chime in, pushing me to publish.

Journalists don't want to crank out a sludge of meaningless and con-tradictory stories, but they're forced to when clicks reign supreme. It's a lot

---

[††] In some instances, "all natural" does mean organic, as the farmer does abide by organic practices but hasn't completed the lengthy and costly certification process.

like a factory farm in that if you ever saw how the media sausage is made, you'd likely put your fork down.

But this trend has been going on for a long time, and across media. Listening to the radio or reading a magazine without being bombarded with the latest nutrition discovery or a debate on keto vs. paleo is near impossible. We're subjected to a constant tug of war over what we should and should not consume, with experts duking it out under sensationalized headlines.

At the Goop conference, I listened to panelists who depicted one's refrigerator as a nutritional minefield. According to one Goop expert, certain fruits, vegetables, and beans are reportedly harmful to the body because they contain "toxic" plant proteins called lectins, which supposedly do not want to be eaten. Lectins are apparently plants' clever answer to predators (that is, us) and cause inflammatory reactions that result in extra pounds and serious health conditions, such as "leaky gut syndrome." This panelist had written a book about how plants are quite literally trying to kill us with poisons, essentially likening the produce section to *Little Shop of Horrors*. Lentils, edamame, and eggplant are some of the many forbidden foods that over time will make you "very, very sick." And tomatoes—watch out, they're inciting "chemical warfare in our bodies."

After this talk, women were discharged into a food hall featuring twenty booths from L.A.'s top health restaurants. It was a cornucopia of bountiful vegetables, spruced-up fruits, and berry chia pudding cups— Willy Wonka's factory for Erewhon devotees. Alas, all the ingredients they were *just* warned about awaited them. Tomatoes! Edamame! All the big no-nos! What hell hath Gwyneth wrought?

Some attendees wondered aloud: "Should we, as we just learned, not eat?" Another sighed audibly to her pals, "Wait, what's safe here?"

A relentless torrent of food rules doesn't simplify women's lives but clutters their minds, drains their wallets, and confuses them to the point of paralysis. Roughly 80 percent of all Americans wrestle with conflicting nutrition information, and of those, nearly 60 percent admit that it makes them doubt their choices.[56] They stand in the grocery aisle pondering: Which frozen entree will do the least amount of damage? (Those who counter with "get out of the frozen aisle!" should keep in mind that many working women might not have the time or resources to cook from scratch.)

The conflicting information compounds "nutritional schizophrenia," a new-findings ping-pong that propelled the *Washington Post* to declare even back in 1984, "Nothing lasts. No assertion has a shelf life of more than 11 months."[57] There's no consistently reliable source of information. No definition of healthy is fully agreed upon. Depending on whom you talk to or even what culture you belong to, a variety of different definitions exist.

If people feel like they can't rely on magazines or soup cans, they'll latch on to strong leaders who do seem worthy of our trust. Or those that, at the very least, cut through the crap and just tell us what to do already.

Taking Definitive Direction from Overnight Gurus

Food Babe blogger Vani Hari has an enticing story and stark before-and-after photos to go with it. She tells the tale of a busy working adult too time-strapped to eat anything but takeout and junk food until her typical American diet—"candy addict, drank soda, never ate green vegetables"—landed her in the hospital. She then spent "thousands of hours" researching chemical production in popular items and changing her diet.[58] Hari learned how to cook, ditched processed food, went organic, and says she eventually saw health issues like eczema clear up. She also lost thirty pounds.

Hari credits the changes in her diet for the transformation. She's become an advocate for investigating what's in your food and detecting "the lies we've been fed about the food we eat."

She proclaims she's no longer duped "by big business marketing tactics" or confused by complicated labels. Offering similar salvation to fans, Hari tells them precisely what to avoid, calling out specific brand products and entire ingredient categories. Like Beautycounter, she's also on a mission for more transparency, placing pressure on conglomerates like Anheuser-Busch to divulge or remove what she considers hazardous ingredients. Through online activism (namely, mom-fueled petitions), Food Babe tries to get the "bad" stuff off shelves.

Hari has amassed more than a million Facebook followers, also known as the "Food Babe army." She built this legion by hitting moms where it hurts: their children. In 2015, Hari led a petition for Kraft Foods to ditch "dangerous" artificial food dyes in its iconic macaroni and cheese. These additives, she wrote, were "contaminated with known carcinogens," caused an increase in hyperactivity in children, and were linked to long-term health problems such as asthma. After the petition garnered 360,000 signatures, Kraft begrudgingly obliged. Hari comes across as a health-conscious David taking on the Big Food Goliath, a crusade that's catnip for moms.

Even those of us without kids started paying attention when Hari began making the rounds on morning news shows and cable TV stations like CNN. The activist grew to be the face of *women who care about food.*

Hari, like many successful influencers, understands the obvious: Outrage works. Fear sells. Here are just a few of the headlines that led her lifestyle website over the past several years:

Is This Weedkiller in Your Favorite Hummus Brand?
Do You Eat Beaver Butt?
Don't Poison Santa!
Does Kale Destroy Your Thyroid?
Sparkling Water Contaminated with Chemicals Linked to Eczema, Immune Suppression, Cancer, and Birth Defects
Are You Getting Conned by Cheap & Toxic Chocolate?

The point isn't to convey a nuanced scientific argument. It's to tap into the public's fear of "chemicals." Or as she once told ABC News, "When you look at the ingredients [in food products], if you can't spell it or pronounce it, you probably shouldn't eat it."[59]

Most famously, Hari started a petition against Subway to remove the chemical azodicarbonamide—which is used to condition and whiten dough during the baking process—from its bread. Hari warned it was linked to a who's who of health issues: respiratory issues, allergies, asthma, tumor development, and cancer. She then dubbed azodicarbonamide the "yoga mat chemical" because it's something that is also found in rubbery objects. "North Americans deserve to truly eat fresh—not yoga mats," she railed.

Calling it a "yoga mat chemical" leaves the impression that we're munching on gym products, which is presumably what Hari intended. But chemicals can have multiple uses across industries, and that in no way invalidates their safety—in the same way that we don't stop drinking water just because it's also found in dish soap. It's an irrelevant fact, but as soon as readers saw that exaggerated association, it was hard to undo. Then the media ran with the "yoga mat chemical" line because, well, it makes a darn good clicky headline.

Hari painted a vivid scene of just how "dangerous" this chemical is, citing a 2001 incident in which an overturned truck carrying azodicarbonamide prompted city officials to issue a hazardous materials alert and evacuate nearby residents. "Many of the people on the scene complained of burning eyes and skin irritation as a result," she wrote. First of all, this was a large spill, and therefore heavy exposure to a raw chemical, which is not comparable to the minuscule amounts found in food production. Furthermore, Hari conflated the chemical's use in products with aerosolized exposure. Those accident bystanders and factory workers who might be subject to direct airborne exposure are at risk when raw azodicarbonamide is *inhaled*. That has no bearing on its physical use in bread baking. You could launch the same attack on flour: that too is a respiratory irritant that can cause lung damage.[60]

The tiny, nearly negligible amount of azodicarbonamide used in the processing of bread does not pose a health risk, according to scientists I interviewed. I'm not insisting on a need for azodicarbonamide, but what's problematic is how influencers present these facts and terrify the average

American. This is why Hari is controversial: though she might be well-intentioned and justifiably mistrustful of the food industry, her calculations miss the mark, devolving into nothing more than worry porn.

Hari claims many common ingredients will "destroy your gut" and cause a host of health problems. If, as she suggests, American pantries can increase risk of cancer, reproductive problems, and thyroid dysfunction, then the onus is on her to prove that. As it stands, the "worrisome" ingredients she cites are generally heavily tested and proven safe in their intended use.

And it's not just food that Hari goes after: she had also previously lambasted the flu vaccine as "a bunch of toxic chemicals and additives that lead to several types of cancers and Alzheimer disease over time"—an accusation without adequate substantiation.[61]

Hari is one of many influencers targeting "toxic" grocery carts with not always proven claims. With the death of the expert and nutrition information descending into chaos, wellness gurus and cookbook authors swooped in, sticking their flags in the ground to claim authority. Problem is, a lot of the information they offer is skewed.

Hari has defended her extreme views by arguing that moderation never leads to change. (Or fortune, one might argue.) "People chastise me for being too simplistic," she told the *Atlantic*, "but it's like, okay, how are you getting through to people?"[62]

Food rules give us order. Like Karl Lagerfeld committing to starched white shirts and fingerless gloves, taking out whole food groups or abolishing sugar (but, oddly, permitting monk fruit or agave, sugars by another name) offers simplicity in what's become a complicated nutritional mess. You can devote precious brain cells to anything but your dinner plate. Having someone else figure it all out for you provides a mirage of safety, as does the ease of tuning out whatever debatable information comes down the six o'clock news pipeline.

But there may be another motive at play in telling people exactly what they need. Like plenty of other bloggers, Food Babe makes money with affiliate marketing. When Hari recommends "clean" or organic brands, she gets a cut of the sales. As for products for which she professes not to have found a suitable alternative elsewhere—such as snack bars or deodorants—she offers replacements from her own organic brand, Truvani, made "with ingredients that you can trust."

Her biggest line is that of supplements meant to round out what is supposedly our crappy diet. She sells turmeric tablets to "support" healthy joints and weight loss; plant-based pills to "support" immune health; and ashwagandha that "supports" brain health, among other supplements and powders.

You sure see the word "support" an awful lot in wellness branding, but never the words "treat," "cure," or "fix." There's a reason for that (and it's not because influencers don't have a thesaurus). "Support" is vague enough for them to promise you something without really guaranteeing anything. It's a clever marketing term that helps brands evade full responsibility, because how can one define support? What measurements could one use for that? The same goes for ambiguous terms like "ease," "stimulate," "boost," or "promote," which do not specifically claim to prevent or treat a health condition.

Sneaky terminology is one of many issues plaguing the behemoth that is the supplement industry, which feeds on those who believe they're at a loss with just a sensible diet alone. So many supplements either hint to an edge on average health, or they invent reasons for people to assume they are, on their own, not healthy *enough*. The more we're marketed to, the more we believe we're "not well."

"There's a Pill for That"

Paving the road to nutrition with supplements has generated big business not just for the likes of influencers such as Vani Hari, but for the industry overall. The $50 billion supplement industry went from 4,000 available products in 1994 to 50,000 in 2019. More than 75 percent of all American adult women take a multivitamin or supplement regularly, despite ongoing skepticism from the scientific community.[63]

Now, some people have legitimate nutrient deficiencies and are prescribed very specific supplementation by a health professional, such as during pregnancy (folic acid) or for conditions like osteoporosis (calcium). Vegans might need some extra B_{12}. People certainly have gaps that require supplementation. But that's not the average pill popper.

The general consumer doesn't seem troubled by the fact that many of their over-the-counter vitamins might just be mere placebos or that "energy" pills often owe their effect to stimulants like caffeine—hardly miracle pills. Supplements notoriously lack the more rigorous regulations imposed on pharmaceutical drugs because they don't require FDA approval before being marketed. The FDA does not monitor whether these products work; the agency just flags whether they're safe to consume. Manufacturers can therefore make vague health claims, like "boosts digestive health," that are not well defined and lack accountability.

In a 2018 study published in the *Journal of the American College of Cardiology*, researchers compared clinical trials over five years to determine whether regular vitamin intake protects against cardiovascular disease. In evaluating multivitamins, as well as vitamin C, vitamin D, and calcium supplements (the most common supplements), "none had a significant effect," reported the authors.[64]

Numerous researchers cast doubt on this American morning ritual. A 2019 NIH-funded study analyzed data from nearly thirty thousand U.S. adults over a six-year period. The subject population was generally healthy: they ate a nutritious diet and were physically active. They skewed white, female, and with a higher level of education and income.[65] Researchers concluded that popular dietary supplements—multivitamins, vitamin A, vitamin K, magnesium, zinc—had no measurable benefit and no influence on their mortality. Any nutrient boosts came from food consumption.[66] "It's pretty clear that supplement use has no benefit for the general population," noted Fang Fang Zhang, the study's senior author and an associate professor at the Tufts University School of Nutrition Science and Policy. "Supplements are not a substitute for a healthy balanced diet."[67]

Plenty more studies have investigated whether supplements impact chronic conditions and just overall health. Too many come up short in proving substantial benefits. As Steven Nissen, the chairman of cardiology at the Cleveland Clinic, concluded, "The concept of multivitamins was sold to Americans by an eager nutraceutical industry to generate profits. There was never any scientific data supporting their usage."[68]

Many consumers don't even know what's in them. Due to a lack of sufficient oversight, supplement ingredients are often not accurately reflected on the label. One 2018 study published in the journal *JAMA* analyzed the FDA's tainted supplements database between 2007 and 2016. Researchers found 776 instances in which supplements were tainted with unapproved pharmaceutical ingredients, steroids, or other contaminants. (Some contained sildenafil, the active ingredient found in Viagra.) The FDA issued voluntary recalls for a little under half of them.[69]

Or better yet, a *Quartz* report discovered that Goop supplement ingredients were awfully similar to those sold on Infowars, the far-right website owned by "Sandy Hook is a hoax" conspiracist Alex Jones. They're branded differently—Goop vitamins go by Why Am I so Effing Tired? while Infowars prefers the more aggressive-sounding Brain Force Plus—but both rely on Ayurvedic-heavy ingredients like the medicinal plant herb bacopa. Unfortunately, bacopa doesn't score too high on efficacy: "The science, based on animal studies, shows some preliminary—but contradictory—evidence of improvements to memory and brain function," read the report.[70] "There is minimal support for the claims about epilepsy and anxiety."

The general supplement consumer is bewitched by the marketing because it sounds great: supplements are easy and promise faster results. Taking them sounds better than what's actually necessary: eating nutritious meals and committing to big, concrete lifestyle changes. We are prone to buying what we want to believe, and we want to believe in quick solutions.

But no magic pill can replace a solid diet, stresses Craig Hopp, the deputy director of the division of extramural research at the National Center for Complementary and Integrative Health, part of the NIH. "You can't eat crap and take a multivitamin and expect to be healthy. It just doesn't work that way," says Hopp. Vital stuff like fiber shows up in what we eat, not what we pop out of a bottle. Hopp sees this insta-quick mentality stemming from a pill that does indeed promise fast, revolutionary results: "You took antibiotics and poof, you were better. It was magic. And I think the incredible success of antibiotics really contributed to people thinking that, well, there is a pill for everything."

Dr. Danielle Ofri, an author and a clinical professor of medicine at NYU, views the supplement industry a bit more suspiciously. The physician believes the industry preys upon desperate patients who don't feel as though they have other options. Many supplement companies take advantage of the fact that medicine is complex, ambiguous, and imperfect and that we don't have cures for all chronic illnesses. "It's never that easy in real life," says Dr. Ofri, "so it's hard, as a physician, to explain that our options for your diabetes are actually quite complicated."

Dr. Ofri's clients, mostly women, are typically very suspicious of taking prescription medication, but that initial suspicion drops to zilch when it comes to supplements grabbed off a Whole Foods store shelf. Dr. Ofri tries to explain that you should be suspicious of anything you take, "whether it's from a health food store or that I prescribe. You should ask the same questions, have the same concerns." These patients do their homework, but they either don't know how to interpret research or it gets muddled by effective labels like "clinically proven." That sounds good, but what does that mean? Who conducted the research? (Was it the brand?) Was there a placebo group? Where were the results published in a peer-reviewed journal?

"The vast majority of dietary supplements, if they had to be a hundred percent truthful in their advertising, wouldn't sell anything," says the clinical exercise physiologist and nutritionist Bill Sukala. Terms like "promotes good health," "detox," or "gently cleanses" have no real medical definition, while "clinically proven" is not regulated. They can mean anything and are therefore meaningless.

It's not just supplements. If you, like so many women today, are indeed concerned with the microbiome, you might opt for probiotics, which quadrupled in use between 2007 and 2012 and propelled kombucha into a billion-dollar industry. Most likely you've done so because brands like GT's Kombucha promise to not only "support gut health" but also "rejuvenate, restore, revitalize, recharge, rebuild, regenerate, replenish, regain, rebalance, and renew" your overall well-being. This is part of the growing "better for you" food trend, in which botanical extracts, probiotics, or "immune-boosting" ingredients supposedly greatly improve our health.‡‡

There's some exciting new research on the microbiome, but it's not *there* just yet. Nutrition experts will tell you a probiotic-infused cookie or bottle of kombucha won't do much of anything. A healthy gut needs fiber—fruits, vegetables, and whole grains.

Kombucha lacks scientific evidence for its aggressive claims, thereby receiving a thumbs-down from medical professionals. Even the alternative health scene isn't fully sold on it: celebrity doctor Andrew Weil downplays the hype, concluding, "The sugar and caffeine may be responsible for the energy some consumers claim they feel . . . I do not recommend kombucha, but if you like it, drink it."[71]

Fantastical marketing is not an anomaly, nor is it new. Jamie Lee Curtis told us we'd poop better in those probiotic-endorsing Activia commercials (parodied by Kristen Wiig on *Saturday Night Live* in 2008). Then suddenly the ads disappeared. Ever wonder why? Well, parent company Dannon had to settle charges brought by the Federal Trade Commission for deceptive advertising. The yogurt maker agreed to pay $21 million for advertising that Activia is "clinically proven" to relieve irregularity—claims that it could not substantiate.[72]

---

‡‡ GT's Kombucha's parent company settled a 2016 class action lawsuit that alleged the brand's products contained "misleading statements" regarding kombucha's antioxidant content and ingredients.

Sukala doesn't have too many kind words for the wellness industry's tactics. As he says, "the business is money. The storefront is 'health.'"

Taking Definitive Answers from
Inconclusive Ideas

Today, three-quarters of consumers are actively cutting back on sugar,[73] and an increasing number of shoppers say they check the sugar content of food labels before they buy a product.[74] Overall, this new consumer behavior is a good thing. The wellness industry (for all its flaws) encourages individuals to take a closer look at what they pile into their shopping cart. And that fast-food chains, airports, and vending machines now offer more fruits and vegetables is not something to gloss over.

But there is a spectrum of nutrition, and it deserves a bit more moderation than is currently being touted. Food has become an utterly fraught ordeal for the average woman. A *Fear Factor* episode that never ends. If you're to take extreme wellness gurus and fad diets at face value, you cannot consume any sugar, gluten, pesticide residue, dairy, "chemicals," and more. But these kinds of stark restrictions do more harm than good. We don't need thirty lollipops. But one won't kill us. Have that cake on your birthday.

Where we do need to focus more is on the big picture of whether we're meeting our overall nutritional needs. The thing is, we basically already know what to eat. We're aware we should lay off too much processed food and increase our vegetable intake. All these specialty diets and strict rules are essentially debating the minuscule percentage of what could be a *wee* bit better in our diet, but they're overblown. Often they're gateways to some hawked product.

All the conflicting, extreme advice has gotten out of hand, which is why experts increasingly weigh in to redirect the conversation. Trailblazers like the registered dietitian Vanessa Rissetto are expanding access to sound, relatable information. As the co-founder of Culina Health and the director of New York University's Dietetic Internship Program, Rissetto shares budget-friendly recipes and practical tips on her Instagram account, incorporating accessible foods that appeal to underserved communities, including vegetables and boxed macaroni. As she advises, if your culture prizes collard greens or rice with beans, go with collard greens; don't feel pressured to eat kale. "It's not so easy if food is where you connect with people and then someone is telling you that the food that you're eating is 'not right.' And oh, by the way, I don't have the money to make those changes."

A far cry from the hardcore purity tests of certain wellness influencers, Rissetto doesn't stress a restrictive orthodoxy. Instead, she advocates doing the best with one's abilities and resources. Not that it stops online critics from lambasting her over the "gall" to recommend a yogurt cup. "It's just the way that society views things—we want it to be hard," says Rissetto. "We want to feel like we worked harder than everybody else."

We are responsible for what we eat (though certain factors certainly don't make it easy). But the hypermoralized mandate to eat well induces guilt whenever we're simply unable to adhere to such regimens.[75] Most Americans barely get the time to take a proper lunch break away from their desk, yet somehow they're held to Alice Waters–level expectations. America is bending toward a healthier future, though it needs a push in the direction of being less confusing and more widely accessible to other groups. You can bend only so far before you break.

Chapter 8

Crystal-Clear Futures:
A New Take on New Age Spirituality

"Close your eyes and bring to mind one thing you're calling in from [the universe]," instructed Lacy Phillips, a former TV actress and model in her midthirties, now a self-proclaimed manifestation expert. "Boil it down to the essence of this thing that lights up your soul."

Wearing a ruffled white shirt and black gaucho hat, Phillips exuded approachable confidence. Over the next hour, she taught the 250 women assembled before her in a sparsely decorated industrial space the basics of attracting their chief desires—which, for most of them, was a better and more meaningful career. The women in the audience soaked in how to find their one true passion and "pass tests" from the spiritual beyond. These tests can come in the form of subpar job offers or being rear-ended in traffic. But more important, the women learned that increasing their self-worth would draw in love, happiness, and a raise. Phillips's presentation was a live version of the lessons she shares on her content platform To Be Magnetic, which sells on-demand manifestation workshops starting at $68.

"How many of you can raise your hands if you feel that you are deserving of what you want?" asked Phillips at the event. An overwhelming majority of hands shot up, and Phillips motioned as if she was counting them. "That's a really *beautiful* number," she cooed.

Following a lecture on establishing confidence to fish for rewards from the great beyond, Phillips proceeded with a Q&A. Participants stood up and stated their astrology sign before explaining their career dilemmas: Can my energy fuel my start-up's success? How do I attract the right kind of clients? Is a disrespectful work colleague a test from the universe? Is my soul "settling" if I go on a reality TV show? Phillips wasn't surprised by the intensity of their frustrations, noting they were experiencing Mercury retrograde. "You guys should have some shit going down right now," she laughed.

Charismatic, attractive, and personable, Phillips comes across like a cool, more successful older sister. She is one of many female manifestation coaches reinventing the law of attraction—the belief that you attract what you focus on—for a new generation. Phillips spreads the philosophy that self-worth is the law of attraction and that we can manifest anything that's in alignment with "our current state of subconscious worthiness." Basically, you need to reprogram your subconscious—rewiring childhood trauma, fixing damaging perceptions, and the like—to break the mold of limiting beliefs.

Through live events, digital platforms, and podcasts, these teachers present a nondenominational spirituality that promises to work in their favor, like a heavenly personal advocate.

Manifestation holds that there's a tangible connection between the mind and cosmic workings. Spiritual influencers' messages of overcoming personal struggles hold that you need a *belief* in yourself since "the universe has your back." That and with talk of modern-day issues—body image pressures, noncommittal boyfriends, sexist bosses—they're instantly relatable.

Dressed like fashion bloggers, these new leaders speak of "calling in" unseen powers to materialize new homes, jobs, or maybe just that perfect pair of jeans. On the To Be Magnetic website, one happy customer detailed manifesting a discounted white Le Creuset tea kettle. Other leaders skew more ambitious, selling $2,000 money workshops that reportedly draw in tenfold the class fee, thereby offering their own spin on the prosperity gospel. Each influencer has their own tweak on the philosophy and the work required.

Many of the more famous manifestation coaches predominantly preach to a group that has their basic needs met, which inevitably sets the tone for the issues addressed. Although some have scholarship programs, it's hard to imagine these experts delivering their advice to those living in poverty or war-torn countries. There are no Manifesters Without Borders. Followers, mostly women, are drawn to the idea that whatever good energy you put out into the world inevitably comes back to you. When I ask, however, whether the Jews in the Holocaust lacked the right energy to escape Nazi Germany, some seem legitimately stumped. "Huh, I didn't think about that," one college-aged manifester replied.

To be fair, manifestation does not entail only thinking good thoughts; the process involves determination, effort, and "co-creating" with the universe. Followers must put in hard work and make sacrifices to be worthy of divine abundance. Essentially, they have to get their lives in order. And Phillips, for one, does not gloss over trauma, racism, and abuse. Nor does she advocate controlling specific outcomes.* "We're certainly very open about how much work has to be involved in this," says Phillips. "It's not a magic show and your life won't change overnight."

At times though, manifestation could also prove a blame-proof strategy: If you get something you wanted, you manifested it. If you didn't, it just wasn't meant to be. Or maybe you didn't do enough on your end to produce the vision to fruition.

---

* To Be Magnetic's workshops offer a disclaimer stating, "It's important to recognize that there are systems of oppression, injustice, marginalization, and abuse that are out of your control. Understand that you did nothing to negatively attract these situations—it is not your fault. Please know that we are not insinuating that you are attracting negativity or being punished because of these situations or events."

While manifestation might have its shortcomings (to be fair, which faith doesn't?), there's no denying people get real value out of it. Three years ago, a Californian named Heather was brutally attacked and held at gunpoint by a stranger. Overwhelmed by the experience, she rarely left the house for a year. Heather credits Phillips—in addition to a therapist—for empowering her to ultimately lead a more conscious, fulfilling life. In the last few years, she said she's manifested her dream job, house, fiancée, even the exact diamond ring and wedding location she envisioned. Her new role as a senior consultant at a health company pays more, aligns with her values, and permits her to do what she always wanted—work from home.

"I would have taken this job before for less money but I have the confidence now to say no, I deserve more," said Heather, who shared her story during the Q&A portion. She was so compelling that Phillips invited her on stage to co-host the rest of the evening. Later, Heather told me she manifested the stage debut, having pictured herself speaking to the audience. "Things just come naturally now because I'm more magnetic," she mused. "I used to use the word 'lucky' but I don't believe that anymore." Phillips was touched that she gained yet another satisfied customer: "I genuinely believe that everybody is worthy of having what they want."

Phillips treads lightly in her role, readily acknowledging that she is not a religious leader or guru. Instead she calls herself a "mold breaker." Phillips says she reminds her audience, 'I'm shoulder to shoulder with you doing this work."

In the wellness world, manifestation joins a medley of other mystical trends that have grown as popular as detox diets. If New Age services were once a scattered industry of solo practitioners, outdated websites, and 1-800 numbers, modern offerings are light-years beyond the Miss Cleo of the nineties. You can now book an on-demand chat reading with a live astrologer. You don't even need to speak to the seer: just *text* them a zodiacal inquiry.

There's also ambiguous spiritual lingo wherein belief in one's personal power takes on a nearly religious narrative. Social media influencers post nondenominational, ego-boosting affirmations such as "I am magical" and "the universe wants me to have the best," which don't align with any specific philosophy but add up to a holier version of the self-help industry. The messaging encompasses radical approval: each individual is special, powerful, and divine. *We are all Beyoncé!*

Influencers got the memo. Suddenly all the style bloggers, fashion founders, and tech stars—choice vocations of the late aughts—became wellness influencers, imparting their self-worth platitudes and yoga wear ensembles like the Dalai Lamas of pop psychology. With an emphasis on maximizing capabilities (à la Tony Robbins) with a sprinkling of fluid superhuman powers ("cosmic intelligence"), they are life coaches turned prophets. You can't scroll through Instagram without these former fashionistas telling you to "trust in the universe," all the while hawking protein collagen powders. Instead of Fashion Week or SXSW, they're reporting from a retreat in Bali.

It's not entirely surprising that the growth of wellness and the explosion of what were once considered "woo-woo" convictions have gone hand in hand—or that they are so intertwined. There's plenty of research indicating the psychological benefits of believing in a higher power. Spiritual involvement has been shown to help individuals cope with stress and is associated with better mental health functioning (like being more optimistic).[1] But this pillar of wellness has since expanded to better include crystals, tarot palm readings, aura photography, and a zillion astrology apps that divulge what Jupiter has to say about asking your boss for a promotion.

These beliefs and practices are certainly not new (as many were popularized during the counterculture movement of the 1960s). But they have since been tweaked and are available everywhere. Urban Outfitters hawks millennial-pink tarot card decks ("cute AF" reads the top review). Boutique fitness studios sell sage bundles to ward off "toxic energy." Spas offer Reiki healers who can massage the bad juju out of your muscle knots. Women's magazines treat these things like essential components of a healthy life. "We all need to take good care of ourselves," reads an issue of *Cosmopolitan*. "And who understands what you *really* need better than *you*? Well, the stars."

"Mystical services" grew 53 percent between 2005 and 2019 into a $2.2 billion industry. Roughly six in ten American adults believe in at least one New Age belief such as astrology or reincarnation, and 40 percent believe in psychics or that spiritual energy is hiding in physical objects.[2] But exactly what kinds of solutions are the new New Agers seeking? A deeper look at manifestation and crystals reveals a great deal about the precise nature of our current spiritual quests. Unsurprisingly, as with the other areas of wellness, a common thread is the frantic attempt to regain control over that which we fear is no longer in our hands.

Working with the Universe to Set Things Straight

The law of attraction didn't start with Madewell shoppers. The concept dates back to the nineteenth century's New Thought movement, and it has seized American popularity at different points and in various flavors, incorporating health, wealth, personal development, you name it.

In the late 1800s, the spiritual pioneer Mary Baker Eddy founded Christian Science, a religion that combines Christianity with metaphysical healing. Pain and disease were all in the mind, she preached. Correct religious thinking could heal sickness. All that separated the afflicted from a cure were prayers and belief.

Hers was a countercultural movement. One of its precepts was that female intuition was better at tapping into divine power. It was an empowering message in a time when society considered women delicate and prone to illness. Their femininity—traditionally treated as a liability—became a sort of superpower. As a result, women made up a strong percentage of Christian Science adherents and leadership.[3]

The movement also had a darker side. Some believers shunned medical intervention for cancer, appendicitis, mushroom poisoning, contagious diseases, and diphtheria. Parents in the sect denied their children essential medical care. People died.

(Mark Twain penned a tale in which he sought the healing services of a Christian Scientist after falling off a cliff in the Alps and suffering several broken bones. He was, naturally, told his pain was but an illusion. When it came time to settle the bill, Twain noted, "I gave her an imaginary check, and now she is suing me for substantial dollars. It looks inconsistent.")[4]

In time, religious leaders adopted the law of attraction to reimagine a God who badly wanted you to be flush with cash. After the Depression, the author Napoleon Hill used positive thinking to sell a vision of capitalist success with *Think and Grow Rich*. It even trickled down to children's education, with an early-twentieth-century story about a small-time locomotive who willed his way into pulling heavier loads. In 1930, the publisher Platt & Munk released *The Little Engine That Could*, about a character who feverishly repeats "I think I can, I think I can," thereby teaching America's youth the treasured values of optimism and hard work. Yet no one ever stopped to consider whether the little engine should risk stress fractures by biting off more than he could choo.[5]

The law of attraction saw a reemergence in the mid-2000s with Oprah and Hollywood celebrities salivating over *The Secret*. The bestselling spirituality self-help book, which sold more than 30 million copies worldwide, claimed that positive thoughts can draw a bounty of enviable good things because the universe has a currency, and that currency is positive "energy." Then, as always, the offshoots came. In 2010, Marianne Williamson, one of Oprah's spiritual advisers, published a book that melded manifestation, naturally, with fat-trimming: *A Course in Weight Loss: 21 Spiritual Lessons for Surrendering Your Weight Forever* advised that "your perfect weight is coded into the natural patterns of your true self." You just need to accept complete dependence on God. Then you can reconcile "your relationship with Not-Thin You."[6]

Today, Jessie De Lowe, a manifestation coach and co-founder of the lifestyle site How You Glow, likens manifestation to life coaching. The former art therapist implores followers to take responsibility for all the issues in their lives thus far, then adopt healthier habits. "It's not promising someone their life is not going to have challenges—in fact, it's the opposite," explains De Lowe. But if the stick is the taking of responsibility for one's life, the carrot is that doing so will help you gain control of an existence that seems increasingly unmanageable.

The majority of De Lowe's clients are young, female, and college-educated. Though they possess countless advantages, she describes an unsatisfied group gripped by peer competitiveness and unrealistic expectations fueled by social media. They aren't comparing themselves to the millennial next door. They're comparing themselves to start-up founders and the globe-trotting friends clogging their Instagram feed. "They feel inadequate, like they're never where they should be [already]," says De Lowe.

Add an unpredictable job market, rampant employee disengagement, and tales of male-dominated workplaces, and it's no wonder young women find themselves searching for ways to hack the universe. It's an appealing concept for those raised to believe that if they follow certain steps, they could get what they want. They were led to trust in a meritocracy, that good hard work always wins. And that, of course, they were special, as told to them 1,001 times by their parents and kindergarten teachers.

Millennials had a hyperstructured upbringing that gave them a false sense of control, says the clinical psychologist Goali Saedi Bocci, author of *The Millennial Mental Health Toolbox*. Raised on happy Disney endings and American exceptionalism, they struggle with the anxiety of not getting what they were promised. "They grew up with the idea that if you want to get the best grades, you do the extra credit," she told me. Apple-polishing millennials got straight As, went to college, then graduated into a recession and found themselves saddled with student debt. Those who secured good jobs later felt stifled by what they considered meaningless positions or weren't adequately prepared for the mundanity of corporate life.

Workplace stress is particularly painful for a percentage of millennials who define themselves through their employment. "Do what you love and you'll never work a day in your life," they were told (much to their grandparents' confusion, who warned that work was to pay the bills). They were naively brought up to "follow your passion," and they just did that. If Americans once clocked in and out at the office, today you'll hear them speak of their life's "calling" and their job as a "mission." In that sense, their job becomes far more than a job—their heart and soul are poured into it. Work-life balance becomes impossible because the self and work are intertwined.

For those who are not living their calling, it's a different sort of pressure—one in which you're forced to endure hearing about cool start-up jobs while you draft legal documents. And if you failed to succeed, the American creed of meritocracy insinuates that you simply didn't try hard enough—*you weren't passionate enough*—despite a flawed and at times unfair employment market (or the loss of nearly 9 million jobs during the 2007–2009 recession). You believe you have only yourself to blame.

The San Francisco–based psychotherapist Tess Brigham sees midcareer patients trying to make sense as to why they can't afford a down payment or why they're still stuck in middle management. Manifestation dangles the promise of speeding up their career—tangible tactics to improve their chances—but also comfort in that it will all work out. "If you say the universe has a path for me, there's something to hold on to," Brigham told me.

Or, as Joseph Baker, an associate professor of sociology at East Tennessee State University and the editor of the academic journal *Sociology of Religion*, explains, there is a natural human tendency to impute purpose to our experiences, to interpret a larger plan in place. If we can't find that framework of agency, we'll create it ourselves: "What we do find pretty consistently is that when organized religion recedes the paranormal often fills that gap," says Baker.

Manifesters essentially adopt a spiritual version of the growth mindset, the Stanford University psychologist Carol Dweck's theory that one's abilities can be cultivated through effort, dedication, and perseverance.

Dweck's research stresses that brains and talent are not the be-all and end-all, rather that optimistically putting in time and diligence leads to higher achievement. On the flip side, a fixed mindset is a belief that you lack the right traits, leading you to adopt a defeatist attitude that holds you can't influence your future.

From this perspective, manifestation makes sense. Followers simply take a resilient can-do outlook on life—that how you view yourself can determine success. Most psychologists will tell you that you're better off keeping your chin up and taking actionable steps to build the life you want. As one manifester told me, it's about expelling negativity "to get shit done."

Manifestation serves as a mix between self-care and self-help, according to manifestation expert and bestselling author Gabby Bernstein, a former nightlife publicist who now leads $1,999 online courses on clearing psychological blocks to increase magnetism. Bernstein readily admits "it's hip to be spiritual," but she also acknowledges a climate that bred a need for her messaging. "The collective feels out of control. People are traumatized . . . Millennials want a sense of security, but they also have the sense that I can do anything and create my reality. That belief system is actually what makes manifesting work."

Positivity is beneficial, but some manifestation leaders teach their flock to block out the negativity that hampers their pursuit of unrealistic dreams. Simplified versions of manifestation propel the idea that we can all reach our potential to draw in success or riches. But that shouldn't disregard structural, social, and irrefutable challenges. As Steve Salerno argues in his book *SHAM: How the Self-Help Movement Made America Helpless,* all of us can't prosper in the free market. "In any competitive closed system, there must be a loser for every winner. By definition then, self-help cannot work for everyone, and the more competitive the realm, the more this is so. Two wonderfully optimistic women who both desire the same man or the same job cannot both succeed . . . [it] could conceivably help some of us achieve our goals. But not all of us."[7]

The issue of how much we can truly control becomes even more readily apparent as manifesters attempt to conjure up larger gains: a rent-controlled apartment, a bigger bonus, or a romantic partner. In Facebook groups, some are downright frustrated and confused, lamenting unemployment or broken relationships. Some try to manifest better health or to heal diseases.

Nitika Chopra, an affable and upbeat Manhattanite, was besieged by pain when she was in her late twenties. She suffered from multiple chronic conditions that interfered with her work and social life. At times it was head-to-toe psoriasis. Other days it was psoriatic arthritis—a painful inflammation and swelling of the joints. So she turned to those who promised blessed relief from the agony: spiritual influencers.

Chopra started following and buying products from gurus like Deepak Chopra (no relation). She sat in a manifestation expert's living room, soaking up the promise of positive thinking, which she took to believe could cure her medical conditions. At one manifestation meeting, Chopra divulged her excruciating pain, only to be scolded by an instructor who interrupted her with, "I'm going to stop you right there. I need you to take that negative language out of your mind. You are not sick, okay?"

"I was so impressionable," reflects Chopra. "And I was so desperate. I thought, these people are all telling me that if I just believe I'm going to get a check in the mail and I just believe that I'm going to be healthy, then it'll happen." Looking back, she acknowledges how devastating and harmful it was. "It is the definition of gaslighting."

The more Chopra listened to these experts, the sicker she became. Not only were her physical symptoms getting worse, but her mental health was on the decline. "I was constantly trying to fit myself into this world of 'You should just be able to meditate twice a day, you should just be able to say these affirmations . . . And then you should be fixed.'"

Chopra was not "fixed." Soon the pangs of failure started. She believed there was something broken with her thought process. In the ensuing months, Chopra berated herself if she ever felt negative or sad or uncomfortable. "[I'd] think, what's wrong with you? Why can't you just feel positively?" This continued for years, to the point where she avoided medication entirely, hoping to attract a healthier future. All the while, she suffered. Chopra couldn't descend a flight of stairs without debilitating pain. Some nights she would scratch herself so hard her sheets were bloodied.

Chopra's experience shows why manifesting health is a tricky issue that most gurus distance themselves from. (Probably because they're also aware of something called a lawsuit.) Lacy Phillips readily admits she hasn't figured out manifesting a medical recovery: "We can't help you with that." Phillips notes that manifestation teachers have a responsibility to be transparent. "This isn't a cure-all," she says.

It all came to a head for Chopra following the 2016 election. Amid the political chaos and "alternative facts," Chopra decided to take a hard look at everything, including her wellness habits. If it wasn't the truth, it just wasn't gonna fly anymore. She realized that multiple complex factors account for our circumstances, and that thinking can't overcome all of them. Shortly thereafter, manifestation got the boot, kicked right back to the universe's return center.

Chopra ultimately founded Chronicon, a digital community for women with chronic illnesses—like Crohn's disease, fibromyalgia, lupus, or endometriosis—to come together to share their pain without judgment or false promises. Most members have similar stories, having seen far too many doctors who didn't believe their symptoms or gurus selling snake oil. It's not so much "solving" anything for them as it is facilitating friendships. "You can tell us what is going on," Chopra told me. "And we'll be like, 'Yes, girl. I was just dealing with that yesterday. I totally get you. I'm so sorry. I'm here for you.'"

There's no harm in a growth mindset. It's important to believe you can accomplish new tasks. But when that optimism is taken too far—when a growth mindset blinds you to obstacles (including very real medical ones)—problems arise. These new modes of spirituality can at times, if left unchecked, devolve into delusional thinking on steroids.

A Talisman for Healing:
Spiritual Lucky Charms

If manifesters take their ability to influence their lives with the utmost seriousness, crystal collectors have a lighter touch, if not any less of a belief that their practices guarantee positive outcomes.

I investigated the crystal craze for *Fast Company* after noticing that glistening rocks once better associated with covens and Stevie Nicks were flourishing in a massive mainstream business market. Crystals showed up everywhere: at yoga studios, in juice shops, on influencers' social media accounts. In Malibu, some residents hand them out for Halloween. And like any trend worth its (mineral) salt, it hit Hollywood, fortifying a bastion of celebrity acolytes. Gwyneth Paltrow, Victoria Beckham, and Katy Perry publicly swore their allegiance to the stones. Adele even attributed her performance hiccups at the 2016 Grammy Awards to the fact that she'd lost her beloved totems. "I got some new crystals now and everything's been going well," she later assured fans.

I was interested in the financials, but more than anything, I was curious what people got out of crystals. Was it just an artistic appreciation for nature's minerals? Or did they hold more religious weight?

This is how I found myself sitting cross-legged on the floor of Colleen McCann's Venice Beach home. Colleen is Goop's in-house shaman and a self-described "spiritual influencer." Blonde, fashionable, and smiley, the former fashion stylist resembles a young Goldie Hawn. McCann is booked months in advance for her services, for which she charges $100 to $1,500 per session. She sees predominantly young and female clients for garden-variety therapy sessions, and she might perform the occasional crystal-assisted exorcism. ("You never forget your first exorcism," she said.)

But McCann's specialty is using quartz, citrine, and other chunks of minerals for what she calls "intuitive business building." With assistance from the great beyond, she helps CEOs, executives, and Silicon Beach professionals make decisions about their business just by, as she put it, "reading their energy." She weighs in on everything from org charts to investment opportunities to redesigning company logos. "I may close my eyes and say, 'Hey, you're thinking of starting a new division,' and they say, 'How did you know that?'" McCann explained. "Or I'll say, 'I see a girl with red curly hair coming in—that's the girl you need to hire.'"

Her loft was filled with crystals, many of which were organized into parallel lines to my left and right, as if I was stationed in the middle of a spiritual runway. McCann blew on multicolored stones and recited a blessing rooted in shamanism. She then closed her eyes and meditated as she listened to the spirits among us. But before she could foresee whether I'd ever land on a *Forbes* cover, she expressed concern. "What's up with what you're eating?" McCann asked me. "They say there's something weird you're doing every day at a certain time." I confessed to my Sour Patch Kids consumption ritual. McCann nodded as if she and her ghostly helpers were already aware. (To be fair, she had a pretty good chance of predicting that any L.A. woman had an eating issue, so I wasn't blown away.) As part of the $250 package I selected, my healer "prescribed" a few amethysts to control my sugar urges, then wished me luck in resisting my temptation.

My experience might inspire eye rolls and snickers, but for a growing number of consumers, crystals are no joke. McCann's business is lucrative for a very simple reason: she sells solutions, much like the one she sold me to curb my sweet tooth. Whatever your problem is, there's a crystal for that. Her book is called *Crystal Rx*, prescribing rocks to calm, energize, and heal everything from fatigue to a broken heart.

For McCann, the reason for surging crystal popularity is obvious. "What we're doing right now as a people isn't working," she said. Our fraught political climate, work overload, and tech dependency leave people "sad, scared, or nervous." She believes crystals can "help people get back on track." The practice of just sitting down and touching an element that comes from the earth, she said, produces a positive, calming effect.

And for the people building businesses around them, a pleasing *ka-ching* sound.

McCann isn't the only one benefitting from the mining mania. I've reported on newly formed crystal galleries, which are like art galleries, drawing Silicon Valley honchos who buy hundreds of thousands of dollars worth of rare, five-foot-high crystals. One crystal e-commerce business watched business double with $88 "money magnet" bracelets that sold out whenever the financial market dipped. All echoed the same sentiment: Demand increases when people are anxious. Bad news means good business.

When I asked Colleen McCann if crystal therapy is just a case of the placebo effect, she was cagey, replying, "There are many ways to skin a cat."[8] Whatever crystals are or aren't, these tools can be extremely powerful, and not something to be discounted. Women I interviewed say they can have a grounding effect. "It gives me something to focus on when I'm anxious," said one who sleeps with crystals in her bed.

In a period of uncertainty, such spiritual beliefs can provide reassurance. They serve as a coping mechanism, where you can count on something when at the whims of an unfair, chaotic world. This proves both compelling and comforting, not unlike a *TV Guide* to the blessings or misfortune about to unfold. They're also widely available.

People can easily join these belief systems because there's a low barrier to entry, a far cry from in-depth study of a centuries-old book or lengthy conversion processes. No need to understand complex philosophies: to get started, one simply needs to feel ready to "transform" their life, then hop onto YouTube, Instagram, or TikTok, all flooded with twentysomething gurus.

It's hard to tell how many spiritual seekers fully believe in what they're adopting. Some find it fun and exotic, not unlike an interest in style fads. For Gen Z, the more untraditional, the more the social cachet, proving just how anti-establishment you are. That which is foreign and uncommon might seem more appealing than what's available in their backyard.

Once I reported on Summit Series, an invite-only event series dubbed a "young TED meets Burning Man" or "Davos for millennials." This community of start-up founders and successful professionals built their own utopia in the ski resort area of Eden, Utah, drawing entrepreneurs like Netflix CEO Reed Hastings, WeWork co-founder Miguel McKelvey, and others who could afford either to build a home or to pay the $2,000+ weekend attendance fee. It's the type of place where you'll see a Mercedes G-Class parked alongside a giant yurt, where high-powered networking commences during dynamic breath work classes.[9] You meet people who think of themselves as spiritually inclined and "enlightened" capitalists, though they would never use the dreaded C word; they instead say they're vehicles for change, or "creative disruptors."

While I was there for a wellness-themed weekend, talk revolved around "influential astrologers" and manifesting investors. No fewer than three strangers asked what my meditation "practice" entailed. One even opened the conversation with the question, replacing the more traditional "So what do you do?" I responded truthfully: I don't meditate. When I need to recenter myself, I open up a Jewish prayer book and recite the prayers I have repeated since childhood. Sometimes, I'll channel my most treasured intentions when lighting the Sabbath candles on a Friday night. That, I explained, was my version of mindfulness.

One looked at me like I just admitted to marrying my dog. Another nervously chuckled and quickly changed the topic. The third didn't respond for five seconds, carefully weighing his response. "I really don't know what to say to that," he finally offered, slowly removing his Warby Parker sunglasses. "*That's* different."

I had committed a taboo. I had, in their eyes, pledged allegiance to a backward regime, to that which they had so independently rejected. I had veered from the now acceptable answers within wellness groupthink, that which prizes the new and unique and the exotic. There I was expressing, of all things, an acceptance of the traditional—*of religion*. I should have just as soon introduced myself as "basic."

I'm not insinuating that uniqueness is the driving force, just that some truly dislike organized religion. Many people take their newly adopted spirituality quite seriously, including those who plan trips and base life decisions around their horoscope. On Twitter, astrology followers consider the ancient art a useful tool for self-knowledge, "an external thing [to] confirm something you already knew about yourself." Tarot helps individuals tap their intuition and analyze their life path. (Some say it's cheaper than therapy.) For the anxious, astrologers offer solace when life feels too complicated—and a rare occasion when they get sole attention. As one Gen Zer tweeted, "It may not be real but it's comforting. [To] have someone tell me that there's always something positive coming makes me feel okay."

Manifestation, crystals, and a host of other spiritual initiatives require individuals to reflect, to retreat from volatile emotions, and instead focus on their innermost needs. Believers rely on the universe and tarot cards for supernatural guidance or influence—to change the hand life deals them. It sounds a lot like religion, frankly. So why aren't these people turning to more traditional faith when they want some help? Why aren't they just going to church when they want to light up their soul?

Because the big three monotheist traditions, as they'll tell you, just ain't cutting it.

Flashback: When Astrology Went to the White House

It was lightly raining in 1952 when a Southern California housewife named Jeane Dixon entered the historic St. Matthew's Cathedral in Washington, D.C. She prepared to kneel before a statue of the Virgin Mary when suddenly, she was overcome by a vision. Dixon saw the White House in its pristine glory, the majestic white compound across a lush green lawn. The numerals 1960 formed above the building like skywriting. Then slowly, the numbers emitted a dark cloud dripping down "like chocolate frosting on a cake," quickly reaching the bottom before a still man. He was young, tall, light-eyed, and had a head of thick brown hair. A heavenly spirit insinuated that he was a Democrat. And that a violent death awaited him.[10] "God showed it to me," she would later recall.[11]

Four years later, Dixon reportedly told *Parade* magazine that a Democratic president elected in 1960 would be assassinated. The disturbing prediction wasn't taken seriously, but following President Kennedy's assassination, word of Dixon's prophetic prowess spread, catapulting her to national fame. She soon snagged a regular seat inside the very same house she once saw in her visions.

Nicknamed "the seeress of Washington," Dixon carried her crystal ball straight into the oval office. Richard Nixon sought Dixon's advice on future terrorist plots following the 1972 Munich Olympics massacre in which a Palestinian terrorist group kidnapped and killed nine Israeli athletes. White House tapes confirm that Dixon counseled the president on numerous issues, spanning the Panama Canal, nuclear arms talks, and even the Watergate scandal.[12]

Dixon eventually became a household name with a syndicated newspaper astrology column, thus offering an air of legitimacy to her spiritual talent. Her biography, *A Gift of Prophecy*, sold more than 3 million copies. But Dixon wasn't just interested in politics and fame. During the World War II era, she visited Navy hospitals and servicemen parties, counseling Army amputees who had given up on any semblance of normal life. Dixon supplied handicapped veterans with the confidence to keep going, to put faith in better days ahead. She gave them hope.[13]

Dixon got some forecasts right, such as her prediction that a pope would be harmed in the twentieth century and that Oprah, who consulted with her in 1977, would enjoy great success. But many more of her predictions were wrong—among them, that the

Soviets would be the first to put a man on the moon, that World War III would erupt in 1958, and that a cure for cancer would be found by 1967.

Dixon also claimed the world would end by 2020.

Pop culture mostly forgot Dixon, but her name lives on in academic circles. The mathematician John Allen Paulos coined the term "the Jeane Dixon effect," which refers to the psychological tendency to remember successful predictions while ignoring the far more frequent failures—which helps explain the prevalence of paranormal beliefs.[14]

In 1997, Dixon passed away from a cardiac arrest. It is rumored that the last words on her deathbed were "I knew this would happen."

Rise of the "Nones": Seeking Meaning in an Agnostic World

"The spiritual wisdom of the ages is openly accessible as never before, and we are free to craft our own spiritual lives," writes Krista Tippett in her bestselling book, *Becoming Wise: An Inquiry into the Mystery and Art of Living.* The author and host of the popular radio program *On Being* says she has no idea what religion will look like a century from now, "but the evolution of faith will change us all."[15]

Tippett soared to stardom for her spiritual investigative work, calling on listeners to explore the meaning of life during their morning commute. In her radio program and podcast—downloaded more than 350 million times—the gentle, folksy host takes on a soft inquisitiveness that mixes Mr. Rogers with Meredith Vieira, if not the occasional motivation of Oprah. Tippett asks big questions of celebrities, politicians, and thinkers surrounding faith, humanity, and purpose. Her show attempts to answer: What does it mean to be human? How do we want to live? She gets attention. In 2013, President Obama awarded Tippett a National Humanities

Medal for "embracing complexity" through hundreds of conversations about faith.

Tippett started her radio program in the years following 9/11, a period in which she observed a societal pull to explore deeper issues but with few available outlets. The world had changed, and so had everyone's priorities. She is among a long roster of talent ushering in a new realm of spiritual life sparked by the "seekers" of the sixties. Each of them boasts their own specialty: the podcaster Brené Brown stresses vulnerability, the bestselling author Glennon Doyle concentrates on feelings, *The Power of Now* author Eckhart Tolle has a Buddhist-slash-mystical approach, and the onetime presidential candidate Marianne Williamson preaches the power of love.

Though their philosophies differ, all echo an "awakening"—a brave journey of inner work that shapes meaning in a world that increasingly divests from former conventional paths to purpose. For the spiritually aimless, they offer up a spiritual life that transcends labels, rules, or hard distinctions. Living an examined, ethical life, they say, does not require an overarching organization. Values are not restricted to orthodoxy.

Tippett grew up with Southern Baptist parents in Oklahoma. Her grandfather was a Southern Baptist evangelist preacher. But even though she too felt spiritual and graduated from divinity school, she struggled with inflexible, cast-iron religious tenets. How could, she wondered, "every Catholic and Jew, every atheist in China and every northern Baptist in Chicago, for that matter—every non–Southern Baptist—be damned?" In a pluralistic and open society, it didn't sit right.[16]

"We are among the first peoples in human history who do not broadly inherit religious identity as a given, a matter of kin and tribe, like hair color and hometown," writes Tippett, writing in a tone that doesn't sound the alarm so much as open the door. "But the fluidity of this—the possibility of choice that arises, the ability to craft and discern one's own spiritual bearings—is not leading to the decline of spiritual life but its revival."[17]

Tippett's moderate, rational, intellectual doctrine appeals to a growing number of Americans disenchanted with the God of their parents, be it for political or personal reasons. Some women reject organized religion for equity or bodily autonomy reasons. Parents recoil after reading of multiple sexual abuse scandals. Young progressives object to any institution that does not welcome their LGBTQ brethren. Some liberals take issue with what they consider objectionable politics or party affiliations.

Many Gen Xers and millennials never really grew up with a strong faith in the first place. They showed up once a year for services to blankly stare into the distance in boredom. Christmas meant Santa and matching pajamas, with Jesus pushed to the periphery. Hanukkah constituted maybe one night of candle-lighting and an Adam Sandler song, though few could tell you the history of the holiday. For most secularized millennials, their connection to a priest, rabbi, or imam factors only into big milestones like a wedding, thereby equating a religious leader with just another hired vendor. Florist, caterer, pastor . . .

Since 1990, when just 8 percent of Americans said they had no religion, the abandonment of organized faith has accelerated.[†] Four out of ten American millennials now identify as religiously unaffiliated, identifying more with a Harry Potter house than a Catholic saint. Called "nones," they constitute the fastest-growing religious demographic. And they are well represented among highly educated and politically liberal women; according to a Pew Research Center survey, "nones" among women rose by 10 percentage points between 2009 and 2019.[18]

To give an idea of Americans' shifting views—in 1998, a *Wall Street Journal* and NBC News survey asked Americans which values they most valued. The majority cited hard work, patriotism, commitment to religion, and having children. In 2019, the same outlets asked the same question, but got different results: patriotism dropped 9 percentage points, religion was down 12 points, and having kids took a 16-point beating.[19]

Religion lost its stature because people feel free to choose alternatives

---

[†] This is not just a U.S. phenomenon. Individuals are drifting away from organized religion in other countries as well.

that accomplish similar goals. Which is partially why a little less than half of Americans today belong to a church, mosque, or synagogue—down from 70 percent in 1999, according to a 2020 Gallup poll.[20]

Perhaps most telling, the current president of the Harvard Chaplains, Greg Epstein, does not subscribe to any one religion. He doesn't necessarily even look to any higher power. He is a humanist who penned a book titled *Good Without God.* "We don't look to a god for answers," Epstein told the *New York Times.* "We are each other's answers." This tracks with the wide market of spiritual suppliers who forgo a literal God in favor of human connection and emotional satisfaction, like feeling welcomed, happy, appreciated, or nurtured. The sociologist of religion Wade Clark Roof put it best when he wrote, "more and more Americans are making religious decisions on the basis of their feelings."[21]

And yet, however independent we humans believe ourselves to be, we still crave a universal order to the chaos. One of many reasons people historically turned to religion was because it was seemingly in their best interests. When limited by our mortal power, humans—with our imaginative, narrative skills—find creative ways to reassert it. In his book *Religion: What It Is, How It Works, and Why It Matters*, the sociologist and University of Notre Dame professor Christian Smith defines religion as both a belief and a set of practices to connect with superhuman powers that can help people avoid misfortune and garner good things. That's not the sole reason religion finds audiences—people also endeavor to make sense of their lives—but it's one of the strongest.

That's why the overwhelming majority of Americans—90 percent, in fact—are not becoming atheists. Atheism, in our typically optimistic society, feels too final. Too negative. A real Debbie Downer. Americans want to believe in *something.* More than 50 percent believe in God as depicted in the Bible, but 33 percent believe "in another type of higher power or spiritual force," according to a Pew Research Center survey. Maybe it's not King Triton flanked by angels on a bed of clouds, but nearly half of U.S. adults believe that God or some other cosmic puppet master is in charge of what happens to them. Two-thirds think the Almighty goes out of his (or her) way to reward them.[22]

Universally, women are more religious than men.[23] Christian Smith suggests this is because women are more likely to be aware of their vulnerabilities and therefore seek additional resources, including those of the superhuman. Women face more violence, discrimination, and poverty, so they're more inclined to prepare strategies to confront bad situations. It's the same reason why some in lower socioeconomic levels are more religious; they objectively need more help.[24]

Organized religion may no longer hold the same authority, but the quest for spirituality is alive and well—on podcasts if not in SoulCycle studios. As Oprah told Stanford University students in a 2015 graduation speech, "I'm not telling you what to believe or who to believe, or what to call it. But there is no full life, no fulfilled or meaningful, sustainably joyful life without a connection to the spirit. You must have a spiritual practice."[25]

In 2020, "focusing on spiritual growth" made its way into Americans' most popular New Year's resolutions.[26] That focus skyrocketed at the start of the COVID-19 pandemic, since, as always, a crisis awakens religious fervor. One survey found that nearly one-quarter of American adults reported their faith had strengthened amid all that sourdough bread baking. *What did the pandemic mean? Was this God or the universe sending a message? How do you make sense of all the deaths?*

But in much the same way that millennials prefer their tech or sneakers, they want their faith customized—a curated reflection of who they think they are. They mix and match a privatized, pluralistic assembly of traditions, grabbing shamanism here and Buddhism Lite over there, with a touch of cultural Judaism for good measure. Islamic symbols and zodiac charts live side by side in equal coexistence, proving one doesn't need to fully ditch one to latch on to the other. "There's sort of been this liminal in-between position where they're outside of organized religion, but interested in religious and spiritual pursuits," explains the sociology professor Joseph Baker.

Bit by bit, a new generation stitches together an eclectic patchwork of practices that supplies them what they sorely lack in modern American culture: guidance, meaning, and a place to belong in a fractured society. A context to shape their eighty-plus years on this Earth. These are things religion offered, but faced with a deficit, they now need to find new sources to frame their standing in the world. If mankind once fasted on a mountaintop to appeal to a higher power, so too can the modern woman flank herself with crystals to summon good energy before a work presentation. And if not with a spiritual alternative, people might venture out to other tightly held ideologies, finding religious convictions in nationalism, identity-based movements, social justice, or, yes, even health—all of which can offer purpose and structure. America is a deeply religious country. As Smith explains, "if religion goes away, at least in this culture, it's going to have to be substituted with other things."

Is believing in manifestation more or less rational than belief in Jesus? Is meditating the same as saying a prayer? That's not the point. (Honestly, very little of what mankind holds religious contains hard evidence.) The point is that people choose it. They get to redefine their faith in a way that feels far more authentic to them. As one college student told me of her newfound conversion to manifestation and crystals, "I'm on my own: if I don't like something, *I don't have to* practice it."

But in the ongoing quest to nail down the right kind of faith, when do you know that you hit upon the right one? How do you decide what propels self-growth? There's no easy answer. If you discard traditional faiths, you still have to wade through a marketplace of gurus. Some are more honest than others. While Krista Tippett and Brené Brown sincerely aim to forge new paths in spiritual engagement, other influencers are ready to twist faith into something that isn't all that different from what people were fleeing in organized religion. It comes down to the leader in question, and what people are specifically searching for.

Which raises some issues: What if in seeking a solution to their problems people are actually aggravating them?

Spiritual Marketplace: A Deeper Connection
or Self-Oriented Ideology?

In 2018, the trend forecasting group WGSN declared that "spirituality is the new luxury."[27] And it sure was apparent.

Columbia Business School offered a certificate in spiritual entrepreneurship. Instagram saw a rush of "purpose-driven soulpreneurs" (chakra beads on top, Lululemon leggings on the bottom) hawking pricey Tulum vacations. Then Amazon Prime's newsletter started sending monthly shopping horoscopes to its members, aligning specific product suggestions to the stars. This is how I found out that communication is reportedly quite hard for Geminis in April, so they ought to practice giving and taking feedback with . . . an Amazon Alexa.

To put it crudely, there's money in selling *to* your soul. Not that it's anything entirely new: many religions also try to sell you something (whether it blatantly has a visible price tag is another story). The difference is that spiritual wellness, as marketed today, is easily digestible, entertaining, and often dolled up in memes or pastel-hued branding. It sure helps that tarot cards and crystals are instantly Instagrammable. (A communion wafer, meanwhile, leaves a bit to be desired in the aesthetics department.) Better yet: it promises super-fast results.

Products like crystal facial rollers are now sold at Anthropologie. These $28 rose quartz beauty accessories claim to encourage "a renewed sense of self," help "aid in the detoxification of your body," and promote a sense of "connection to the universe." That such products lack clear clinical evidence doesn't mean we should completely discard them as spiritual tools, though retailers should not suggest health benefits. (A conflation between spiritual well-being and health crosses the line. By claiming physical health benefits, we therefore put the wellness bar quite low—at the unscientific level.)

Tarot card sets and crystals are just a few of many spiritual objects sold at popular retailers. Urban Outfitters sold smudge kits (a sacred Native

American practice), while Sephora planned a $42 "starter witch kit." But the idea of purchasing and picking only what you want from different faiths, like some sort of spiritual Sizzler buffet, can also be a way to avoid pricklier issues like a faith's controversial beliefs and instead select just the fun, self-serving parts. Very few seem to pick the more communal aspects, like service, charity, and responsibility. Or it divorces an ancient tradition from its larger context or wisdom to pulverize it down to . . . athletic yoga.

The new wellness marketplace caters to self-oriented spirituality. On Instagram, spiritual influencers encourage people to "celebrate" themselves and seek a never-ending journey of self-love with few calls for humility or consideration of others. These posts contradict themselves in that they stress constant self-work, then proclaim we're perfect as we are. "Never apologize for who you are," they impart, but then demand, "become the best version of yourself." Remarkably, for all of the influencers' talk of empowerment, they encourage you to rely on them, because repeat business pays the bills. Workshops, crystal kits, and horoscope subscriptions are codependency with a price point.

Worse, these spiritual concepts can serve as a hall pass to do whatever the hell you want because self-love is your actual God. Inconsiderate behavior like flakiness is excused in the name of "listening to intuition." Harsh feedback becomes "releasing bad energy." "Don't feel guilty for doing what's best for you," reads an Instagram post posing as spiritual advice. "Dismiss what no longer serves your soul," advises another. College professors tell me of students who manipulate the zodiac like a mental health diagnosis. How can they be expected to accept criticism on their essays when they're a Pisces, known for being sensitive? *This is who I am,* they argue.

Modern spirituality has been a refuge for those alienated by organized religion, most notably those ostracized by it and even individuals who lack the money to participate in certain religious lifestyles. But these belief systems also have their blind spots: self-exploration can devolve into self-centeredness if left unchecked. Conversations revolve around how some life force is always sending signs—in dreams, through Netflix algorithm recommendations, or via Bumble flirtations. The universe, as Regina George would say, is obsessed with these people. And nothing is more important than their needs. That's what it sometimes comes down to: self-love, self-compassion, self-improvement. *The self.*

Also, as the famed social scientist Robert Putnam wrote, privatized religion might feel more psychologically fulfilling "but it embodies less social capital." As people surf from practice to practice, they might be less committed to a specific community and less inclined to be meaningfully involved over long periods of time. That's likely because new denominations have been "directed inward rather than outward."[28]

Not to mention, when everyone has their own mix of practices that shape them, "it's very rare that you get a fullness of experience—of community—because everything is somewhat itemized or bite-sized," says Casper ter Kuile, a Harvard Divinity School fellow and the author of *The Power of Ritual*. That might have unintended effects. "I think that's what contributes to this sense of cosmic loneliness—that sense that nothing fits completely, like something is always missing."

Wellness—*real* wellness—emphasizes communal well-being and social support (not to mention, reasonable expectations about the future) to thrive. But as religious tradition eroded, so did its focus on communal unity, replaced with striving for capitalist success and emotional soothing. We seem far more focused on *feeling* good, seeking acceptance, and dwelling on our innermost lives.

If you are only concerned for yourself, is there room left for others?

Too often, one might choose self-serving spirituality because that's human nature. If deciding between a practice that demands real self-examination, communal sacrifice, intellectual study, and giving back or one that lets you hustle your way to prosperity, you might just choose the latter. You are busy, stressed, and overwhelmed as it is anyway. Why not pick that which suits your immediate needs?

Again, it's not that traditional religions are exempt from similar issues. They too can breed egotistical characters or self-centered behavior.

But spirituality alternatives that focus on success, consumerism, and narcissism create their own meaning crisis. Now some turn to belief systems that seem to fixate on those exact things, in an almost circular cycle of pressure. Or we lean in to a spirituality-lite that argues everything we need stems from me, myself, and I: scribble in your gratitude journal, concentrate on manifesting, squeeze your crystals . . . they all are done alone, in the privacy of one's home.

When a family member dies, crystals do not offer a communal ritual, nor does manifestation soothe collective grief or solidify memorial rites. Belief is one part of the equation. But we can't just prioritize the self, because that puts us back where we started: unwell.

Chapter 9

You're Not Working Hard Enough

Gasping for air, I struggled to keep up with a fast succession of push-ups. This was after what felt like an eternity of jumping jacks. I took a five-second rest, which quickly drew the attention of the instructor. Dressed in a branded sweatshirt and sweatpants, he approached me with a booming voice.

"This isn't SoulCycle!" he shouted, as I insecurely tugged at my leggings. "Get working!"

At CONBODY, a prison yard–themed boutique gym run by ex-convicts in New York, there is no rest for the weary. In this intense cardio class, I, and my fellow gym rats, worked diligently using only our body weight, just like prisoners do. It was all part of the theme: In the basement-level space, mugshot printouts of celebrities—O. J. Simpson, Zsa Zsa Gabor, and three of Lindsay Lohan—lined the entrance hall. At the end of the hall, a metal gate featured a graphic of barbed wire. Further in, a cement wall fenced in the check-in desk. CONBODY offers an "inmate experience" for young professionals intrigued by prison. Their clients watched *Orange Is the New Black* or *Prison Break* and are, by the gym founder's account, curious what lockup feels like.[1]

The trends only got tougher. I've also tried out trampoline cardio, aquacycling (like SoulCycle but in waist-deep water), and super cold HIIT workouts stationed in giant bespoke walk-in refrigerators. By early 2020, I found myself in a Tribeca fitness studio that specialized in electrical muscle stimulation (EMS). I took a high-impact cardio class where I had to wear a powersuit, much like a wet suit, that emitted electric shocks to cause involuntary muscle contractions. Throughout the workout, an instructor would press a button that sent electrical currents through my body, paralyzing me in my tracks as I tried to complete a burpee. Each time I was zapped, it felt as if I had suffered a heart attack.

I thought, *This has all gotten insane.* I'm getting nearly electrocuted or literally pretending to be so fit as to survive prison life. I can't work this hard. The Physical Activity Guidelines for Americans recommend at least 150 minutes a week of moderate aerobic activity (brisk walking, pushing a lawn mower) or 75 minutes of vigorous aerobic activity (running, swimming laps), with two days of muscle-strengthening activities (lifting weights, power yoga).

When did we decide that the average Joe needs to exercise like an American Gladiator? Why does it feel like everything requires so much effort? Or perhaps the better question is: Why do we feel the need to work so hard?

"Crush" Your Workouts:
Hard Labor for Hard Abs

Fitness is important, yet it's become increasingly demanding and performative. Among the trendiest of boutique studios across the country, you'll find Rise Nation, which is pure stair climbing. Crunch Gym launched a class called X-Treme Firefighters Workout to train students as if they were first responders and firefighters (the goal is to become strong enough to carry an unconscious human being out of a burning building). Big cities are home to plenty of popularized boot camps that employ former marines who force paying customers to endure "punishing" exercises like barbed wire crawls. These are all workouts in which we're told to "torch," "burn," or "crush," as though we're gripped in the clutches of war.

The trendiest of fitness regimens, it seems, run on good old American fuel: hard, hard work. When Peloton's internal marketing documents were leaked in 2019, we learned that to differentiate itself from other fitness brands, Peloton suggested that the brand isn't for everyone. It's for the ambitious, those who put in the effort to achieve greatness. "[We're] not a party on a bike," read the materials.[2]

To be sure, there's a market for this. For many, the appeal of a tough workout goes beyond body sculpture. They're attracted to the intensity and the need for endurance—*the sacrifice*. Call it achievement, transformation, or mental resilience, but the discomfort and perseverance required to vanquish "weakness" offer a real high. Some say this paves the path to self-actualization. Others say pain is character-building—a metaphor for overcoming life's many obstacles. And a few will readily acknowledge it as a tool for spiritual awakening.

This is not to suggest there isn't value in becoming strong. Acquiring strength is valuable for obvious reasons: A woman might feel more confident, attractive, and capable. She might feel powerful. She might draw on her physical strength to accomplish more tasks at home or feel more at ease in the boardroom. And that's all great.

But the perception of popularized fitness trends can backfire if it intimidates the average person. "Super high-intensity workouts inadvertently shame people into thinking that if they're not doing high intensity, beat-your-body-up workouts, then you're not really working out and you're wasting your time," says Carrie Myers Smith, a fitness industry expert and the author of *Squeezing Your Size 14 Self into a Size 6 World*. Experts instead offer the most commonsense advice: just go with what feels good to you. If people find walking boring or CrossFit too strenuous, they should find whatever will motivate them, be it tennis, jogging, or dancing in the dark to Robyn. "It's unfortunate that as a society, we seem to feel that more is better, including with exercise," says Heather Hausenblas, a professor of kinesiology at Jacksonville University and the co-author of *The Truth About Exercise Addiction*. "As a society, we really have a warped image of what health is."

If the greater fitness industry isn't pushing strenuous workouts, then they're promoting the idea of optimal fitness—that you need to squeeze every last bit of sweat out of a class. Time is a scarce resource to be managed, and is best handled by fitness trackers or health apps to track "progress" and log weekly "streaks." We keep score of our commitment to our bodies, tinkering with sleep stats and steps taken, guaranteeing we don't fall off the given path. We're besotted with data. By engaging in constant external monitoring, we surrender our own assessment. We let the machines judge, control, and optimize our actions.

HIIT workout franchise Orangetheory, for example, uses heart rate monitors to track your anaerobic threshold during cardio classes. Creator and co-founder Ellen Latham incorporated the idea after speaking with fitness enthusiasts who believed they were underperforming in comparison to those around them. Latham wanted to emphasize individual progress—backed by data. "I'm very much into the belief of competing against yourself," she told me, "specifically your last best self."[3] The goal, therefore, is to strive for *the next best you*.

Goals are great, there's no arguing that. Yet the quest for one-upmanship can taint our view of fitness, or worse. Lee, a mother of one in her late thirties, started running in her early twenties. Her mission, like that of many young women, was, as she describes it, to meet "the fitness standard." She worried that a few extra pounds would jeopardize her ability to achieve the American dream. "I [thought] if I look like that, I will be happy. I'll meet a man, I'll get married and I'll have all the things that I want to have and that society tells me I should have," she explained.

In 2013, Lee bought a Fitbit. At the start, tracking the data was fun. Lee could analyze her runs and daily calorie intake, using the numbers to push herself further. But the new gizmo didn't aid her runs as much as pinpoint all the ways she was falling short. Lee began to obsess over her stats. She punished herself if she underperformed or didn't hit new goals. Lee started planning her meals the night before, calculating exactly how much she would burn off with any given cardio exercise. "So I have to go for a forty-minute run and this is my only food for the day and I can't deviate from that because if I do then I'm probably gonna gain a pound and that's going to make me slower," she reasoned. If her then boyfriend asked her to go out for a meal, she would panic because she would need to schedule an activity to precisely cancel out the calories. "It's rearranging your life to fit with your [fitness] plan."

In time, exercise no longer served as a stress outlet, rather as a nerve-racking chore—an obligation. "It took all the joy away," reflects Lee. The situation came to a head when her fertility shut down due to overexercising and doctors warned her she was headed for a health crisis. In 2018, she finally recognized that she was suffering from fitness OCD, and Lee deserted her Fitbit. "That's when I started to dig into the actual damage that I'd done," she says, "years of depriving myself."

A quarter of American women use fitness trackers. Many indeed find them motivating. But for all the buzz, about half of users will tire of their shiny new tech toy and shove it into a drawer within six months.[4] Some stick with it, though some research isn't all that encouraging. One 2016 study found that while quantifying our every move might increase health consumers' tendency to engage in an activity, it can also simultaneously reduce how much we actually enjoy that activity. "This occurs because measurement can undermine intrinsic motivation," reads the study. "By drawing attention to output, measurement can make enjoyable activities feel more like work, which reduces their enjoyment."[5]

Top-tier gyms, meanwhile, offer a suite of coaches, treatments, and services meant to remedy any issue that might be standing in the way of achieving Halle Berry's body. In 2018, Equinox announced the debut of "sleep coaching," where personal trainers solely focus on improving snooze habits to benefit exercise performance. While sleep coaching isn't anything new, it's often used by professional athletes.

Now it is being rolled out to the general consumer to help them reach their "potential."

Perhaps Gwyneth Paltrow explained this endless quest for self-improvement best when she exclaimed on her Netflix series, *The Goop Lab*, "It's all laddering up to one thing: optimization of self. We're here one time, one life. How can we milk the shit out of this?" And hence we need fitness trainers, gadgets, and strenuous workouts to reach this magically hidden but tappable perfection. Our enhanced self is all there, simmering under the surface, just waiting for us to unlock it.

Flashback: Productivity Through Pumping Iron

In mid-nineteenth-century England, a movement dubbed "muscular Christianity" propelled believers to pump iron in the name of heaven. At a time of a "crisis in masculinity," society sought to uphold man's supposed God-given nature in an overcivilized world. Exercise was performed in the service of a higher power: it was a way to build character, avoid immoral pursuits, and ultimately "protect the weak." Physical prowess not only exemplified a commitment to God, it also made you more useful in service to others. Like a missionary He-Man.

The Protestant work ethic heavily influenced the popularity of fitness. As industrialization quickened, emerging middle and bourgeois classes found themselves with far more leisure time at their disposal. The idea of free time was so novel that they needed to find a purpose for it. Sports and outdoor activities were therefore encouraged as a means for righteous self-improvement, rather than pure amusement, which they deemed lazy and wasteful.

Up until that time, physical discipline—be it fasting or abstinence—was more or less delegated to the clergy. With this new era, the merger of sport and religiosity was touted to the masses as an expression of piety and servitude. This ethos evolved into team sports supported by local churches. Momentum hit a tipping point with the introduction of the first Young Men's Christian Association (YMCA) in London circa 1844, followed by New York City in 1869.

But such an emphasis on strength inherently maligned any form of perceived weakness, insinuating that the less fit were less than devoted to their creator. As one American pastor at the time wrote, "He who neglects his body, who calumniates his body, who misuses it, who allows it to grow up puny, frail, sickly, misshapen, homely, commits a sin against the Giver of the body . . . Round shoulders and narrow chests are states of criminality. The dyspepsia is heresy. The headache is infidelity. It is as truly a man's moral duty to have a good digestion, and sweet breath, and strong arms, and stalwart legs, and an erect bearing, as it is to read his Bible, or say his prayers, or love his neighbor as himself."[6]

You can hear echoes of this sentiment a century later in James Fixx's 1977 manifesto, *The Complete Book of Running*. The jogging enthusiast detailed the need for mastery over ourselves: how exercise cultivates qualities such as "will power, the ability to apply effort during extreme fatigue, and the acceptance of pain." Running takes work, and maybe we *need* more work, he proposed. "Too many of us live under-disciplined lives," wrote Fixx. "By giving us something to struggle for and against, running provides an antidote to slackness."[7]

The Fitfluencer Effect

From the nineteenth century to today, the fitness industry—like the diet industry—has glommed on to wellness to sell us an aesthetic ideal.

Publications like *Shape* and *Women's Health* publish piece after piece promoting how to "drop two sizes" or achieve a "bikini body." They imply that body modification in pursuit of the beauty ideal is the ultimate goal of getting active. Models' and celebrities' bodies are airbrushed to a flawless degree, projecting a surreal and sensual fantasy that consumes the reader. As one former *Women's Health* editor told me, these magazines simply continue a long, complicated legacy of women's aspirational (read: unrealistic) beauty standards because "that's what people want," whether they admit it or not. If magazines won't deliver it, then Instagram or TikTok will. In fact, social media does deliver it—and better—which is why they've stolen the mantle from declining traditional outlets.

Social media networks have exploded with imagery of people working out, via brands but also just peers bragging how they beat their last record. (Far rarer are people posting about being too tired to exercise and resigning themselves to the couch.) On Instagram, the hashtag #fitness has been used nearly 500 million times, which is separate from the 230 million #gym posts. At the top of the heap, often generating those hashtags, are the social media fitness stars—also known as "fitfluencers." The Tracy Flicks of exercise sell us on peak physicality: that hot, ripped body with zero percent body fat and chiseled abs. The most recognizable of this group is Kayla Itsines, "the Internet's undisputed workout queen," a fitness app founder with 14 million Instagram followers.

Just how big is fitfluencers' reach? *Forbes* reported that the top ten combined have an audience of more than a hundred million people—and that was back in 2017. Fitfluencers are only gaining more traction online, with some able to earn up to $30,000 per Instagram post. Fitfluencing has evolved into a real industry: Equinox partnered with Hollywood agency William Morris Endeavor to launch a fitness talent management practice to develop personal brands and score large-scale sponsorship deals.

Most fitfluencers aren't exactly pushing health, even if they look like it. "Be healthy" or "get strong," fitfluencers parrot, understanding full well that "fit" has replaced the space once afforded to "thin." They wear little clothing, ensuring that fans see perfectly sculpted body parts, as they stress workout plans that are more linked to fat reduction and visual appearance than cardiovascular health.

One study of Instagram, Facebook, Twitter, and Tumblr found that "fitspiration" imagery overindexes thin, toned women. These women were far more likely than men to be under twenty-five, have their full body on display, "and to have their buttocks emphasized."[8] Other researchers discovered that while fitspiration posts were "less extreme" than thinspiration (imagery encouraging thinness), there were no differences "with regard to sexual suggestiveness, appearance comparison, and messages encouraging restrictive eating."[9]

During the COVID-19 pandemic, a number of fitfluencers doubled down on the importance of a challenging daily exercise regimen, beating the drum that fans had better start sweating before they couldn't pull up their sweatpants. Suddenly women had to contend with pangs of personal inadequacy while dealing with stay-at-home orders. They feared their peers would emerge from isolation "as the body beautiful" while they barely found the time to shower.

Is this fitspiration or more like fitpressure?

Even athleisure upholds a specific body type. Some women feel that the uniform of women's fitness—the ubiquitous leggings and sports bra—mostly flatters the svelte and toned. *Who else can wear skintight spandex and flash their midsection?* Meanwhile, activewear brand marketing doesn't rely on realistic imagery of an average-sized woman, save for a few images every so often. Bigger-sized models have entered the fold, but they're still a minority that feels more like tokenism. Instead, we're treated to a medley of beautiful twentysomethings—flat bellies and all—that we, in turn, expect in our local gym.

What this all means is that today we are saddled with two equally unrealistic depictions of the female body: lean fitfluencers and perfectly curvy celebrities such as Kim Kardashian. One shows up on your television screen, the other in your Instagram feed. In a way we have triple pressure riding on women today—we need to be thin, curvy, *and* toned. The goal is a big butt, a teensy waist, and feminine musculature. It almost makes you yearn for the days when we simply needed to starve ourselves.

It's discouraging and relatively new, says Steven Loy, an exercise physiologist at the kinesiology department at Cal State Northridge. "Twenty years ago, a thin body was what was being pushed, but you didn't see the muscle. Now you see the same thin body, but it's got muscles that you can see." So basically, society added new bells and whistles to the unachievable ideal. "They've raised the bar on you." One health expert I spoke to reported a steady stream of young gym-goers with the same exact lower back pain, an ailment that usually afflicts an older segment of the population. The culprit? Too many booty-building exercises were performed with poor form.

Fitfluencers would have you believe that a rock-hard body (and booty) is just a matter of scheduling in a daily workout, of "committing to yourself." The audience is not privy to the amount of work that goes on beyond the iPhone screen, where fitfluencers spend hours every day exercising. Not to mention, imagery might be airbrushed and the influencer's poses manipulated to enhance their best angles. In comparison to traditional media, fitfluencers fuel more feelings of inadequacy because these individuals are not supermodels or Hollywood stars; they play up being real, "average" people, which then makes you feel worse for not rising to their bench-pressing level. It *looks* achievable. But fitfluencers fail to disclose that bodies react differently to specific exercises: genetic diversity cannot guarantee exact results.

On the surface level, #fitspo might seem like progress: Why shouldn't we promote fitness? It's healthy! But an onslaught of aesthetic fitness imagery isn't motivating the average American to get moving. On the contrary, it's intimidating them to the point of quitting before even starting. Carrie Myers Smith hears from self-conscious women who believe they need to lose weight and firm up *before* joining a gym. "We're not inspiring [the majority of] people to be fit," she told me. "We're just continuing to support the ones that already are fit, and shaming the ones that aren't." By 2020, 56 percent of Americans experienced this "gymtimidation," according to a Mindbody survey.[10]

The ones opting out of an unwinnable race aren't wrong. The likelihood that anyone can achieve influencers' level of fitness without time, money, and good genes is slim to none. The right kind of body is the product of the right classes, the right clothes, the right sneakers . . . the right effort. Our flesh is thereby an expensive project we must funnel more and more money into, forever iterating on Frankenstein's buff monster.

Aesthetic fitness doesn't necessarily equal health. Being fit looks like many different things. "The images that people are bombarded with are these hyperfit individuals, which I would tend to argue may not even be that healthy at the end of the day," says Heather Hausenblas. "Individuals internalize that and say 'that's what I need to look like to be healthy and to be fit.'"

You don't have to push it to the limits to be within health's reach. But there's no pride in gentleness, right? As with clean eating, extreme fitness yields extreme results—and maybe some respect. That's because moderation isn't prized in our culture.

Likewise, why do fitfluencers harp on rigid aesthetic ideals when science allows for far more body diversity? Because social media incentivizes it. Algorithms reward posts that garner the most likes (or controversy, for that matter), not those that align with medical advice. If someone wants to grow their following so that they can snag partnerships or get invited to live in a TikTok mansion, then they'll follow suit. "[It's] a vicious cycle, because when you're promoting content, the stuff that performs the best is usually the least factual stuff or the terms that aren't scientifically correct," Charlee Atkins, founder of the fitness lifestyle brand Le Sweat, told *Well+Good*.[11] "What sells is 'toning,' 'lengthening,' 'burn,' 'booty'—all of these words that didn't have definitions until the fitness industry created them . . . And so those of us who are in the fitness industry and promoting our products, for us to reach a larger market we're almost forced to also use those terms."

The algorithms don't do any wonders for women's self-esteem. In 2021, a leaked internal research report revealed that Facebook was made aware that Instagram (which it acquired in 2012) is harmful to girls' body image. The company was warned that 32 percent of girls said Instagram worsened their insecurities, blaming the photo sharing app for increased anxiety and depression. As one eighteen-year-old told the *Wall Street Journal*, "When I went on Instagram, all I saw were images of chiseled bodies, perfect abs and women doing 100 burpees in 10 minutes." Facebook, according to the report, made "minimal efforts" to address these mental health issues.

One study, though very small, further analyzed social media effects on young women. After twenty university students viewed fitspiration for one to four hours a day, they experienced greater body dissatisfaction and their self-confidence plummeted. These same individuals, however, had also spent years, like all of us, consuming advertising and traditional media. What was the difference, then? Fitspiration was potentially more potent because "perhaps women do not process fitspiration images *as critically* as they do thin-ideal images, or perhaps adding tone and strength to thinness cumulates to provide women with more ways in which to feel inadequate."[12]

While men also face pressures brought forth by a shirtless Chris Hemsworth, it's far more acute with women. Unsurprisingly, researchers found that women are more inclined to exercise for weight loss and toning, whereas men are more inclined to do it for enjoyment.[13]

Women are far more targeted in body culture, in part due to how gender intersects with social identity—and how it's both constructed and enforced, explains the *Body of Truth* author Harriet Brown. Traditionally, men's social power and reputation stemmed from the things they did, whereas women were typically prized for how they appeared. "It's deeply, deeply baked into our culture," says Brown. "I don't think it's possible to be a woman in this culture and not feel these things . . . We still seem to believe that so much of our value comes from how we look, how thin we are, and how sexy we are, whereas men have a lot of other avenues."

In recent decades, social standings have shifted, but the blueprint remains intact. A 2017 Pew Research Center poll found that society differs over what it values in men versus women. The top traits revered in men were honesty and morality, followed by professional success. For women, it was physical attractiveness, followed by empathy and being nurturing.[14] Women are told from multiple touchpoints that their body matters, that their physical attributes determine their success.

You can't blame them when they simply give in.

Productivity Tentacles Grow Longer and Stronger

It's not just our fitness we need to crush. Nowadays, you also need to leisure better.

Vacations have shifted in recent years. Burned-out Americans popularized wellness travel, one of the leading trends in the hospitality sector. Vacationers seek getaways filled with fitness classes, yoga, surfing, and guided meditation—in that order. They're not as interested in getting wasted in Vegas. (Although even Vegas is looking to reinvent itself as a wellness destination.) "When you have such little time off, you really can't afford to come back from a vacation where you drank too much, stayed up all night, and ate really horrible food," explained Beth McGroarty, the director of research at the Global Wellness Institute. "You can't afford coming back feeling worse than you did when you left."[15]

One poll found that 40 percent of millennials reported they'd rather go on a fitness retreat with their favorite instructor than attend a five-star relaxation resort.[16] I am guilty of this. I will sign up for a surf camp or stay in a fitness-class-focused hotel before ever staying in a regular resort. I just can't let that precious time go to "waste." Heaven forbid I sit by the pool and order a steady stream of grilled cheese sandwiches, which is what I actually want to do.

Like me, women might also fear gaining weight on vacation, aware that one too many midday margaritas might undo all the pre-trip starvation endured to fit into that bikini. As the writer and eating disorder survivor Gina Susanna recounted, to prepare for memorable (that is, Instagrammable) moments, "We need to make sure we are thin enough to enjoy them."[17] Susanna had heard from women who were "terrified" of going on vacations because they feared being surrounded by unhealthful foods or without exercise access. "I was just so sick of the constant diet culture voices telling me I needed to 'look perfect' to enjoy myself," she wrote.

Now, some people truly relax by exercising, and the idea of spending hours moving the body excites them, especially if they never get to be active during their sedentary day-to-day life. For them, hiking for six to eight hours a day is fun. They enjoy the exhaustion—"the good kind"—and clarity that comes from the end of an active day outdoors. Rigorous activities in nature are the ultimate reset for them.

But others feel that their vacations or any free moments require efficiency—a subtle pressure to always be *improving*. They need to maximize their time, no matter the occasion. Bodily obligations are not afforded a PTO reprieve. In an interview for *The Cut*, the Boulder-based physical therapist Nicole Haas said that an urgency to stay in shape on vacation is leading to an increase in injuries. One persistent client of hers blew out her back by attempting crunches in a compact hotel room, among other bad decisions: "I had someone do a thousand squats on that one hotel chair. Well, now your knee hurts! And I'm like, *Seriously?*"[18]

We also just respect hard effort more. There's a hierarchy of relaxation activities, and certain ones get pushed to the top. For Fiona, a full-time elementary school teacher and married mom of two, exercising guarantees a short period of time when no one bothers her. It's a mini-escape built into the workday. She wakes up an hour before the rest of her family to slip down to the basement and engage in a streaming cardio class. Fiona notices a massive difference in her mood if she doesn't get this one sacred hour: a missed class unleashes the Irritable Hulk. "It's definitely 'me time,'" says Fiona. Everyone knows that should they rise early, they can't ask for a snack or help in finding a misplaced sweater when she's working out. "I don't have any other time when I'm alone," she sighs.

In some ways, self-care offers a cover for whatever a woman needs to do to feel sane. For example, if a wife tells her husband to watch the kids because she needs to apply a facial mask, he might roll his eyes. If, however, she changes her terminology, saying she needs to "engage in self-care," she has invoked mental health, and therefore the activity is fully sanctioned. It's much the same way men might train for a marathon "for charity." As some men admitted to Jason Kelly in his book *Sweat Equity*, it's an acceptable way to escape familial obligations. "When you're riding your bike for five hours on a Saturday, it's harder for anyone to argue with you when you say you're helping cure cancer."[19]

Fiona concedes that less active hobbies, like reading, don't quite pan out in her household. To start, "you don't look as productive to other people," thereby inviting family members to interrupt whatever novel she's engrossed in. Although she can't fully blame those around her: she too will interrupt her reading to do some light cleaning. She just cannot convince herself that being immobile earns the same kind of deference as breaking an early morning sweat. Reading just doesn't feel worthwhile *enough*. She was raised to be a high achiever who never slacks off or "takes it easy." So why would her relaxation efforts be any different?

If you listen carefully to American media or scroll your Instagram feed, you will notice a hustle culture that dictates you should always be doing *something* even when that something should potentially be nothing. (Or, as Peloton's Ally Love puts it: "Hustle never sleeps!") We just can't stop indulging our inner high-achiever. The productivity mandate stares down on you in every aspect of your life, requiring you to be more mindful with your kids, get more fit, or become more Zen. It's easy to feel lazy if you're not actively "bettering" yourself at all times. So much so that 54 percent of women feel guilty when they need to take a break or rest.[20]

There's an actual term for this feeling, where you can't ever fully relax because you feel pressured to be productive: "Sunday neurosis." Believed to have been coined by Hungarian psychoanalyst (and friend of Freud) Sándor Ferenczi, it refers to the anxiety we feel when we attempt to be idle instead of, say, training for a marathon. It's the restlessness that comes with being free of structure, duty, and work. Freedom might just feel like emptiness. Or guilt.

Workaholism pervades everything, including, oddly, fashion. Take the famous athleisure brand Outdoor Voices, which popularized over-priced color-blocked workout attire. The company's motto is "doing things," pushing the idea that it's better to be doing things than not doing things—and somehow, these things should be done in $88 leggings. Outdoor Voices floods social media with this doctrine, encouraging young women to photograph themselves hiking, exercising, or buying smoothies with the hashtag #doingthings, thereby communicating, "Look at me! I invest in my health!" Fans' attire, therefore, is not best suited for sitting on the couch watching TikTok. Outdoor Voices shoppers are doers; *they're more active than the rest.* To date, more than 225,000 images include this productivity hashtag.

Fitness culture is also everywhere. Employers build onsite gyms to inspire healthier habits (or, more likely, to lower rising healthcare costs and boost productivity). Gyms are popping up where you least expect them, even inside the supermarket. Orangetheory, the fastest-growing fitness franchise, partnered with the Iowa-based grocery retailer Hy-Vee. ShopRite opened a fitness studio in New Jersey that offers yoga and Zumba classes. Some Whole Foods stores offer a range of workout classes on their premises. CVS Health is testing "health hubs" where customers take a yoga class as they wait for pharmacy refills.[21] There is no escape. Our culture will remind you at every single turn that you should be in the gym.

It's great to have so many opportunities to get moving, don't get me wrong. But it's starting to feel like perseverance and efficiency have invaded our personal lives: hard work, sacrifice, effort . . . these are what get our engine going in our overly ambitious, goal-oriented society. Here's the thing about productivity: it's always a means toward an end goal. It's in service of something you want—or need.

Perhaps we feel compelled to constantly improve our bodies because we know full well what health (or more likely the appearance of health) signifies in our culture. We know we need to effectively compete in a cut-throat market. It seems practical: If you are up against dozens of women for a job, a partner—heck, any opportunity—in our society, you might consider anything that gives you a leg up. And that toned body might very well suggest that you are *self-disciplined, hard-working, and fully in control*, as it's come to mean. It's a survival mechanism to some degree because society upholds the body as a representation of ability.

We live in a culture that preaches you alone are responsible for your success, and that ethos spreads to more than just our career. Such a culture creates a lot of pressure, if not body-shaming. It's also indicative of healthism—a concept connoting a moralized view of health that stresses the responsibility of the individual ("lifestyle choices"). This belief system holds that it's your fault if you fall ill or embody what society considers unhealthy, like being bigger bodied. By this logic, certain people are better than others, with those falling behind likely "deserving" of whatever comes their way (despite extenuating circumstances like budget, access, ability, or genetics). So no wonder we're trying to ensure that we never fail: No one wants to be the deviant. No one wants to be judged.

It sounds like we're working so hard to be perfect.

Although, no matter how hard one tries—you can squat, down-dog, and stage beautifully positioned acai bowls on Instagram all you want—it won't ever be good enough. Unattainability is the leading tenet of perfection. More than anything, perfectionism says a lot about what we crave—it is, at the end of the day, an anxious need for control over our lives.

Girl, Get Happy!

"Six things mentally strong people do," read Gwyneth Paltrow's Instagram post. In bullet point format, the black-and-white text laid out precisely what constitutes the psychologically blessed: They don't waste time feeling sorry for themselves, they "welcome" challenges, and they don't exert energy on that which they can't control. Most important, "they stay happy."

It wasn't long before a mob of women flooded the Goop guru's comments section with critiques of such reductionist advice. "Real life adversities can be incredibly difficult to overcome," wrote one follower. Others noted that though Paltrow had good intentions, the post minimized human adversity and ignored mental health issues. One angry woman wrote, "Feelings buried alive never die." Another simply demanded, "You need to take this down."

What Paltrow was really saying was this: *You should work to make your brain right.* Society constantly emits this kind of low-frequency messaging, but it's turned up high in wellness culture. Herbal supplements allude to fixing your gut *and* your brain. Svelte social media influencers pose with functional beverages as they babble on about their inner peace, beckoning followers to follow their lead. Framed by idyllic backdrops, they promote "quieting the mind" and "choosing" to commit to contentment, repeating that sheer determination cures all ills. They ask us to overcome mental hurdles through gratitude or to imagine a laugh track scoring daily challenges.

It's talking heads and celebrities but also average moms who repeatedly talk of calming themselves into states of bliss. It's everyone on Instagram only uploading their highlight reel without proper disclaimers: these are filtered, calculated depictions. We're led to believe that positive emotions are all under our own control, that happiness is but a "choice." Never mind that many other cultures view happiness as a collective goal, a social endeavor that connects you with other people. Instead, we are asked to shoulder this lonesome burden in a *Truman Show* facade of mental health. And yet Americans are the unhappiest they've been in fifty years: only 14 percent of adults say they're "very happy."[22]

Emma Anderson, a psychologist and senior lecturer at the University of Brighton, has researched the gendered nature of self-help and finds several similarities to the current self-care discourse. Much like how self-help books bang the drum on how we are flawed and can always strive to be "better," wellness posits that we are forever improvable. If historically women were expected to be demure, modest, and subservient, today they're held to idealized femininity dictating constant positivity and resilience. Though self-help and wellness are quite different, "they have a similar impact in disallowing other ways of being—disallowing anger, for example," says Anderson. "'If I can just try to be more positive, practice gratitude, and be more mindful.' These are all aimed at a kind of quiet, pacifying state of mind."

Unsurprisingly, being commanded to be happy often sparks the opposite reaction. Journalist Ada Calhoun, the author of *Why We Can't Sleep: Women's New Midlife Crisis*, spoke to hundreds of women across the country, and nearly all echoed the same sentiment: they are stressed and continually on edge, they are socially obligated to be calm, cool, collected, and they should always be giving and never demanding. "It's the equivalent of being told to smile by somebody who is catcalling you on the street," says Calhoun. "For a lot of women I talked to, it's making them very, very angry."

These expectations soon permeate how we express ourselves. Stacey Rosenfeld, a psychologist and the author of *Does Every Woman Have an Eating Disorder?*, finds that her female patients are socialized to suppress their negative emotions. We're conditioned from a young age to be polite, agreeable, patient, serene, giving—a new anvil of ideals dropped on our head at every stage of life. "And so being angry doesn't really fall into the expectations set forward for girls and for women," says Rosenfeld. Our bad moods and (often justified) anger are simply personae non gratae. Basically: Put that shit away. You are expected to hide your dissatisfaction and instead figure out a way to lessen it for those around you.

Negative emotions are crucial to feeling better. A 2017 American

Psychological Association research study found that people are much happier when they are given the freedom to express their emotions, even when those emotions are resentment, anger, or despair. Yes, we can practice gratitude—which has shown to be remarkably beneficial to mental health—but why not make more room for expressing what ails us?

Maybe because America has long emphasized rugged self-help, which is a decidedly American phenomenon, born of Puritan values. This idea of people venturing out to secure their own happiness rather than passively hoping for it goes as far back as the eighteenth century. (Indeed, a Russian adage attests that "a person who smiles a lot is either a fool or an American.") We're a country founded on meritocracy; she who works the hardest wins. Now we've applied that philosophy to our emotions.

In America, there's this idea of this great happily ever after out there on the horizon, explains Ruth Whippman, the author of *The Pursuit of Happiness* and *America the Anxious*. "That if you just keep trying and keep doing another self-help class and another wellness program, you'll eventually get to this glittering ideal." And self-help targets more women than men. We have to improve ourselves to meet an unattainable standard or a default male ideal, says Whippman, who sees gendered expectations exemplified throughout modern society. For example, many women's co-working spaces offer onsite amenities and programs which center on self-improvement: meditation sessions, fitness classes, vitamin shots, or nutrition lectures. Male-dominated clubs, on the other hand, get to have *fun*. They incorporate real leisure, with arcades or activities like ping-pong tournaments and whiskey tastings. There is simply not the same imperative for men to improve themselves in the same way.

"It's kind of ironic because all of these things which are supposed to be about relaxing and taking the pressures off modern life just end up actually piling the pressures on," says Whippman. "It's just another thing that you have to do and be and achieve. It's just an extra state that you have to get to." These are not necessarily new trends, though they are amplified by social media, which trades on the currency of perfection.

The tides are shifting. Once the COVID-19 pandemic hit, women started to question these unsustainable pressures. They couldn't do it anymore. There's a desire to understand the underlying issues at play: Why does everyone seem so utterly depleted? Why are we forcing ourselves to feel better about it all? And what do we need to feel better that doesn't add *more* pressure?

Charting a Chiller Course

The pandemic pushed Americans to reassess their priorities and aspirations. Millions quit their stressful jobs, while 42 percent of workers in a LinkedIn survey said they were taking a break for their well-being or to spend more time with loved ones.[23] More and more people recognized widespread suffering, with mental wellness growing into the dominant lens. There was a far greater honesty about stress, psychological woes, and day-to-day struggles spurring collective vulnerability. In fitness too: a 2021 survey of 16,000 Americans found that over a quarter of adults surveyed work out to reduce stress.[24] It's why, anecdotally, when you asked people why they exercised, you were more likely to hear them say it's for their "sanity" than desiring Kayla Itsines's physique.

A societal emphasis on mental health is moving the industry outside the framework of productivity and aesthetic goals, says Beth McGroarty of the Global Wellness Institute: "The new compass point is one of healing and forestalling crisis," she says, noting that serious health management is overtaking the "bionic woman model."

In her research, Whippman found that the single biggest factor affecting happiness across the board is social support. Calhoun, meanwhile, witnesses groups of women coming together to discuss long-avoided issues and reassess impossible ideals in a way that feels both constructive and therapeutic. She launched a monthly social club for women to be "in each other's presence with no filters." Attendees, she reports, find it far more healing than any spa or yoga class.

Progress is slow but growing. Young women protesting the deluge of toxic positivity on social media have turned to digital communities like Sad Girls Club, which counts more than a quarter million Instagram followers looking for authentic emotional support.[25] Even who women have turned to for advice has changed: there are influencers who advocate compassion and moderation, not a six-pack and an emotional lobotomy.

One body positivity advocate changing the face (and shape) of fitfluencers is self-described "fat femme" Jessamyn Stanley. Stanley, who is Black, tries to widen the appeal of yoga by posting intricate poses and inspirational advice on Instagram for people who feel excluded from wellness. She'll photograph herself doing the splits upside down while clothed in a sports bra, exposing her belly and stretch marks in an industry that's generally exemplified, by Stanley's account, by a "perfectly slender, usually White [woman who] obviously has some kind of money to afford all those leggings."

Stanley's repeated use of "fat" is to reclaim a word she believes undeserving of its negative connotations. "The only way you can let go of a weapon, especially in the form of a word, is to take the weapon back," she told me. Stanley took her efforts beyond social media, launching her own fitness app, The Underbelly, where she invites yoga learners to access their feelings in an authentic way. "You don't have to omit the sadness, the anger, and all of the other 'ugly' emotions that flavor our lives,"[26] Stanley wrote in her book *Every Body Yoga*, meant as an amuse-bouche for intimidated yoga beginners who "don't feel comfortable walking into a studio."

The radical fitfluencer's insistence to fight for the further inclusion of various body shapes struck a chord within the Instagram community. Fans learn, for example, how to tailor yoga poses for all body types, with tips on how to move around with larger thighs or breasts. A sweep of her account shows thousands of likes and hundreds of comments from followers comforted by her honest depictions of pursuing wellness activities in an idealized climate. Some cry watching her videos. "You are an inspiration to the ones that don't look like the so-called 'model type,'" wrote one fan.

Stanley wasn't surprised. "[People] want to see another person that's like them," she said of her 470,000 followers. She believes a large swath of Americans want to exercise but feel put off by traditional instructors and the mainstream media's unattainable depictions. "I was overwhelmed by people [who responded] 'Wow, I didn't know that fat Black people could practice yoga, I thought it was only skinny women," she said, adding, "There were a lot of people who think that I'm a unicorn."

Stanley does not consider herself any sort of mythical creature. If anything, she said, "I am the norm, I am not the minority."

• • •

You can get sucked into the culture of it all. With wellness, you'll see yourself on a constant quest of betterment, the ideal always on the horizon. We bow at the altar of excellence with our hard-earned effort, be it a meticulous meditation regimen or Olympian-level fitness classes. You would think everything should propel you to great new heights—to self-conquest—for there is no glory or virtue in the neutral. And people don't always realize it's work because of the way it's been marketed—as a "lifestyle."

But make no mistake, we are striving for perfection, not unlike our religious ancestors working toward salvation. We have an image of what perfection is in our head—it can be super fit, calm, or free of any ailment—and it is reinforced like propaganda even when built on shaky premises. I'm not against self-improvement, rather that we have internalized a silent imperative: that we must continually work to upgrade our bodies and brains.

The pressure, ironically, can have the opposite effect. Fitness enthusiasts can push themselves so hard that an entire industry sprouted *in response to it*. One of the leading industry trends, with double-digit growth, is that of recovery: big-box gyms have hired recovery coaches and set up dedicated areas with self-massage tools.[27] One-on-one assisted stretching studios—like a spa for your overworked muscles—have opened across the country.[28] This means that for some, salvation isn't always promised as much as what eventually awaits us: burnout. Then the cycle starts all over again, reverting us through the rhythms of self-care. It's one big reinforcing complex: work hard, fall apart, then buy some stuff so you can get back on the horse. A snake eating its own tail.

If it's not mental upgrades and strenuous sweat—the productivity mandate—then it's another powerful doctrine embedded into trendy wellness doctrines: level up your health with technological advances. With cutting-edge science at our fingertips, why wouldn't you want to go further? These are two sides of the same coin, assuring us we can maximize just about everything.

But can we?

Chapter 10

Chasing Golden Unicorns: Biohacking the Future

The small back room of the InterContinental hotel in downtown L.A. was bursting at the seams. Roughly a dozen chairs were set up for a lecture. Instead, almost a hundred people showed up. Most of the casually dressed millennials at the 2017 ideas conference Summit L.A. either sat on the floor or stood shoulder to shoulder. Those in the back stood on their toes, struggling to catch a glimpse of the speaker, the biohacking leader Dave Asprey.

Other than Gwyneth Paltrow or Lacy Phillips, Asprey was the closest I've witnessed to guru status. The participants bombarded the founder with health questions: What should I eat for breakfast? Can I have a glass of wine at dinner? Should I be taking the psychedelic drug ayahuasca? What sleep tracker do you use? Fans shot their hands in the air, each competing for a morsel of his wisdom.

Asprey, a tall, elegant man dressed in leather alligator boots and a chambray shirt, handled their questions with ease. He answered all inquiries with the air of a "cool" college professor, at times readjusting his orange-tinted glasses while applauding their curiosity. Equal parts peer and educator, Asprey peppered his answers with personal anecdotes and preferred products. The crowd's iPhones lit up as they googled his advice.[1]

Popularity wasn't new to Asprey. He first catapulted to fame through his high-performance coffee brand called Bulletproof. The caffeinated drink was infused with two tablespoons of grass-fed unsalted butter and MCT oil (a supplement sourced from coconuts and made of fatty acids). Clocking in anywhere from 250 to 450 calories (based on butter added), the beverage is claimed to boost energy, increase cognitive function, and help shed pounds. Asprey came up with the unorthodox recipe after traveling to Tibet and tasting traditional yak-butter tea drinks that locals consumed to keep warm. In 2011, he sold his own version as a self-optimization tool.

Over the next few years, Asprey's fatty cup of joe received coverage in everything from top-tier business publications to morning news programs. "It's a gateway drug for taking control of your own biology," Asprey told the *New York Times*. On *The Tonight Show*, host Jimmy Fallon shared a warm mug of Bulletproof coffee with actress Shailene Woodley and declared, "It's good for your brain."[2] Bulletproof became a curious cultural phenomenon, hailed as a "miracle drink" and drawing fans ranging from Halle Berry to Tim Tebow. Today, the creamy concoction is sold at Whole Foods, among other retailers, including Bulletproof's own brick-and-mortar Santa Monica coffee shop. Bulletproof has now evolved into a lifestyle concept, expanding to books, a podcast, conferences, and a whole suite of self-enhancement products like memory strengthening supplements and "amplified energy" bottled water.

But Asprey's biggest success was popularizing the term "biohacking." It's a concept borrowing research from bodybuilding, biotech, anti-aging science, and nutrition to make you look, perform, and feel way better than the average bear. Asprey describes biohacking as "the desire to be the absolute best version of ourselves," but it's more like an attempt to use cutting-edge science to overcome physical limitations. His company's mission? To tap into the unlimited power of being human. And according to recent industry reports, biohackers will become "the new wellness pioneers," heralding a new era where we can shortcut our way to optimal health.[3]

Asprey was once a mere mortal, a cog in the American lifestyle wheel. The former cloud computing executive was unhappy with his weight, sluggish, foggy, and moody and dealt with a host of issues, including ADD, OCD, and chronic fatigue syndrome (among other diagnosed and self-diagnosed disorders). He adopted one fad diet after another. He exercised every day. But still, the scale barely budged, and he didn't feel any better. Asprey's doctors were not helpful. They assumed he was secretly munching on candy bars. The entrepreneur recalled thinking, "I'm going to troubleshoot this myself, because I am not getting help from the medical establishment."[4]

So Asprey became his own guinea pig. He imported European "smart drugs" (cognitive enhancers). He tested brain-boosting contraptions. He committed to intermittent fasting routines.

Asprey spent fifteen years and over a million dollars to reportedly lower his biological age. In the process, he lost a hundred pounds and, by his account, increased his IQ by more than 20 points.

Today, Asprey lives like a health-obsessed Iron Man. He swallows fifty supplements every morning, recovers in a cryotherapy chamber he built in his house, and plans to get an injection of stem cells every six months. He says he no longer needs the eight hours of recommended sleep, making do with precisely six hours and ten minutes.[5] Every day he does some sort of biohacking exercise: "I could do red light therapy. I could do neurofeedback. I could just do some squats on a vibrating platform. I could do a resistance band workout with blood flow restriction," he told *GQ*.[6]

At this rate, says Asprey, he'll live to be 180. He thinks you can too. "I can tell you firsthand that you're not condemned to live with the body and brain you were born with," Asprey proclaims on his website. The Bulletproof website reads like a rundown of things people can regulate: stress, energy, mitochondrial clocks, risk of cancer, biochemistry, collagen production, sexual performance, and clarity of thought. (My favorite promise-filled headline is the one on daveasprey.com: WANT TO LIVE LONGER? BREW YOUR COFFEE THIS WAY.) DIY augmentation takes the form of neurofeedback devices as well as cold showers and fasting regimens.

In some ways, Asprey sees his work as a humanitarian effort: "We're helping people—we're empowering them by giving them control of their biology so that maybe they might see their doctor less." The entrepreneur envisions a future in which individuals become their own body experts and less dependent on medical professionals.

With help from Asprey, biohacking became synonymous with Silicon Valley, a sector that welcomes disruptive experimentation in the name of productivity. This is how Asprey became a star attraction at Summit, a conference heavy with tech founders, entrepreneurs, and ambitious creatives. But I was rather surprised to see that nearly half the room were women, if only because the biohacking scene skews male. Asprey said his Bulletproof conferences boast 50 percent female attendance, a significant uptick since he started. "My experience is that women are, on average, better biohackers than men because they have far more body awareness," Asprey told me. "Women are under tremendous pressure from a career perspective, and they are often even more constrained for time than men are."

Biohacking resonates because we're all frustrated, says Asprey, noting that complaints extend beyond the scale. Its appeal is motivated by exasperation at not having enough time, and therefore not enough energy, for work, relationships, or personal pursuits. Asprey gives one such example: "You're frustrated that every day after you've finished your commute home, you just need to lie down and put your feet up, that you don't want to play with your kids . . . It all comes down to what I want my body to be—to support me and be my servant."

At the conference, I approached a few women, curious about what they were looking to take charge of. Most of the answers included ordinary grievances such as fatigue or weight loss. One petite thirtysomething told me she was intrigued by Asprey's fertility research. This was news to me. Does biohacking cover reproduction?

"It covers *everything*," she replied. Indeed, Asprey's books explain how to safeguard one's fertility in addition to sharing how he personally cured his wife, who was diagnosed with polycystic ovarian syndrome and declared infertile. He says he did so with biohacking techniques—not through medical interventions like IVF.[7] They now have two children.

"Whether or not you choose to have kids, to become Super Human you want your body to be as fertile as possible because our bodies are designed to get out of the way as soon as we can't reproduce," Asprey writes in his *New York Times* bestseller *Super Human*. "No matter how old you are, you don't want your hormones telling your body that you're past the age of reproduction. A much better signal from your hormones is that you are young enough to have kids and therefore worth taking up room on this planet."[8]

To that end, we need to reboot our bodies, hike up our supplement intake (Bulletproof's supplements, that is; "First things first, throw away your multivitamin," reads the website), and detoxify our surroundings.

I was captivated by all of these biohacking ideas. It was as if they'd come from a wizard's spellbook to magically force the body into submission. I too wanted to know how to manufacture more energy at the office (or heck, even at dinner with friends). I too am frustrated by having to work super-long days and feeling like I can't get ahead. I too wanted to extend my fertility as my biological clock thumped ever louder. I wanted it all: stamina, youth, and focus. I was just as tired and over it as everyone else in that room.

But it also made me wonder: To what extent can scientific advancement bend nature to our will?

The Illusion of Control

In 1976, two researchers set out to understand an age-old human question: How important is our sense of control?

Ellen Langer (Harvard) and Judith Rodin (Yale) conducted an experiment on older adults. They separated a nursing home into two floors. The residents on the "agency" floor were told they'd have free rein to do what they wished with their room furniture, go where they pleased, do what they wanted during their free time, and independently care for a plant given to them. The patients on the "no agency" floor were notified that the staff would take care of every last detail and decision for them, including watering their new plant.

In reality, both groups had the freedom to do as they pleased. No one would stop an individual on the "no agency" floor from seeing a friend or watering the plant. The *perception* of what was permissible was all that differed. After eighteen months, the researchers discovered that those in the group that was granted more individual control and personal responsibility were happier. They also showed improved health. The "no agency" group had more deaths.[9]

Langer eventually made groundbreaking research progress in what she called the illusion of control, which is the tendency for people to overestimate their ability to control or impact events over which they actually have no influence. This impression makes us feel more confident and at ease. We hit elevator buttons that are already lit and wear "lucky" jerseys to a baseball game for the same reason: we want to feel that we contributed to the solution, that we matter. "Our biology is set up so that we are driven to be causal agents; we are internally rewarded with a feeling of satisfaction when we are in control, and internally punished with anxiety when we are not," writes the neuroscientist Tali Sharot in her book *The Influential Mind*.[10]

Most of us know and appreciate the comfort of taking action instead of waiting around and just hoping things will pan out. In the face of chaos, you can exert some influence. Plenty of people benefit from a similar placebo effect, by which the perception that something is working provides a certain amount of relief.

When it comes to health intentions, most people would probably seek effective benefits, not just a placebo. But in making decisions, we can overestimate our odds at achieving the desired outcome. Part of this stems from what's called a positivity bias or "the Pollyanna principle": a tendency for the mind to focus on positivity more than negativity. When we think we have more influence than we do, the obvious danger is that we might fall for a solution that is easy and simple versus taking the time and effort to analyze the situation, which is likely more complex than we assumed at first glance. Pollyannas might not anticipate potential problems.[11]

The wellness industry capitalizes on this bias, similar to how casinos enhance players' perception of control over the risk of gambling. Brands know this bias is psychologically beneficial: a sense of control reduces anxiety, fear, and stress levels, all things that contribute to overall mental health. When we believe we might be more in control, we're much more likely to buy something.

It's an open industry secret. The guidebook *Marketing to the New Natural Consumer* reads, "Note that the use of natural products as a way of regaining control over one's physical and emotional self is *not* contingent upon efficacy . . . It is not necessary that a treatment (such as reflexology) or a regular maintenance plan (taking Vitamin C) necessarily works. Simply engaging in these behaviors brings a regained sense of control to the individual." The co-authors go on to deem it a coping strategy—an antidote—to the stress of modern life, similar to partaking in body-modification rituals (like tattooing) as an "attempt to reclaim part of their self from the larger institutional structure."[12] So brands may not sell you an actual solution, but rather the illusion of a solution. A psychological exercise with a sticker price.

The biohacking movement is perhaps the most brazen example of harnessing our physiology to grasp this illusion of control. Not long after hearing Asprey speak, I visited the physical embodiment of his movement: Bulletproof Labs (now called Upgrade Labs), a futuristic "human upgrade center" in Santa Monica filled with space-age pods and curious contraptions better suited to NASA astronauts than SoCal residents. Somewhere between a gym and a science lab, its mission is "to help you achieve the highest state of physical and cognitive performance."

Inside, young and fit people seated in plush leather lounge chairs quietly flipped through magazines while receiving IV nutrient infusion drips.

An "atmospheric cell trainer" resembling Superman's pod reportedly "massages cells from the inside out" to balance out stressors. An "oxygen trainer," which looked more like a gas mask hooked up to a stationary bike, supposedly increases circulation. Then there was a tanning bed–like contraption that exposes your entire body to red and infrared LED light to "boost mitochondrial function." It was a dystopian Disneyland—or an Equinox designed by Christopher Nolan.[13]

"When you apply technology to your body there are so many things you can do that have a higher return on your investment of time and energy," Asprey told me. One of his favorite machines reportedly lets him get two and a half hours' worth of cardio in just twenty-one minutes. Asprey has all these toys at his own home, but he wanted to share them with busy professionals looking to sneak in a brain tune-up or ultra-quick workout.

In much the same way, supplements claim you can quickly master your fate. Companies like Elysium Health sell "revolutionary" at-home kits that test your biological age, then suggest their line of pills to reduce it. Their tagline? "Get ready to take control of your future." This simplistic marketing works. Goop promoted the kit on Instagram, writing, "A DNA test that can determine your rate of aging? Sign us up."

The trendiest supplement label in wellness circles remains Moon Juice, which sells powdered adaptogen (that is, herb and mushroom) blends claiming to fix your brain, sleep, stress, energy, *and* love life. These pills and concoctions, aptly named Power Dust and Sex Dust, harness the "power of plants" to "deliver beauty, balance, and vitality as a daily practice." The majority of the herbs—touted to improve immune functions or reduce stress—are backed up by little or contradictory evidence. But that doesn't stop Moon Juice from claiming on the Nordstrom website that their "elite" powder fuels "your physical and entrepreneurial feats."

Here's one overall distinction worth thinking about: health versus self-improvement. Over the decades, we've dialed up self-enhancement in various sectors like beauty (plastic surgery) or fitness (steroids). We've always sought individual interventions, though not always to heal as to boost, and now that optimization creed has come for wellness. You could argue there's a big difference between contact lenses and Botox: one solves a medical problem, the other perhaps less so (depending on your beauty philosophy). And so a chunk of late-stage wellness, for all its talk of health, seems more like Botox—a nice-to-have—than anything resembling a must-have.

This is likely what Fran Lebowitz meant when she made headlines by declaring "wellness is greed" in the Netflix documentary series *Pretend It's a City*. "Extra health," is how she described it, lamenting, "It's not enough for me that I'm not sick. I have to be 'well.' This is something you can buy." She has a point: it's how we've been sold on sleep trackers and overpriced magic pills, not to mention $118 Lululemon leggings. These were all hardly necessary until they were introduced to us, then marketed ad nauseam.

It's all subjective though, no? Botox (or acne treatment, for that matter) can be part of someone's mental well-being; it can make someone feel less insecure about their appearance. Maybe it helps them leave the house with confidence. That's why so much of wellness is debatable: what you might call "improvement" might be another person's "necessity." On one hand, there's an instinct to shun anything that's overly consumerist and lacking scientific evidence. On the other hand, there's something to be said for helping people feel better, or more "like themselves."[14]

We can't solely blame marketers for offering up new modes of self-improvement. They simply respond to a consumer demand that has its origins in the (far more regulated and science-backed) healthcare industry. There is an expectation—a sense of near entitlement—that if we have the technology to elevate our well-being, why don't we?[15] *Why aren't companies doing more to enable that? Why can't they solve all of life's problems?*

People are demanding more health solutions, and that's something the pharmaceutical and medical industry hasn't fully been able to address. So they turn to the wellness industry.

It should be noted that healthcare branding, which is not to be confused with wellness marketing, helped bring awareness and legitimize ailments that long affected women. Complaints ranging from pain to mood swings might have once been discounted before the industry named and publicized them as perimenopause, anxiety, and other recognized conditions. That helped ease the stigma. But wellness doesn't function like healthcare branding—it's not beholden to the same standards of efficacy or regulations on what you can and cannot promise the consumer.[16] That's how you end up with a bunch of fantastical-sounding supplements and optimization gizmos.

But still, why do we fall for the quick and simple solutions, or as the clinical exercise physiologist and nutritionist Bill Sukala calls it, "chasing golden unicorns"?

Research shows that stressful environments and highly competitive situations spur a desire for control. This makes sense: when you need to achieve something, you spring into action mode (without necessarily thinking through all the potential outcomes). This natural reaction is precisely why biohacking gained a loyal audience in Silicon Valley. Overwhelmed tech bros were desperate for a leg up. This is a work culture where workhorses survive and leaders look up to Steve Jobs, a man who once fired 25 percent of a team with parting words such as "You guys failed. You're a B team. B players."[17] Being number one reigns supreme in this industry, so anything that offers even the slightest competitive edge can mean rising to the top or snagging that promotion. A pill or drink that promises you can work longer, harder, and with less sleep? Contraptions that will cut workout time in half? Catnip to the overworked and undersupported.

Over time, seeing how biohacking resonated with men, those same companies started coming for women, who, to be fair, are just as overwhelmed.

Asprey's female fans have the same frustrations as men, just perhaps with different origins. They were compelled by his assessment: society mandates that people either have superhuman stamina or work like a dog to keep up. In contrast, he was suggesting, *Hey, it's okay, I know a way for you to keep up with what the world demands.* Biohacking isn't necessarily about becoming Superman, I learned; it's focused on spending "more time enjoying the fruits of [one's] labor and less time sweating it out in the field."[18] So if a buttery, textured coffee promises sustained energy, women are all for it. They've undoubtedly internalized the idea that their current skills aren't enough for them to succeed in our competitive society.

If only it were guaranteed. A portion of Bulletproof's peddled lifestyle advice and product lines relies on studies conducted on animals or studies with such small test groups that it would be hard-pressed to find definitive takeaways. According to the UK's *Daily Telegraph*, these claims aren't as strong as you'd believe:

> Another paper—"Switching from refined grains to whole grains causes zinc deficiency"—is a report of a 1976 research project featuring a study group of just *two people*. A third study—"Diets high in grain fibre deplete vitamin D stores"—is a 30-year-old study of 13 people.
>
> A fourth—"Phytic acid from whole grains block zinc and other minerals"—is based on a 1971 study of people in rural Iran eating unleavened flatbread. Another is about insulin sensitivity in domestic pigs.
>
> In other words, the research upon which the Bulletproof Diet stands is not exactly cutting-edge.[19]

As for buttered coffee, it promises to give you energy. It's supposed to banish hunger pangs, jump-start fat burning, and sharpen mental focus. Bulletproof suggests having it in place of breakfast—a meal in itself—thereby competing with our treasured avocado toast.

Much of the drink's fanfare stems from the butter, which is high in omega-3s, and also in MCTs (basically coconut oil), which some studies suggest improve cognitive function in Alzheimer's patients—a promising start. But MCTs don't necessarily have an impact on the healthy, and the studies supporting MCT benefits are mixed. As critics have pointed out, there's no evidence to presume this is a superior breakfast or that its ingredients induce fat burning. In fact, critics say it's a low-nutrient replacement—yet clocking in at 450 calories and 50 grams of fat—for what could be a better-balanced meal. Nutrition experts warn that it decreases your nutrient intake by about one-third,[20] whereas you could get healthy fats from foods like avocados or salmon.

Bulletproof offers big, vague claims without always the evidence to back them up. Also, as far as I'm concerned—though clearly this isn't a study either!—their fatty coffee doesn't suppress hunger. I tried it, and by 11:00 a.m. I was aching for a bagel. By noon, I was eyeing my dog's food bowl.

Another potential downside of biohacking is that it makes people *feel* more proactive about their health than they actually are. It's a psychological effect that researchers refer to as "illusory invulnerability." If you believe you're already taking action, you may be less compelled to pursue actual healthy habits. Or you may even engage in unhealthy behavior. In one study, those who took supplements were more likely to neglect activities such as exercise or eating balanced meals than those who didn't. Consuming supplements also spurred unhealthy indulgences, like choosing an all-you-can-eat buffet over a healthy meal. Taking that magic pill gave them "license" to slack off.[21]

Sometimes individuals do see a positive effect after taking a supplement. But can they prove it's causal versus coincidental? If someone decides to commit to a healthier lifestyle and couples it with a vitamin regimen, then yes, they will likely experience physical changes and start feeling better. But who's to say the pills are doing anything?

Maybe every industry sells control, whether that's beauty, automobiles, or tech. Sure, but you can't quite equate nutrition to cosmetics. The stakes are higher. When it comes to our health, there is no place for deceptive marketing tactics or faulty science. But the promises are just so alluring: Who doesn't want to believe they can live longer, better, and stronger?

Flashback: "I'm Gonna Live to Be a Hundred"

In June 1971, health guru Jerome Irving (J. I.) Rodale appeared on *The Dick Cavett Show*. Dubbed Mr. Organic, he was a pioneer of the natural health movement, having founded *Prevention* magazine and authored books such as *Happy People Rarely Get Cancer*. Semiretired at age seventy-two, Rodale felt fit as a fiddle and ready to divulge his secret to longevity: a nutritious diet. "I never felt better in my life," exclaimed Rodale with a smile. "I'm gonna live to be a hundred."

Following a commercial break, Rodale moved over on the couch to let the next guest take center stage. Suddenly, the audience heard Rodale let out a sound that resembled a loud snore. Assuming it was a prank, the audience erupted into laughter. But this was no gag. Cavett took one look at his guest—mouth agape, head thrown back—and knew something was wrong.

Rodale was pronounced dead on the spot. He had suffered a fatal heart attack.

Years later, while recounting the incident, Cavett joked, "Who would be the logical person to drop dead on a television show? A health expert."

Jokes aside, Rodale remains an important figure in the modern wellness movement. Like his predecessors and successors, he was quick to promise an Eden of health. Rodale penned columns full of practical lifestyle advice. He sat at the forefront of healthy and organic food. Rodale also harbored a mistrust of government, medicine, and industrial powers. His dogma centered on questioning accepted health tenets both big and small.

While skepticism is warranted (and necessary), reformers can sometimes get it wrong. Rodale pushed a slew of unconventional ideas, some far more experimental than scientific. He believed in exposing the body to shortwave radio waves to boost the body's supply of electricity.[22] Sugar, in his mind, was so toxic it could severely impair judgment and even lead to crime. (Rodale even supposedly suggested that Hitler was a sugar fiend addicted to whipped-cream-topped cakes, implying that a sweet tooth turned him into a genocidal maniac.)[23] Rodale was also an anti-vaxxer, advocating a dietary cure for polio. "Isn't there a better way of conquering polio than jabbing all the children in the country with a needle?" the publisher wrote in a 1955 issue of *Prevention*.[24]

At one point, the Federal Trade Commission targeted Rodale's book *The Health Finder*, which claimed to help people add years to their lives and free themselves from colds, among other promises. The agency deemed the book not only inconsistent with modern science but engaging in deceptive advertising. The FTC took Rodale to court, and he defended himself on First Amendment grounds throughout the 1960s.

Rodale, Inc., grew to become one of the world's largest health and wellness publishers, printing popular magazines such as *Men's Health*, *Women's Health*, and *Runner's World*, before being acquired by Hearst. In addition to the empire Rodale established, he endures as the pinnacle of dissent both from centuries past and the wellness gurus yet to come.

Can I Truly "Own" My Biological Future?

In 2018, I started receiving invitations to check out a mobile clinic offering on-the-spot ovarian egg reserve testing, which measures the anti-Müllerian hormone (AMH)—just one marker of a woman's remaining egg supply. The traveling clinic was run by the femtech start-up Kindbody, dubbed "the SoulCycle of fertility" by *The Verge*. Here, I and other women could learn for free about what might convince us to buy their core service: oocyte cryopreservation, also known as egg freezing.

So one spring day, I visited an egg-yolk-yellow bus parked in a busy mid-city intersection across the street from the Los Angeles County Museum of Art. It held court among other transportation vehicles, namely food trucks, UPS trucks, and Uber pickups. This bus, however, saw a steady stream of women jumping in, then exiting fifteen minutes later to pick up free lip balm and water bottles from a nearby table. A line formed in front of the splashy vehicle—a revolving door of fashionable parishioners in high-heeled sandals and work-appropriate attire.

Unlike stuffy OB-GYN clinics, Kindbody had confidence-boosting "girl boss" mottoes like "Own your future" lining the bus's walls. In addition to free testing, the fertility buses offered a "wellness lounge" where women could indulge themselves with spa-like skin care consultations. This was no drab affair. It was all smiles, catchy hashtags, and swag—like a midday Sephora dash.

What would generally be regarded as a hard sell was rebranded as wellness. The company compared their services to other areas of proactive health care, such as nutrition or exercise. "Egg freezing is absolutely a form of self-care," declared Gina Bartasi, the founder and CEO of Kindbody.[25] In an interview with *The Verge*, she said, "What we want to do is help women live a life of no regrets, and have children when they want them, on their own timeframe." Kindbody's website read, "Freezing eggs is like freezing time."

Kindbody is one of many fertility start-ups that emerged in the last decade to counteract new societal shifts: in 2019, following a four-year downward trend, U.S. fertility rates hit a thirty-five-year low. In addition, more women in their thirties and forties are having babies, which inevitably increases the need for medical intervention for those impacted by age-related infertility. In 2009, 475 women chose to freeze their eggs. By 2017, there were 9,042 women.[26]

Egg freezing start-ups sell peace of mind from knowing that you can store your eggs this winter, then gather them when a future spring arrives. And why not learn about it with a little bit of levity? The appeal is obvious, if not seductive: Who doesn't want more time? Time to travel, time to solidify a career, time to buy a house, time to pursue Timothée Chalamet. The more time the better.

Kindbody's roaming reproductive tour hit major U.S. cities, with an emphasis on women in their midtwenties. When deciding where to go next, Bartasi asked: *Where is SoulCycle opening up? What is Drybar doing?* They ended up rolling through the Hamptons.[27] Throughout the tour, the brand kept it light, upbeat. By using trendy terms like "self-care," Kindbody transformed a medical procedure into something more empowering. They destigmatized fertility treatment.

The Kindbody tour proved a bona fide success, drawing new clients to their upscale brick-and-mortar boutique clinics that looked more like Instagrammable coworking spaces than sterile medical clinics. Women froze their eggs and believed: They *could* have it all.

But missing throughout all that optimistic talk might have been a reality check. It's posted in FAQ sections and perhaps quickly addressed during an introductory session, but if you look at the overall marketing messaging, you might take away more promise than medical realism.

Thawing the Painful Truth

"It was more painful than I was ready for." "It's a serious thing." "Be sure to buy truckloads of ibuprofen." I received these and other cautions from my friends and online strangers when I first looked into the procedure.

Egg retrieval is an intrusive process of daily hormone injections, multiple ultrasound appointments, and blood tests as well as an invasive procedure usually performed under general anesthesia.* On rare occasions, it can result in painful complications. I know: I've done it.

Not to mention that it's wildly expensive. Egg freezing starts between $6,000 and $10,000, though some of my friends spent closer to $15,000

---

* Patients undergo the same hormone injection and egg retrieval procedure as IVF, but IVF is defined by fertilizing the extracted eggs into embryos.

following the number of tests and drugs required. And costs don't end at gathering the eggs.[†] The eggs need to be stored (usually $600 plus a year), then survive being unthawed, fertilized, and implanted back into the uterus via IVF. How much, on average, does it cost for the whole soup-to-nuts menu for having a baby? Clients often need more than one IVF cycle, hiking the average cost of successful egg freezing and IVF to somewhere between $40,000 to $60,000.

With little state and insurance aid, it's one of the largest out-of-pocket health expenses millennials face. A 2015 survey found that more than one-quarter of women aged twenty-five to thirty-four accrued an average of $30,000 of debt after undergoing fertility treatment. Some raid their 401(k)s, take out loans, borrow money from relatives, or start GoFundMe campaigns. I once reported on how cash-strapped millennials were forced to turn to their parents for IVF treatment costs. But as you can imagine, mixing family, money, and reproductive health has its own complications—for example, grandparents who believe they wield certain rights over a child they personally paid for.[28]

The procedure is worth it if it means a little bundle of joy at the end though, right?

Well, that's where it gets tricky. Success highly depends on an individual's age when they freeze their eggs and on the freezing technique. While egg freezing boasts its share of success stories, it also involves numerous eggs that don't survive the thawing period, fertilization, embryo progression, implantation, etc. The chances of a single frozen egg resulting in a live birth for women under the age of thirty-eight is between 2 and 12 percent, according to the American Society for Reproductive Medicine.[29] One stat you won't see on a peppy social media post: of the approximately 2.5 million IVF cycles performed annually,

---

[†] On average, egg freezing patients will spend between $30,000 and $40,000 on treatment, medication, and storage, according to family planning resource FertilityIQ. Women average 2.1 cycles, each of which can cost up to $20,000.

a staggering 2 million do not succeed, which puts the global IVF cycle failure rate at nearly 80 percent.[30]

A lot of confusion exists as to what constitutes "success" in this sector. Are we discussing the success of retrieving and storing eggs, of getting pregnant, or of actually having a baby at the end of the process? A lot of accurate but misleading numbers are floating around. Rates are hard to analyze because egg freezing is still so new—many who put their eggs on ice haven't retrieved them yet. But there's no confusion about the fact that fertility takes a nosedive as we age, something we might prefer to ignore.

In 2014, a marketing executive named Brigitte Adams graced the cover of *Bloomberg Businessweek* with the headline FREEZE YOUR EGGS, FREE YOUR CAREER. Wearing a black dress and heels, and with her hand defiantly positioned on her hip, the blond professional became the "poster child for egg freezing." At age thirty-nine, Adams spent $19,000 icing her future plans as she continued searching for Mr. Right. She later started an egg freezing educational website and digital community called Eggsurance.

Six years later, at forty-five, Adams picked a sperm donor and cashed in her coupon—to disappointing results. Some of her eleven eggs didn't survive the thawing process, while others failed to fertilize or turned out to be genetically abnormal. Only one egg produced a normal embryo. That one resulted in a chemical pregnancy, which is a very early pregnancy loss shortly after implantation. By then, there were no more eggs to retrieve.

"I never imagined that my egg freezing gamble would end this way," she wrote on her website, lamenting how long she'd waited to start the defrosting process. In an interview with the *Washington Post*, Adams noted that there wasn't enough discourse about "part two"—what happens when women try to use their thawed eggs—and that the "huge marketing hype" crumbles in the face of biological reality.[31]

Egg freezing technology is certainly improving, and doctors I interviewed note that many traditional clinics' messaging and approach differs from that of startups. Still, women are starting to take a harder look at what's a more complicated medical process than they might have initially assumed, but usually only after having invested considerable financial and emotional effort.

Grace Clarke, a marketing and content consultant in New York, spent four years saving up enough money to freeze her eggs with Kindbody at the age of thirty-two. But the experience proved less than optimal. Clarke says there wasn't nearly enough emphasis on educating her on probable outcomes—that is, how many harvested eggs might result in a live birth. In the end, she felt she did nothing more than buy uncertainty. "The biggest issue is that Instagram and social media have trained us to not dig deep and explore the truth, to take marketing slogans at face value," Clarke holds. "I would do anything, anything, anything, to help other people understand what it took me four years, nine thousand dollars, ten pounds, tons of shots, and a breakup to learn: Egg freezing is not a calendar date. It is an expensive marginal increase on your odds."‡

Now, I am not invalidating the miracle of modern reproductive assistance, which I myself have sought. No one can deny that reproductive technologies help couples start families. For women diagnosed with infertility, endometriosis, or undergoing chemotherapy, these new technologies have been a lifeline.

But we need more acknowledgement that many individuals put their faith in the process only to meet heartbreaking losses. There is concern that young women are not sufficiently informed about the odds they might not get a baby in the end. Success is dependent on an individual's biology; there's a lot of variability in outcomes. No one should consider it an "insurance policy"—insurance policies offer guarantees, while egg freezing does not. This misconception is also a testament to how uninformed some American women are about their own bodies, or how they're advised to brush off fertility until it's too late—or both.

---

‡ The exact measure of increased odds is hard to determine because it is so individualized and impacted by age. There's also little long-term data.

Not all women are educated enough about fertility, which means they are also not armed to make the right decisions during pivotal years. So, at the very least, egg freezing start-ups are inspiring individuals to learn more about their bodies. But some might question: Should they be the ones doing this?

But also, what in our culture has led us to a point where egg-freezing clinics are rolling through cities? We've revered cultural milestones—homeownership, career success, and paying off student debt—without always aligning them with childbearing years. Our society doesn't always make it easy for many women to have kids at a biologically preferable time. America inadvertently incentivizes the delay of motherhood: women who reproduce before age thirty-five never see their pay recover relative to their partners' pay.[32] Paltry work-life support structures, as evidenced by the lack of subsidized childcare, limited parental leave, or more flexible opportunities for working moms, are designed to make women wait. But fertility won't.

There are other reasons too. Hopeful grandparents might accuse women of being workaholic careerists who won't supply them with a grandchild until they've reached the C-suite (a charge never directed at men). *Obsessed with work*, they complain about their ambitious daughters. But according to one Yale research study, the chief reason women wait is that they're still looking for a committed partner.[33] Many women report that potential mates are unwilling to settle down or are uninterested in parenthood anytime soon. Of course, they can forgo a partner and seek a family on their own, but that's not easy; raising and affording a child is hard even with two parents in the picture these days.

The reason behind the interest in egg freezing is that people feel they don't have very good options, says Josephine Johnston, a bioethicist at the Hastings Center. "They're trying to gain some modicum of control, even if it's imperfect and even if it's not a guarantee," she explains. When they don't feel they're in a position to have a child during their childbearing years, then at least they can do *something* to try to preserve their fertility.[34]

But—echoing the clean beauty issue—the impetus is on women to preplan a solution for a culture they feel isn't looking out for them. With so little support, it's up to them to empty their pockets to fix the problem, and the problem is women's bodies. When Kindbody's website includes "facts" such as "You'll never be more fertile than you are today," the company sends a rather alarmist message: a responsible woman needs to take medical action now before her fertility further declines.[35] Our biology is therefore something that must be *managed*.

Egg freezing is generally available only to those who either pay for it on their own or receive financial assistance via a top-tier workplace benefit. Companies like Apple, Facebook, and Google offer egg freezing at the request of female employees (thereby setting industry standards), but Johnston believes we need to identify the root causes of involuntary childlessness. "People say this [workplace benefit] is what women want. Well, why do they want that? Because everything else is against them. 'This is the only choice because I don't have the options I want.'"

Younger generations hear horror stories from women who waited too long and simply want to avoid any heartbreak. Their motivation is better described as future damage control. One egg freezing hopeful told the *New York Times*, "I wear sunscreen to protect myself from future sun damage. I work out to keep off my weight. Why would I not do something to prevent future emotional pain and suffering?"[36]

Others worry about how casually some marketing treats egg freezing. They're concerned that it propels younger women to believe they don't have to worry about fertility until later in life—a luxury usually afforded only to men. *Come flex your feminist muscles, flex your workplace independence* is the potential takeaway, according to Miriam Zoll, the author of *Cracked Open: Liberty, Fertility, and the Pursuit of High Tech Babies*.

Liberation—from conformity, authority, biology, or "the patriarchy"—has become a mainstay thread for the advertising and marketing industries, infusing consumerism with cherished American ideals. Carl Elliott opines in his fantastic book *Better than Well*, "Americans have a hard time resisting anything that can be phrased in terms of self-determination. Autonomy, liberty, freedom: these are among our most powerful words."[37]

Egg freezing companies by no means promise women anything, but there is legitimate concern that the nuance gets lost in translation.

This is not an argument against egg freezing or IVF. We're so very lucky to live in a time in which women have options and the ability to seek reproductive assistance. Instead, the concern is that commercialization promotes a still nascent, complex technology to women. One study published in the journal the *New Bioethics* found that many fertility clinics engaged in deceptive advertising by selling the procedure persuasively, not informatively, all while minimizing risks and the low birth rate.[38]

As most any doctor will tell you, for every success story, there are many disappointed women. Even the most promising breakthroughs can have their limits.

Enhancing Human Potential or Wielding Hope?

Hidden beneath layers of clever marketing, the wellness industry beckons with a far stronger, more seductive message than relief or escape. The carrot it dangles in front of women is the one thing they desperately desire: control. Women are promised they can manage the chaos ruling their life by following a laid-out plan: eat right, exercise, meditate, then buy or do all this stuff. This mass consumerism is a vehicle for harnessing everything that feels turbulent in their lives.

The allure of control is communicated throughout wellness. Fitfluencers transform the sluggish to the masterful. Spiritual influencers hawk crystals to help followers snag a coveted job promotion. "Clean" snacks dangle a disease-free future. Woven throughout lies the message that you can manipulate what is unruly, subpar, or standing in the way of progress. Buy it, use it, think it—and you're back in the driver's seat. All noteworthy goals. We *should* try to take control of our health. We should take responsibility, as much as possible, for what we eat, how we sleep, and how much movement we engage in. But there's a significant distinction between what we can actually manage and what is out of our hands. When it comes to new scientific advancements, at what point do we admit we're denying real limitations? Or relinquishing control to brands and leaders as a costly crutch?

We start to think anything is possible, partially because wellness ads tell us health can be attained, maintained, and elevated. "But every time you reach a milestone, the goalpost moves farther away," says Sarah Greenidge, the founder of WellSpoken, an organization committed to regulating wellness brands to ensure that they provide credible information. "It keeps you chasing wellness, which makes sense—it keeps you always consuming. You can always be more well, more in control." As the market grows bigger and ever more encompassing in all areas of life, organizations like WellSpoken attempt to course correct an industry showing signs of growing pseudoscience.

"The wellness industry has thrived on a very low-health-literate, high-disposable-income consumer," says Greenidge, who hopes to rein in brands and educate consumers. WellSpoken consultants partner with companies, content creators, and influencers to offer guidelines on how to communicate their messaging. Their goal is to crack down on false claims and exaggerated solutions to the very many issues we're now told we can manage.

Most physicians, in contrast, will rarely promise full control or guaranteed results. They won't definitively say they'll cure patients of serious cancer or that you'll live to be 180, which is why they're not the leaders of this movement. Gurus gather the masses with assurance, not probability. Or as the author and biochemist Isaac Asimov once said: "Inspect every piece of pseudoscience and you will find a security blanket, a thumb to suck, a skirt to hold."

It's comforting. When we feel overwhelmed, these rituals—like popping a morning supplement—make us feel safer. But the truth is, life is wild. You cannot control everything. Longevity, least of all from a glass bottle, is never guaranteed. Even Dave Asprey cannot control everything, despite his claims of stalling aging and plans to live past what's humanly possible. On Twitter, biohacking fans observe that the forty-seven-year-old founder is *graying*. His thick mane reveals him to be a biological normie. They ask: What's up with the "perennially haggard" look? Why wasn't he able to fully reverse his hair color? Why does he already "look 135 years old"?

While real scientific breakthroughs and advancements occur, we also need to recognize the limits of science. The way that wellness has been commodified by gurus drawing from science and then exaggerating results spreads the toxic positivity message that you can fully accomplish what is an impossible goal. But bodies, even the best bodies, eventually betray us. No one will ever be completely healthy forever. We can't stop the aging process. At a certain point, our biology breaks down. That's nature.

Chapter 11

Democratizing Wellness: Pushing Back Against "Wellthness"

Nestled on the Sunset Strip, a block from the famous Chateau Marmont, Remedy Place is no mere gym. It is a members-only wellness social club—a place where booze is banned and health is served through IV drips.

Here, L.A.'s richest and presumably healthiest get first dibs on the hottest new workout trends. They treat themselves to "detoxifying" infrared saunas. They submerge their bodies in subzero cryotherapy chambers. They engage in power networking over yoga mats. It is, as the founder and wellness adviser to the stars Jonathan Leary told me, a space for people of a certain status to hang out and be active, not unlike a twenty-first-century country club. It is what he calls "social self-care."

But the kombucha-flowing happy hours don't come cheap. Monthly memberships start at $495, capped at two hundred members. Remedy Place doesn't have to worry about selling spots; before it even opened, celebrities, entertainment industry elites, and pro athletes came calling. Nike sent its executive team to check it out, followed by Goop. As Leary told me when I visited during the week of the club's opening, "in a place like L.A., people do love some type of exclusivity."

I reported on Remedy Place in the context of other new spaces marrying high-end fitness with elite hobnobbing. There is also L.A.'s Monarch Athletic Club, which charges $1,000 to $2,000 *per month* for access to unlimited private training along with a recovery suite, IV therapy, and a nutrition bar.

In New York, an exclusive fitness lounge called GHOST bills itself as an "architectural playground" full of art, boutique classes, live DJ sets, a marble boxing ring, and luxury amenities like Himalayan salt infrared saunas. At $3,000 a year (on top of a $400 registration fee), Ghost is, as the founder describes it, "the Soho House of fitness." It's primarily invite-only but you can try to get in: access entails a thorough application process digging into a prospect's job and lifestyle interests. An in-person interview is required. Imagine the college application process—but with your Instagram account in place of a personal essay. And just like getting into Harvard, membership connotes status, affirmation that you are good enough.

The Manhattan boutique workout studio The Ness permits a small percentage of new clients by way of a member referral system, which means newcomers are vetted and vouched for by those already accepted. "If you're hosting a dinner party at your house, would you just post flyers of the invite and say everyone come over for dinner? No, you invite your friends," co-founder Colette Dong told me of her mostly female clientele. "We feel the same way about fitness in terms of garnering a community . . . [Our clients] feel really comfortable and let loose."[1]

If wellness is already the new luxury signifier, these places have escalated it to a new echelon. It's no longer enough where you work out, but *with whom* you work out. You need to know the right people, be in the right shape, and offer something in return—social cachet—for application approval. It's the next step for those who see fitness intertwined with their personal brand. Wellness, it could be said, is now a doorway to exclusivity.

Makes sense, if only because the wellness economy now mirrors American income inequality, where the middle class gets smaller and smaller, to the point where only a disfigured hourglass remains: democratic models like the YMCA on one end and affluent boutique gyms on the other. You're either going budget or you're going luxe. But the luxe seems to be winning, the hourglass squeezed ever tighter, more lopsided. "It's much easier to target the one percent than it is to really come up with a model for the ninety-five percent," says Beth McGroarty, director of research at the Global Wellness Institute. "Community is now the entrance and aspiration."[2]

While the upper class perfects their downward dog, the communities most in need of physical exercise profoundly lack it. Apart from the limited number of gyms or recreational centers in rural areas, many can't access parks or safe outdoor spaces. A 2018 study found that three-quarters of wealthy individuals exercise on most days, compared to a quarter of lower-income populations.[3] That gap, researchers suggest, will only widen further.*

Wealth and wellness are near synonymous terms these days, morphing the idea of health as a necessity into one of indulgence. Premier health clubs are but a chia seed in the granola bowl of upscale wellness. Fitbit released fitness tracking jewelry. Beboe THC vape pens are referred to as the "Hermès of marijuana." When I did a story on Goop selling $90 vitamin packs, Clare Varga, head of beauty at trend forecasting firm WGSN, summed up the "wellthness" trend: "It's become aspirational," she said. "It's an investment and demonstration of self-value with a healthy body becoming the ultimate must-have fashion accessory." You'll see this

---

* The fix isn't simple. Even if gyms, parks, or digital health trackers are made available to underprivileged groups, it's not a given they'll have time to use them.

reflected in pop culture. If a film wants to connote an affluent Type A woman, she'll, sure enough, be shown furiously pedaling in a cycling class or dressed in head-to-toe athleisurewear.

It's not just what we buy or do, but where we live. Gated health-focused communities and condo buildings compose what will soon be a $180 billion wellness real estate market.[4] The upper crust is scooping up homes equipped with posture-supportive heat reflexology floors, mood-enhancing aromatherapy, and vitamin C–infused showers. Rounding out their in-house staff, they employ a 24/7 "personal wellness assistant" to remind them to exercise, meditate, or to tend to any "emergency" wellness needs, like, I assume, replacing an empty oat milk carton.

Take Troon Pacific, a development company selling sleep-enhanced homes with over-the-top health amenities such as built-in bedroom speakers programmed with guided meditation. It made headlines when it listed a "wellness-focused" mansion in the Bay Area. The 8,350-square-foot estate incorporated "biophilic design" (nature-inspired architecture) and an entire floor dedicated to health and fitness—a gym, yoga deck, massage room, sauna, and steam shower. (The home, of course, also came equipped with a Tesla car charger.) "The greatest luxury in life is your health," Troon Pacific CEO and co-founder Gregory Malin told me, "and so wellness became our focus."[5] The house sold for nearly $20 million.

The wealthy always take trends to the extreme. Once a specific product or idea becomes popular, then people want the fancy version. When everyone has a TV, then comes the demand for sophisticated, voice-activated home entertainment systems. So too with wellness. As the sector grows and technology advances, it ratchets up more and more.[6] That's why you start seeing ads for ethically mined 24-karat gold dildos.

Wellness is more susceptible to scrutiny because of what it stands for, which consumers presume should be afforded to all. But it does make you think: How did wellness, the pursuit of health, become associated with luxury? And though these high-end efforts generally get the most attention, they certainly are not the majority. So who are the new players expanding the reach to more communities?

Drink Your Way to a Better Life

In one Instagram post, the curvy, striped beverage bottle sits on a vanity shelf alongside luxe brands: La Mer, Chanel, and the prestige skin care line Sunday Riley. In another, a manicured and jeweled hand grasps the bottle against a designer floral dress, like the last accessory of a perfect ensemble. There it is again as a model runs with the bottle down a hotel hallway. Sometimes it's the star attraction of an afternoon spent relaxing at a luxury pool. The brightly colored bottles are constantly spotted in posts of good-looking people engaged in fun, chic activities.

Why is Dirty Lemon—a health drink—acting like a vodka brand?

It is, at the end of the day, just water, lemon juice, and a teensy bit of activated charcoal. Yet the beverage brand promises you, quite literally, the world: globe-trotting adventure, allure, mystery, beauty, and sexiness. You could say Dirty Lemon is a line of functional elixirs with big ambitions. Beyond its social media fantasy, the collection of $6.99 drinks promises to transform one's body—it claims to improve digestion, stimulate liver function, and "gently cleanse your system of impurities." Consumers vaguely know the nutritional benefits of this expensive lemon water, but that's not what matters. What matters is that *it's cool*. And cool is the currency.

Dirty Lemon founder Zak Normandin told me he was inspired by skyrocketing start-ups such as the millennial beauty brand Glossier. He wondered: Why can't we do the same for health tonics? So Dirty Lemon incorporated lifestyle photography that spoke "around" the juices. The company also purposely designed the product to stand out on a 2x3-inch screen—bright colors, minimal wording—so it could be the star of an Instagram post. Unlike other product categories—such as a vacuum cleaner—wellness beverages lend themselves to be photographed everywhere. You can shoot them in a convertible, at the beach, in the bath. A mattress, no matter how trendy, can't pull that off.[7]

Almost every wellness brand sells some sort of mythical state of bliss on Instagram, their preferred playground. Their sales pitch is less about health benefits and more about something stronger: a feeling. It's about feeling good, feeling in control, feeling attractive. Brands are counting on you buying a fantasy, not unlike the fashion industry's tactics. Kombucha, supplement brands, and collagen proteins use the same playbook, populating Instagram with imagery of smiling models seemingly enjoying a life of sugarless beverages on an empty stomach. For detox tea, it's flat tummies and opulent white marble kitchens, while collagen powder brands prefer athletic types posing in the lush outdoors.

This is partially because luxury marketers, publicists, and branding consultants now work for the wellness economy. All the PR firms that once pitched me as a journalist on fashion labels and high-end restaurants a decade ago currently represent supplement brands and "natural" food or beverage companies. But that's to be expected when the wellness industry doesn't always lead with science, but coalesces around emotion and consumerism.

Once celebrities entered the wellness fray, the aspiration factor skyrocketed. Halle Berry has a wellness site. Kristen Bell launched a premium CBD skin care brand. Miranda Kerr became an organic beauty mogul. Not to mention the slew of stars either fronting or investing in snack brands or fitness tech. They work in an ecosystem where they send their goods to their other celebrity pals, who then further promote the brand in their glossy kitchens. When you see Oprah hawking Clevr Blends, a $28 powdered instant latte brand advertised as "made with brain-boosting, mind-clearing, mood-lifting ingredients," it *might* be because she believes in all those claims. But it's also likely because her pal Meghan Markle is an investor. Celebs know an opportunity when they see one. They're businesspeople as much as they are entertainers.

The same goes for Goop. While Paltrow and her company do not offer one single answer to being well, a seductive philosophy runs through Goop's veins: trendy experimentation leads to control, and with control comes enlightenment. But enlightenment certainly won't come fast, and it won't come cheap. A dizzying stream of pills, clothing, and accessories is crucial for this mission—conduits for an ailment-free paradise, just within your credit card's reach. These are hopes repackaged in millennial-pink canisters. This arsenal of luxury products, presumably, could help one look and feel just like Gwynnie herself. Or, as Paltrow once explained to Harvard Business School students, "it's crucial to me that we remain aspirational."

This is the magic of Goop's allure—Paltrow looks good on the outside, a mirage presumed to be the consequence of what she consumes on the inside. Goop's leader isn't just selling the pretty millennial-pink canister; she *is* the millennial-pink canister. And she's able to sell it by creating a "culture of lack," wherein you're always on the cusp of missing something to achieve the desired state. By peppering in a few relatable anecdotes, she convinces you there's no distinction between her—a Hollywood megastar—and you, the consumer.

"I do think in my case, eventually always the pros of [celebrity] outweigh the cons because I can go into any market and talk about what I'm doing, and that's a powerful lever to be able to pull," Paltrow told me during an interview on her supplement line.[8]

"We tend to trust the names we recognize," explains Sheril Kirshenbaum, the co-author of *Unscientific America: How Scientific Illiteracy Threatens Our Future*, because we're hardwired to gravitate toward that which we know and aspire to. We're living in an Instagram culture that draws us in, wherein we want to enter the orbit of the beautiful, rich, and put-together. Paltrow presumably lives a lifestyle we want. In contrast, we don't know many scientists or academics personally. So it makes sense we'd honor a connection to someone we, at the very least, recognize from award shows.

"Following these personalities gives us a false sense of connection, but a sense of belonging that many people are probably really yearning for,"

Kirshenbaum points out. "They want to be part of a community. They want to be accepted. They want to feel smart. They want to feel like they're part of something bigger and maybe that they're making these healthy, socially conscious decisions for their own households, families, and children. By following these influencers, they can be part of that."

Molding one's appearance is one of the easiest ways to gain access to this culture, to signify we are "pursuing health." You just need to accessorize with the "right" clothing and accessories. Your attire signifies you have the time—if not the resources—to work out. To be well. It's how we made sleek $50 S'well reusable water bottles—for God's sake, water bottles—a status symbol. Women's magazines, meanwhile, do their part when they position an arsenal of CBD tinctures as a gateway to the cool kids' table. In a culture obsessed with ambition and physical attractiveness, wellness props are the ultimate signal: I'm driven. I work hard. *This is who I am.*

Groups of women in workout leggings flanked by juice bottles are no different from Harley-Davidson biker gangs. They have a distinctly different appearance (Barbarella with a yoga mat), lingo ("Let me meditate on that"), and rituals (sage-clearing a new home). These cultural markers serve as deliberate borders to distinguish them from the masses.[9] To join them, you need to swear allegiance: buy the swag, perform the lunges. Those who do are greatly rewarded—they get to belong. And like anything in life, the more you give of yourself to something, the more "it" defines you. In time, the truth of what we need to live healthily no longer matters because one's whole self-image is wrapped up in these beliefs.

There's a big motivation to join wellness culture because it's fashionable. A woman might feel a surge of self-esteem for participating in the crowned culture. She can feel empowered for prioritizing her body, and by extension, herself. She flaunts her participation on her social media channels, letting friends know that wellness is a core pillar of her lifestyle. These postings affect those in her circle: One study found that exercise habits are susceptible to social influence and peer pressure, which means you take up running to get fit, but maybe also to keep up with your health-centric friends.[10]

If dental care became the next symbol of self-care, I assure you there would suddenly be a flush of women posting pictures of themselves flossing.

Since our culture is based in part on capitalism, the wellness industry has become, in part, reflective of our individualist and consumerist culture. (You're not going to stop Americans from buying stuff—that's how we express ourselves.) The movement may have sprung from revolutionary roots, but it has since divorced itself from an anti-establishment ethos to grow as bloated as the establishments it once rallied against.

Now, I am not one who cannot enjoy a bit of fantasy and luxury. I've subscribed to *W* and *Vogue* since I was thirteen. But what separates wellness (or what claims to be wellness) from other sectors is that health should not be associated with class, image, or five-star hotel pools. Inevitably, the messaging becomes intertwined. We start to conflate health with specific kinds of people or products because that's all we're accustomed to seeing—a very narrow *appearance* of health. If thin, wealthy, and attractive are all we're trained to see, that becomes our automatic factory setting.

Not everyone appreciates this new culture. I spoke with an executive of a popular at-home fitness equipment company that was making inroads with older consumers frustrated by millennial gym rats who made them feel insecure with their flagrant displays of body perfection and Lululemon fashion shows. At home, no one could judge their average arms, let alone a ratty college T-shirt. They said they missed the nineties, when "people weren't afraid to look like crap at the gym."

Luxury wellness marketing is most puzzling when it comes to self-care, which was stripped down to sparkly stuff to lure affluent women. Companies will make you believe that their product is crucial to achieving relaxation and therefore take advantage of your (sleep-deprived) vulnerabilities. But there is no uniformity to stress relief, as everyone has their own particular burden and their own preferred mode of relief.

Barbara Riegel, a professor of biobehavioral health sciences at the University of Pennsylvania and a leading researcher on self-care, considers most marketed solutions merely fleeting self-soothing techniques. Real self-care, by her professional definition, is more aligned with both physiological and psychological health maintenance, including nutrition, sleep hygiene, exercise, and illness symptom management. These are not things that need the snazziest device or hippest boutique class. "Self-care has been taken over by marketing," says Riegel, who adds that her fellow international researchers are confused by all this talk of facials and tech. "This is a U.S. phenomenon."

Other industry experts agree that wellness is indeed a global trend, but what's going on with American women is something else. It is a mania not replicated in certain European countries where they have better work-life balance, more communal societies, and a more attentive (or socialized) medical healthcare system. Some have policies in place that support self-care. Sweden, for example, set up a 24/7 open hotline for registered nurses to respond to citizens' non-urgent health issues. One Italian academic told me, "We take two-hour lunches with friends or coworkers to eat fresh food and we receive four weeks mandated vacation. I'm not sure my country *needs* all this wellness."

Self-care does not require a SoulCycle class, Sephora shopping spree, or Bali spa retreat. Oddly, a large percentage of these pricey solutions were thrown out the window during the COVID-19 pandemic. Women quickly learned they could sometimes get the same results with smaller, more affordable activities, like going for a hike.

On one hand, commodification skews health initiatives and intimidates those who cannot buy fancy products. But on the other hand, the aspirational aspect has inspired more people to participate. I used to go with friends to boozy brunches on weekends—now we go to yoga. It's not a zero-sum game. Whether for the right reasons or not, more women are focused on their health these days. It's fun. It's cool. It's *joyful*. It's no longer the drudgery we once thought it was. Women might buy a meditation app membership instead of a purse, or spend a Sunday at the gym instead of the mall. Maybe because of the market, they become aware of solutions that really can help them. Mental health is probably the best example of this. In the span of just a few years, mental wellness went from taboo to widespread discussion. Then, as technological advancement pushed therapy and support groups to the forefront of convenience, the category expanded well beyond the usual stakeholders.

As wellness gains more traction, more and more people demand access. They, in time, innovate solutions that fit their specific requirements. I've profiled a BIPOC-worker-owned yoga cooperative in South Central L.A. and mental health apps catering to underserved communities with diverse therapists. You can no longer say wellness is strictly for a certain person: more groups have joined the fray. Even that which starts off with upscale circles can be adapted to suit others in need. It is, as one wellness researcher described to me, "trickle-down wellness."

Take Timeshifter, a personalized jet lag app first popular with business travelers, pro athletes, and anyone keen to optimize every hour while traveling. Now Timeshifter is working to bring its wellness app to shift workers who possess unique health risks, including an increased risk of diabetes, heart disease, and even certain cancers due to circadian rhythm disruption and lack of sleep. These are people in manufacturing, construction, mining, delivery, the military, and medical care; nurses, soldiers, and truckers who are more at risk of drowsy driving, which increases the risk of fatal car crashes on the commute home. Many of these professions have a high proportion of women, such as nursing, where the night shift is par for the course.

Luxury is to *some degree* where we're at. In most media outlets, wellness is generally presented through the prism of a very specific lifestyle, potentially spurring ageism, ableism, and elitism. But the average gymgoer does not come from a "sleep-enhanced house," nor do they frequent a fitness studio to flex their superiority muscles. Gyms (and streets) are filled with people of all colors, backgrounds, and professions. Most are just looking to get in some exercise or release some tension from having been glued to an office chair all week.

Flashback: When Female Complaints Made Way for Female Pressures

What would a combination of Oprah, Gywneth, and Estée Lauder look like? Lydia Pinkham, the inventor of the most popular health tonic in nineteenth-century America. Pinkham's face graced newspapers. Her herbal concoctions sat atop every pharmacy counter. She even inspired folk songs.

In 1875, the Massachusetts native created Pinkham's Vegetable Compound. It was advertised as made with "natural" ingredients, and Pinkham claimed it was superior to whatever the medical industry was hawking. Her advice? "Let doctors alone." Each bottle contained life root, unicorn root, black cohosh, and fenugreek seed suspended in 19 percent alcohol. Pinkham was a strict temperance advocate, but the family business had no qualms about selling forty-proof bottles of booze.

Pinkham's concoction promised to cure all female "weaknesses," of which there were many: menstrual pains, headaches, kidney issues, uterine prolapse, labor pains, indigestion, faintness, addictions, "floodings," "irregularities," and flatulence. It was a broad cure-all, but some of these terms had hidden meanings. As Sarah Stage writes in *Female Complaints*, "floodings" and "irregularities" were a wink and a nod to those seeking an abortion.[11]

What separated this tonic from the competition? Each bottle featured a sophisticated profile illustration of the dignified, middle-aged Pinkham. Seemingly wise, compassionate, and sturdy, people compared her to the Mona Lisa or Lady Liberty. Pinkham came across as someone you knew, someone you could trust. Pinkham used this to her advantage when she encouraged women to write to her with their problems, which she would answer and often publish as testimonials. It was a novel concept back then: building a personal connection with a brand. Hundreds of women per month wrote in complaining of issues that Pinkham shrewdly blamed on an era ill-suited for women. Pinkham's ads described how the American woman was "expected to play a complex role of many duties, some of which are entirely incompatible with each other." A woman was made to keep order in the house, bear and raise the children, cook fine meals, do all the shopping, and potentially work outside the house . . . all while looking and acting presentable. "Sometimes a servant and always a lady," is how she put the burden foisted on women. The same copy could run today.[12]

Following Lydia's death in 1883, Pinkham's Vegetable Compound shifted its focus from health to that of appearance. Beautiful women invested in their health, read the new copy. The compound would "cleanse" and beautify the body, thereby restoring women's chief power: their looks. "There is no secret about a woman's beauty; it all lies in the care she devotes to herself, to removing from her system all poisonous impurities, and keeping at bay those fearful female diseases," read one ad.

Shortly thereafter, the marketing shifted again to exemplify upper-middle-class women of leisure. But the marketing illustrations didn't line up with the clientele: wealthy people could afford physicians. It was the working class who resorted to over-the-counter tonics. The new company owners understood that status is aspirational, and that customers would want to believe that they— alongside the gloved and stylish—were *peers* relying on the very same product. They too wanted in on what the respectable and rich possessed, "if not real, then vicarious."[13]

Branching Out Beyond a Narrow Representation

Each morning at six o'clock, Maggie Holub begins her work tending to corn and soybean crops on her five-hundred-acre farm in Scribner, Nebraska. Born and raised here, farming is in her blood. She was raised with hogs and chickens. Tinkering with irrigation systems and fertilizing crops are second nature to her. Although, Holub didn't expect to run a farm in her twenties; her original plan was to join the family-owned farm once her father retired. Unfortunately, in 2014, he passed away from terminal brain cancer at just fifty-one, thereby accelerating the succession plan. Holub went from some-time helper to full-time third-generation farmer. Today, the friendly and approachable Holub operates and fixes all the farming equipment and hauls all of the grain with two semitrucks and trailers.

But Holub has another passion—one that she's increasingly sharing with others: fitness.

Three evenings a week, Holub packs a trailer filled with dumbbells, yoga mats, and other exercise equipment. Her destination? Anywhere that lacks organized fitness in her rural vicinity. As a trained exercise instructor, Holub runs a mobile gym that sets up shop in neighboring small towns that lack not only exercise facilities but also adequate broadband Internet service. These are people who cannot just watch a streaming fitness class or buy a Peloton. "In any large metro area, there's a gym on every corner and you can go there twenty-four hours a day," says Holub. "We don't have that." In the summer months, she leads cardio strength routines outdoors. In the winter, she scouts for indoor spaces like high school gyms or community centers.

Outsiders assume that rural populations don't need group fitness classes or gyms because they have access to the outdoors. But residents in isolated communities are often at risk for health conditions. For one thing, there are no sidewalks, bike paths, or street lamps in some areas, making safety a legit-imate concern. Or it's freezing cold half the year and they cannot comfortably run or walk outside. Not to mention that many people simply don't enjoy walking or running. Some need a communal outfit to hold them accountable.

In farming communities, there can be a stigma against fitness culture. Farmers might presume exercise is unnecessary since they already move their bodies all day on the land. But there's a real need for everyone else around them, such as their partners or kids who lack adequate movement. That Holub shows up in their neighborhood and charges only $2 a class leaves few excuses for them not to participate. Lots of people, many of them women, flock to Holub's classes. They come to exercise and to socialize—interactions they crave when they're often quite isolated. "You have to go out of your way in rural Nebraska to go be with or meet somebody else," says Holub.

Farmers are one group among many trying to better represent their needs. They even have their own influencers who speak to their specific agriculture community. They might not, for example, take an interest in veganism or plant-based diets if they raise cattle and their family loves meat. Social media posts show more barbecues and beer than avocado toast and almond milk. As one dairy farmer fitfluencer put it, "I wanted to show people that you can still consume dairy, achieve the results you want, and thrive while doing so."[14]

Women on farms have concerns that differ from those of corporate career women in metropolitan areas. In place of bad bosses and meeting fatigue, they battle environmental stressors and machinery breakdowns. They juggle a hectic schedule of feeding farm animals and caring for their families. In one post detailing the importance of self-care, one woman wrote, "We pour our hearts into animal welfare, church potlucks, and [the] county fair. Our anxiety is guided by the weather, the markets and consumer demands. Most of the time we leave it in God's hands and pour another cup of coffee. But friends, no matter how many times you reheat it in the microwave . . . you cannot continue to pour from an empty cup."

Plenty of independent trailblazers are charting a new course in health initiatives. Despite a large Hispanic population, hardly any Spanish-led yoga classes were available in Miami. The bilingual yoga teacher Rina Jakubowicz recalled Hispanic women telling her, "It's for white people, it's not for us." Others expressed concern that it was a religious practice at odds with their faith. But Jakubowicz sensed interest. So she established a bilingual yoga teacher training course, which was then accredited by Yoga Alliance. Her first students included a cleaning and cooking crew who worked for her yoga studio employer. "They didn't think they could do anything else in the U.S. besides cleaning houses. It was really empowering," says Jakubowicz, who has since run several training courses. "They were really grateful to have somebody willing to spend time to teach and connect with them instead of just looking at them as labor. Now they can go out and teach."[15]

The landscape is shifting. I hear from Black women who say they're teaching yoga to rap music and not what they deem "dying whale music." They wear baggy T-shirts emblazoned with the names of hip-hop groups instead of Lululemon gear. The Black Yoga Teachers Alliance, a nonprofit and professional membership organization, counts hundreds of teachers, and its Facebook group has swelled to six thousand. Leaders believe there is still a way to go in terms of representation and access, but they sound optimistic.

These are just several of countless innovative contributions in fitness, though maybe you haven't heard of them. One reason you might associate wellness with overpriced juice bottles is because that's what clogs Instagram and mass media. Look at your local news or even hop on neighborhood Facebook groups and you'll notice a plethora of independently led initiatives working to close the health gap. I think that's important to remember before bashing the entire industry. It's nuanced: there's some good, there's some bad. A few steps forward, then one or two back.

Wellness—real wellness—doesn't require all the fancy fixings touted by glamorous stars or pricey social clubs. People are starting to recognize that.

Get Together: New Wellness Communities

What I am most excited about in wellness are the communities being brought together. I feel strongly that connection is one of the most important pieces of the wellness puzzle and not emphasized nearly enough. I think about Ganja Goddess Getaway (now called Glowing Goddess Getaway), the women's cannabis retreat I described in the introduction. At first glance, it might seem just like an outdoor house party. But that retreat has a higher aim: deep connections.

Ganja Goddess Getaway co-founder and CEO Deidra Bagdasarian began hosting the retreats following the birth of her second child. "I was kind of isolated after having a baby," she told me. "I needed a women's event." Bagdasarian wanted to recharge and connect, but not in a superficial way.

Bagdasarian believes cannabis can be used "as a creative and spiritual tool" to help women get in touch with themselves and bond more easily with others. With a joint, new friends can cut down on the small talk and get to the real talk. "Cannabis helps take down our walls and be our authentic selves right from the beginning," she explains. I saw it firsthand as the Getaway participants divulged family secrets, embraced strangers, and swapped phone numbers. As soon as I would introduce myself and extend my arm for a handshake, women would laugh and bear-hug me instead. The slightest I overheard of bad blood was someone saying in a soft, compassionate voice that another member "needed to soak in some positivity." Later I spotted them laughing together by the pool.

What started as a modest retreat series with roughly fifty participants ballooned into one averaging two hundred. Then came smaller regional gatherings—free of charge—held every Sunday at, naturally, 4:20 p.m. (consumables are brought potluck-style). Bagdasarian wants to expand the retreat once more U.S. states legalize marijuana use, with a plan to go nationwide. "We just got so much feedback about how this was something that [these women] were missing in their life," says Bagdasarian. "All women are in need of sisterhood and a safe space—and cannabis, it turns out, works for everyone."

Getting people outdoors in a low-cost, communal manner is a trend gaining traction. Many Americans have limited budgets, barring them from club memberships or expensive at-home exercise equipment. At the same time, they increasingly value experiences, particularly those that put them face-to-face with others. Many organizations engage specific communities by organizing local hikes and nature outings, including Outdoor Asian, Fat Girls Hiking, Latino Outdoors, and others.

Even wellness real estate got a more accessible makeover (or at least more accessible than a $20 million wellness mansion). Haven is a co-living compound in Venice, California, that houses ninety-six strangers brought together by their commitment to wellness. Roommates get to live in a fully furnished adult dorm with a fitness studio, healthy cooking classes, a co-working space, meditation areas, and events ranging from star energy healing ("bring your crystals and water") to sound baths.

Compared to skyrocketing apartment rental prices in L.A., Haven is a far more affordable option (by more than half the cost for a one-bedroom), especially considering the add-on amenities. But residents aren't just here for the slashed rent or a full moon circle ceremony. They want, in their words, to "find their tribe." And many do among this diverse group of yoga mat–toting millennials, most of whom are independent contractors and entrepreneurs. These are yoga instructors, meditation teachers, and cannabis founders.

Residents are equal parts health enthusiasts and spiritually enlightened. They overuse words like "experiences," "energy," and "gratitude" to describe the frustration of sharing a bathroom with a dozen other housemates. "Everything is a journey" is how they described chore duty. When I visited, an upstairs bathroom was plastered in a dozen Post-it notes with scribbled affirmations such as "I trust my intuition fully" and "My life is unfolding exactly as it is meant to be." (This is where I felt a bit concerned for them: *Let them poop in peace.*)

But overall, life at Haven seems idyllic. Residents meditate or quietly journal on a living room couch while aromatherapy vapors roam the halls like calming spirits. They flip through tarot cards or work on their Burning Man project. Small groups grab surfboards and head to the beach, just a few blocks away. Or they bike ride to a nearby health market to buy ingredients for a communal vegan dinner. Residents explained that they were "a hundred times" happier sharing a 350-square-foot pod-style room with six other strangers than when they'd lived alone in luxury condo apartments.

An unorthodox living arrangement raises eyebrows. Haven residents are subjected to inquisitive questioning by friends and family, many of whom scoff at their cramped shared living quarters. Why, they wonder, would any mature adult decide to bunk with strangers? "Most of [the time] it's like, how's the cult?" said one resident. "People don't get it."[16]

Is it a cult? Or more like modern social survival? I asked a twenty-five-year-old yoga teacher named Katie why she decided to live at Haven. Katie said she had hustled her way through school and work, but there was no one to share her success with. "We live in this world where society celebrates getting to the top as fast as you can and doing it all on your own and getting your ginormous apartment and living by yourself," said Katie, "and then sometimes you question, *Why?* Why am I here by myself?"

Katie's new living arrangement changed all that. "The best thing [about Haven] is coming home and there's always somebody here," she said. There was one particular element that sealed the deal for Katie, and when she mentioned it, I realized how crucial something seemingly so small could be. It's likely something many of us who live with others—be it parents, spouses, or friends—take for granted: "You come home and they say 'Hey, how was your day?'" That, to her, was real wellness.

Chapter 12

Guides for the Perplexed

You don't hear much about Food Babe Vani Hari in the press anymore. Mainstream news networks seemingly stopped booking her. She's not as prevalent in women's outlets. Blogs criticized her up the wazoo.

Since her reputation's descent, grassroots efforts have sprung up to combat misinformation and aggressive marketing claims. One influencer who has more than three hundred thousand Instagram followers is a food scientist who has positioned herself as the anti–Food Babe. For safety and privacy reasons, the public knows only her first name, Erin, and she goes by the handle Food *Science* Babe. On social media platforms, you'll find Erin posting in-depth explanations as well as entertaining TikTok videos debunking food myths—everything from outsized concerns about GMOs to why certain ingredients are banned in Europe but not in the United States. "So many times an ingredient is actually not banned in Europe, it's just called something different," she told me with a twinge of exasperation. "In some cases, yes, *it is* banned in Europe, but that doesn't necessarily mean that it's unsafe."

Other times she's called upon to weigh in on whether secreted beaver butt goo is, as Vani Hari suggests, "lurking" in your vanilla ice cream.[1]

That gem keeps circulating on social media, prompting Erin to address it more than once. "I'm really sick of talking about beaver butts, but here we go again," she remarks in one video. Having worked in the food industry for over a decade—in both the organic and conventional sectors—Erin knows precisely when influencers are peddling pseudoscience or fabricating fears. "It's not very obvious sometimes that [Food Babe] is spreading misinformation," says Erin. "So much of it is not outwardly apparent to somebody that might not know. That's why I feel like it's even more harmful."

Approachable and funny, Food Science Babe Erin has converted a mass of women who were once like her. Before taking on her cheeky moniker, she was a strict organic devotee who shopped in accordance with the Dirty Dozen list, ate "clean," and excluded whole food groups. "It is a part of your belief system and almost like your identity to some extent," she says. Erin never questioned her beliefs because the messaging was so rampant. She just assumed it was true. She was so committed she went to work for an organic snack company to craft new products. But in helping this brand secure organic and non-GMO certifications, Erin saw firsthand how food marketing claims often have little or muddled scientific evidence. "I realized how arbitrary certifications were—just submitting paperwork, paying them, and then you get to put this label on your product," Erin told me. "This doesn't really mean it's healthier."

Erin also participated in marketing meetings that singularly focused on one target group: moms of young kids. "[Marketers would say] 'they're looking for these labels, they'll spend more for these labels.' It was never 'we want to make sure it's healthier' because that's not what those labels mean." Erin repeats what all those toxicologists told me about clean beauty: "It's really just marketing."

At the same time, the anxiety over what to feed her family was taking a toll on her health. As a working mom of a young child, Erin wondered: Why make shopping or eating tougher than it already is? Why are we torturing women? "It's just causing such unnecessary stress and fear . . . making somebody think that what they're feeding their kid is going to make them get cancer is just ridiculous." Erin often hears from scientists butting heads with their marketing teams that want to push fantastical packaging claims. "It's difficult when [the marketers] don't have the science background and it's the marketing that's being conveyed to consumers."

Erin quit her job and redirected her efforts to share what she knows with a thirsty public. An increasing number of women have turned their backs on the fearmongers of the Web to flock to her well of knowledge. Food Science Babe has racked up over 3 million likes on TikTok, where she posts hilarious videos of why it's absurd, for example, to say "I don't eat anything with chemicals." She's made inroads with parenting circles by explaining why orange juice cartons with a "non-GMO" label are a scam. (There are no GMO oranges, so *all* orange juice is automatically non-GMO.) "Anytime you create a label that says 'non' or 'free-of,' consumers are obviously going to think whatever isn't in there is somehow bad, because why else would you have that label?" says Erin. "But in reality, GMO crops are just as safe and at least as nutritious as their non-GMO counterparts."[2]

Her motto? "Facts, not fear."

Medical experts also attempt to educate the public on social media, proving: If you can't beat 'em, join 'em. Physicians are going so far as to establish their own influencer groups, which function much like talent agencies. Dr. Austin L. Chiang, an assistant professor of medicine at Thomas Jefferson University Hospital, co-founded the Association for Healthcare Social Media—the first nonprofit society for health professionals on social media. He believes the best way to counter misinformation is to transform doctors into the very thing threatening their authority. "In our medical training, we don't have any sort of marketing or communications training," says Dr. Chiang, "and yet we're expected to impact our communities and the general public."[3]

This rings true. Americans need to schedule an appointment to see a doctor, and few have a daily relationship with their primary care physician. In comparison, they can easily build a relationship with wellness influencers who share tips, then leave their DMs open for two-way communication. So if doctors once were siloed off in medical journals, now they're sharing evidence-based medicine in funny TikTok and Instagram clips. Why should influencers hold all the influential power?

Dr. Chiang believes that if medical professionals are trained as storytellers, it'll be easier to spread accurate science and challenge disinformation. If they need to learn some TikTok dance moves, so be it. During the COVID-19 vaccine rollout, Dr. Chiang could be found dancing in a white coat to "Good Day" by Nappy Roots as he explained the differences between the Pfizer and Moderna vaccines on TikTok. "Won't stop pandemic if not enough people get it," Dr. Chiang explained as he tossed his hair back and forth.[4]

The need for more scientific influencers became evident during the pandemic. Bizarre conspiracy theories about the vaccine—that they contain microchips, alter DNA, or enlarged Nicki Minaj's cousin's friend's balls—grew stronger by the day. Influencers got bolder. And they didn't need mainstream media acceptance to continue their work on social media.

Vani Hari, for one, was busy launching attacks on the FDA and spinning her wheels about . . . sanitizer. Hari worried that disinfectant booths were coming to your local school, airport, stores, and public places. She asked, What are these chemicals going to do to your skin? What do disinfectants do to the microbiome? Food Babe urged followers not to conform to this "madness," to protest those ushering in oversanitization. "If you don't want to be subjected to disinfectant spray booths everywhere you go, it's time to make your voice heard!" she wrote on Facebook. "Please tag your friends and family to warn them what might be coming. Now is the time to speak up, before it is too late."[5]

Hari plays up her unorthodox "outsider" status, no doubt appealing to those looking to join a passionate crusade or community. She consistently plays up the "us versus the rest of the world" rhetoric (literally the title of one of her book chapters), which undoubtedly makes readers feel they're a part of something revolutionary. In a public response to critics, she quoted

Mahatma Gandhi: "First they ignore you, then they laugh at you, then they fight you, then you win."[6] Except it wasn't Gandhi who said that; it was an early-twentieth-century trade union activist.

Aggravating the issue of how to best communicate scientific truth, the Internet serves up the more popular characters, like Vani Hari, with little to no vetting. Online, popularity wins. Algorithms are tailored to our individual biases, which means we read what we want to read. It gets hard to communicate with others because we all absorb different sources of information, says Sheril Kirshenbaum, the co-author of *Unscientific America*. "In many ways, we're all living on the same planet, but we are living in very different realities based on who we're listening to or coming into contact with." We can now, in effect, design our own reality, a kind of magical thinking suited to our desires. A modern-day Tower of Babel.

People also overestimate just how much they *think* they know in science. Kirshenbaum points to the drama over genetically modified foods that have parents clutching their pearl onions. She co-directed a national survey that revealed that despite fears over demonized GMOs, 45 percent of American adults did not even know that all food contains DNA.[7] "That's wild to me," says Kirshenbaum.

When it comes to affluent Americans, misinformation is sometimes even worse, thanks to rampant inaccuracies elevated in Facebook groups, marketing campaigns, or group texts. One survey asked people whether they avoid buying products containing "chemicals" at the grocery store, with 73 percent of higher-income participants responding yes, compared to 65 percent of those from lower-income households.[8] Researchers concluded, "We also observed that even though higher earners have more access to information about food, they are also more likely to be influenced by misinformation and pseudoscience."

It's not that these people aren't smart. It's that they weren't properly trained to understand the scientific process and how to be critical thinkers. "If we give everybody a much more solid understanding of how data gets collected and what's good methodology, what's cherry-picking . . . they would be a little more adept at recognizing when they're being manipulated or when something being reported might not reflect reality," says Kirshenbaum, "because it's very easy to fall for something, especially if you want to believe it."

Science illiteracy does far more damage than inducing stress and unnecessary shopping sprees. By mid-2020, I—as well as plenty of the science experts cited in this book—noticed a growing group of women falling prey to chemophobia. Some women were taught to fear all "chemicals," and in time, that philosophy poisoned their logical thinking. The fear migrates: If "chemicals" are bad in food, then what else are they bad in? Should I not get the vaccine? Should I shun all "unpronounceable" medicines? Should I just eat vegetables instead?

Digital communities help feed these fixations. Countless social media posts repeat "facts" that distort science and scare women. "I'm very nature-oriented and always strive for an organic vibe. [A vaccine] doesn't deliver on that front," wrote one "self-taught physician" on Twitter. Another pleaded, "Let's take our health back from these people who seek to fill our bodies with man-made chemicals."

"In some ways, COVID made [access to information] better, as far as science communicators realizing, 'I need to get out there and debunk stuff.' But at the same time, I feel like a lot of it got worse too," Erin told me. Pseudoscience pushers have gotten more confident, more vocal. It's difficult for science communicators such as Erin because their work is time-consuming: "It's easier to create content when you're just making stuff up and you're not actually having to double-check it or do research." Science communicators generally don't make a lot of money off these educational efforts, nor do they partner with supplements brands or sell a juice detox guide.

Erin is mixed on where we stand moving forward. "I feel like with every new science communicator that decides to start a page, ten more wellness influencers decide to start a page," she laughs. "I'm not sure if it is getting better or not!" And yet she's still out there every day as Food

Science Babe, answering women's questions and debunking ridiculous Pop-Tart ingredient claims. She receives messages "all the time" from women who say they stumbled upon her content, forcing them to rethink their beliefs. They're eager to learn. "I hope that people are seeking out more science communicators, and maybe it's easier for them to find us when we are on social media . . . Hopefully, it's getting better."

How can you, on your own, ensure that you are more scientifically literate when it comes to wellness? There's no easy guide to this ever-growing industry, or to one's health. But here are some takeaways I like to keep in mind:

Remember that wellness isn't one-size-fits-all. It's great that Moon Juice guru Amanda Chantal Bacon starts her morning with calendula tea, green juice, three tablespoons of bee pollen, a shot of pressed turmeric root in freshly squeezed grapefruit juice, and something called "activated cashews." But that might leave one a little hangry. It might not be for you.

Health is specific to an individual's needs. Know that it's quite hard to quantify a lot of preventative medicine because it's based on individual factors, so you shouldn't believe anyone who says a product or modality will definitely work for *you* just because it worked for *them*.

Check your biases. We are all partial to ideas or products that reflect something we already believe in, be it political, cultural, or religious. But the more you practice challenging your biases, the better you get at it. When you see a product (or influencer) claiming "natural" or "chemical-free," ask yourself, Am I buying in to this because I presume natural is better? Do I sincerely want to try this or do I just want to *feel* more aligned with something I value?

Be wary of emotionally manipulative language. Influencers yodeling about how an ingredient will nuke your body are trying to arouse an emotion. The same goes if they say an item will transport you to a purer era, appealing to our desire to run away and live on a farm. Take a step back to consider whether you believe the product's purported benefits (or harm).

Demand evidence. If someone has a striking claim, they better back it up. They can't just make statements like "Your child's American Girl doll is hiding toxins in its ponytail" without evidence. The onus is on them to *prove* that.

Consider your sources. Who are you taking your health advice from? Is it someone with established credentials? What is their expertise? Are they someone other experts refer to and quote? Now that wellness has seeped into the general culture, you'll see it touted by fashion bloggers, celebrities, and (some unqualified) podcasters. Consider rounding out your information diet for a fuller picture.

Analyze intentions. When someone promotes an idea or a product, ask: Is this person or organization beholden to a corporation, brand, or lobbying group? Are they trying to sell me something? For those who blur the line between health and business growth, take their product suggestions with a grain of Himalayan salt.

Is it necessary? Think if you need something or if it's just a shiny "extra" pulling you into the cult of self-improvement. We often make wellness purchases from a place of lack, says the WellSpoken founder Sarah Greenidge. "Explore where that feeling of lack comes from," she advises. "Check in with your body and think about: Is this something that's going to serve me right now?"

Evaluate the root stressors. Analyze what causes you stress, pain, or unhappiness. It could be work, social media, or an overpacked schedule. Before masking complaints with self-care rituals, see whether there's any way you can weed out the fundamental causes. (You can't always: there's only so much we can influence.)

Understand that science is always evolving. Scientists are constantly reevaluating health science research, pursuing further studies that might change what we once accepted in the past. That doesn't necessarily mean that past scientists were sloppy or reckless, rather that science is a continual journey of attaining more knowledge. We do the best we can with the information available at the current time.

Loosen the grip. Control—or the semblance of it—is very much a part of our mental health. We will do anything to possess it, including summoning the spirits to help us nab a dream job. It's the same reason we watch the Weather Channel; we want to manage what we can't predict. But that doesn't get you far down the line. Inevitably, something will come undone. Take a cue from meditation: relinquish a bit.

Much of this also applies to our understanding of how science works, or more aptly, *should* work. As the mathematician John Allen Paulos explains in *Innumeracy*, nearly every activity carries some risk. The question is: How much? And in comparison to what alternative? We're made to believe that science is absolute and iron-clad, thus any shaky ground has us reconsider the whole thing. When in reality, "there are always uncertainties in any live science, because science is a process of discovery."

There are always some uncertainties and elements out of our control.

Conclusion

There's a bigger consideration about our pursuit of health through wellness that goes beyond the science literacy of it all. It comes back to one of the main issues we've covered, which is that with millions and millions of dollars backing the marketing of the wellness industry, it can sometimes be difficult to tell whether our efforts make any difference at all. I'm often asked point-blank: *Is wellness working?* It's a tough question to answer. For one thing, it's too early to tell. We don't have any metrics to make a definitive judgment call on how all these trends impact greater public health. But I'd like to think we're on our way to smoothing the path forward, to distinguishing between the effective and the ineffective.

Granted, the pursuit of wellness is as old as time. Greek philosophers openly extolled the benefits of integrating mind and body—it was Pythagoras who advocated for soulful "me time" in the morning to center oneself before socializing. Ancient Jews observed the Sabbath to reflect and recharge for the week of labor ahead. Buddhist meditation dates back centuries. And America didn't only inherit the political traditions of ancient thinkers, we also got their penchant for wellness gurus.

Our American version of wellness went into high gear alongside the Industrial Revolution, when the rich got healthier and the poor less so. In today's information revolution, we Americans say we can't keep up with modern life. We say technology has moved too fast, the healthcare system is broken, and workplace productivity burns us out. Eating well, moving around, connecting with nature, and even just sleeping normally have been taken away from us. Those things used to be easier, public, or commonly held, but now if we want those things we have to pay for them. And you know what? We will because we're desperate for it.

In the summer of 2021, I revisited The Class. This time, the cardio workout was held outdoors on the Santa Monica Pier. Dozens of women assembled at 8:30 a.m. for a "heart-clearing" session set against the backdrop of the rough Pacific Ocean waves. A peppy blond instructor named Pixie sermonized on gratitude and the importance of expressing emotions between bouts of jumping jacks. After asking us to "pound out" resentment by gently beating our thighs, she told us to get loud when others try to silence us. "You don't need anyone's permission but your own," she firmly instructed. I once again witnessed women showing weighted emotion. They danced with abandon and breathed heavily with intention.

Later, I chatted with one fellow classmate who said The Class was just as relevant then as it had been years earlier. "It's only gotten more stressful," she laughed. There was a raging new COVID variant, a torn country at each other's throats, and so on and so on. The world, it seemed, was irreparably out of balance. The Class, for a moment, helped calm that anxiety.

Like her, I had to admit I was thrilled to be back among my emotional jumpers. Maybe it wasn't a cure-all or the community I had envisioned, but it sure did *something*. That's about as much as I expect these days from most wellness pursuits.

Wellness was initially introduced as a symbol of empowerment and a better way of life, and to some degree it is. If we're talking real wellness—

good nutrition, disease management, and such—then yes. You can't discount the myriad of ways we can live a healthier lifestyle. Quickie marts sell bagged carrots and display as many water varieties as soft drinks. Tech platforms democratize access to streaming fitness classes. Terms like "prevention" and "being active" are part of the American vernacular now.

We openly discuss mental health, far more than our parents' generation did. Look at the sophisticated offerings ranging from affordable therapy apps to inclusive digital support groups. Maybe it's not perfect, but it's progress. Do I wish there was more of an emphasis on community and less on personal intervention? Could we focus more on systemic issues? Of course. But what's the alternative right here and now in our highly individualistic society? You have to appreciate that which is, at the very least, making modern life a bit more manageable.

In the same breath, I must say that there are issues within the greater wellness industry, as covered throughout this book. So much of the wellness movement is built upon critique—a pushback against a disappointing health system, revulsion at pharmaceutical scandals, and a distrust of Big Food. Those are all warranted concerns, but they can come at a cost. Obsessing over "natural" or overvaluing alternatives can obstruct clear thinking. Doctors and manufacturers undoubtedly harmed women in the past, but we can't ignore science or evidence-based medicine in the name of defying authority. The romanticization of fighting the establishment does just that.

Pseudoscience and quacks have always been a mainstay of American culture. But we've entered a new era of uncritically accepting them and their charcoal-infused nonsense. Once supplements and "detox" kits overtook store shelves, we blindly embraced them. Herbal Essences now sells "gluten-free" shampoo, which is ludicrous considering that no one drinks their hair product. (Perhaps the company knows they can make a buck off those who have been taught to fear gluten, presumably, in all forms.) We started going with the flow instead of following the research.

I've seen far too many women—myself included—adopt new rituals and debatable products with nary an ounce of skepticism.

While we might want to just brush off problematic issues in the name of the free market, there is a societal impact to consider. Deceptive marketing has deeper ramifications. It starts small, then gets larger, until eventually it overtakes an entire industry. Even the word "wellness" has become an ambiguous, amorphous term—untethered to anything concrete, with more and more products shoved under its umbrella every day. It's dulling our bullshit detectors.

Wellness is paraded as something anyone can achieve if they just commit to their health destiny. Then, as Arthur J. Barsky writes in *Worried Sick*, "everything seems either healthful or harmful, and life becomes a series of prescribed and proscribed behaviors. Personal habits, diets, leisure activities are all modified to conform to the orthodoxy of the healthy lifestyle, as if there was only one way of life that could assure us of complete and endless health."[1]

So much of the current messaging serves to control women's time and role in society. Our health becomes a catalyst for investment, one demanding negotiations, sacrifice, and performance. We need to purge our figures of excess fat, rid our minds of angry thoughts, cleanse our organs of "toxins," fix whatever is "wrong" with us. It's fueling what can only be called self-absorption, revering our body to unhealthy proportions.

This is why it's difficult to discuss wellness in generalized, absolute terms. There is good, bad, and a whole lot in between. You cannot fully denounce it, nor can you disregard its growing problems. Often you need to discuss each sector individually, since this industry is ever expanding, encompassing more than a dozen subindustries. But overall, experts express optimism. "I feel we're marching in the right direction in terms of awareness and people acknowledging that it's multidimensional," says Ophelia Yeung, a senior research fellow at the Global Wellness Institute. "You can't just fix [everything] with medicine. You have to live [healthily]. I think that message is really out there now."

Wellness will continue to grow because the inherent sentiment remains the same: the status quo isn't cutting it. We shop at farmers' markets to cut back on overprocessed food. We wear a Fitbit because we recognize our lives are too sedentary. We go to yoga because we need a moment to slow down. Those activities in turn help define us—and what we want our lives to be.

· · ·

A 2020 Ogilvy study of seven thousand consumers discovered that a majority of shoppers now expect most brands to provide wellness offerings. Car manufacturers, for example, are reportedly incorporating wellness into vehicle design with features that measure stress levels or emit mood-altering scents (which may be helpful—we'll see). "Every brand can be a wellness brand now," noted Marion McDonald, Ogilvy's Global Health and Wellness Practice Lead. It sounds as if wellness will soon be part of pretty much every aspect of everyday life, in the way that religion was back in the day.

The title of this book is not meant to be taken literally. I am not suggesting that women engage in wellness practices or join a gym as a way to replicate the role of organized religion. That would certainly be pushing the comparison. But I do see ways in which wellness functions as deconstructed religion, a regulatory system instructing us how to move through our lives. It's almost as if it's cementing a new moral order. Wellness has ethical values (healthism). People follow laws dictating what they must ("organic") and must not ("toxic") consume—a quest for purity to sanctify the body. Nature is armed with godlike powers, which then assumes sickness is thereby attributed to the unnatural or synthetic. Wellness has its symbols (a yoga mat) and high priest (Gwyneth), if not false idols (supplements). Rituals can be picking up a turmeric latte before a workout class or instituting a daily gratitude practice.

Wellness even has many of the same sins (gluttony, sloth) and self-denials (food again) as religion. There are significant differences, though: this clergy sermonizes not about the devil but rather the daily environmental threats against which we require amulets (clean beauty).

Worshippers are provided with belonging, whether that's via an identity or community. Eating "right" or working out are imbued with sacred meaning because they all funnel into a promised salvation: a life free of stress, aging, and sickness. True believers—the hardest-working, that is—can gain entrance to this Eden of control. The belief is not necessarily based on science, but psychology.

How are we to interpret this? Well, it depends on how it's used and who's in charge. When the gospel is embraced by well-intentioned, scientific entities, then maybe it can be beneficial. But when it's adopted by the Goops of the world, less so. Pursuing healthy habits in itself is good. It's the pseudoscience, hyperconsumerist ethos that is muddying the waters. That's the distinction I hope I made throughout this book.

The religious treatment of wellness might also be because we've made it harder for people to find aspects of a fulfilling life in modern society. I think a lot about Oprah's Stanford University speech in which she implored students to find meaning. There's one question after she says "You must have a spiritual practice," and it's *What is yours?* I think about those young adults staring at what is essentially a very difficult, existential homework assignment: How do I find fulfillment in this culture? What is the meaning of my life? How do I define myself? It's not easy, especially in a society so obsessed with identity yet in which the familiar road map—with guardrails like religious orthodoxy or strict gender roles—no longer necessarily applies. That people gravitate toward overly marketed wellness makes sense in this day and age if only because the existential dilemma facing us can be overwhelming.

Many want meaning and a guide directing them how to get it. The acclaimed late author David Foster Wallace may have put it best when he said atheism doesn't exist in our culture:

There is no such thing as not worshipping. Everybody worships. The only choice we get is what to worship. And the compelling reason for maybe choosing some sort of god or spiritual-type thing to worship [...] is that pretty much anything else you worship will eat you alive. If you worship money and things, if they are where you tap real meaning in life, then you will never have enough, never feel you have enough. It's the truth. Worship your own body and beauty and sexual allure and you will always feel ugly, and when time and age start showing, you will die a million deaths before they finally plant you. On one level, we all know this stuff already—it's been codified as myths, proverbs, clichés, bromides, epigrams, parables: the skeleton of every great story. The trick is keeping the truth up front in daily consciousness."[2]

If we crave belonging and we increasingly worship good health, how do we ensure wellness is the best it can be? Redirecting the private sector economy is one part of the equation. For what wellness truly sets to cure, we also need systemic solutions and public infrastructure. We need more medical research, improved doctor-patient relationships, policies to support women, and better consumer product regulatory oversight. We need stronger communities. In our individualistic society, we are told that everything is our responsibility (and then often directed toward an app). But we're not supplied with enough support, even financially, to pursue healthier habits. Wellness, therefore, becomes everything that insurance and medicine won't touch. But if institutions want to change the landscape—as they publicly claim—why not incentivize fitness, nutrition, and connection?

Public investment is building. Fitness is a good example: A few state parks now advertise the mental health benefits of nature and attempt to widen access to recreation. Some physicians "prescribe" nature-based treatments, like recommending that patients join organized social hikes. Local governments are building more walking and biking trails to encourage daily physical activity.

Granted, the public sector is generally divided in that parks and rec is separate from the health department, which is separate from social services.

And maybe we need a wellness czar at the city, state, or federal level to coordinate them all. Or perhaps we should look to other countries for innovative ideas. New Zealand adopted a "well-being budget," while the United Arab Emirates employs a minister of happiness. Ophelia Yeung told me there's no one successful model that the United States can readily replicate. "[Wellness] is such a nascent emerging field, and there is no one really thinking about it from such a perspective yet," she said. "Thought leadership is needed." Although, even if there was a model, it would hardly be a copy-and-paste situation: each population is unique in its needs and experiences.

Insurers and employers are shifting too. It's not uncommon for health insurance plans to include gym membership discounts and stress management programs. ClassPass, the fitness class subscription platform, teamed up with Kaiser Permanente to offer thousands of free online workouts and reduced rates for live exercise classes. These are just several initiatives proving, at the very least, that society increasingly recognizes that citizens need help to live healthier lifestyles.

• • •

Early in the writing of this book, I called up Don Ardell, considered one of the architects of modern wellness. In 1977, he wrote a book titled *High Level Wellness*, which was groundbreaking for its time. Ardell wanted to educate the public about the actions they could take to promote their well-being. The individual was meant to ask: How can I feel better? What tools are at my disposal to ensure health and happiness? None of the answers, except for injury or disease, included a visit to the doctor. But his book wasn't *anti-doctor*. "Modern medicine is a wonderful thing," he wrote, "but there are two problems: people expect too much of it, and too little of themselves."[3]

A manifesto for personal responsibility, the book focuses on the stripped-down core pillars of the movement. "Wellness was never meant as an advertising gimmick, a brand, a treatment, a market, industry, or service," he stresses more than forty years later. Self-responsibility and community were equally emphasized. "Making a decision that you want to live a healthy life is not the same as being able to do it," says Ardell. "If you don't have a supportive culture—friends, family members, and your environment . . . your chances are next to zero to be able to pull off."

Voices like Ardell's get lost amid the noise, especially as we elevate the wild and pricey. But I notice pockets of consumers questioning their newfound habits. In much the same way that women pondered the status quo, they now seek to understand why they've gravitated to wellness. I believe consumers want to return to evidence-based solutions, of which there are plenty. They are floating around out there, in the same communities where they drink cold-pressed celery juice.

As for me? I threw out my supplements. I welcomed Neutrogena back into my bathroom. I've learned to pause before buying the hype on a new product, while simultaneously permitting myself to enjoy many products lacking scientific evidence. I still buy kombucha, though I drink it for the taste, not because I believe in some kind of magical gut healing. And though I still spend a fortune on my favorite boutique fitness classes (because they're fun), I try to remind myself that I don't need the fittest of bodies.

Wellness didn't solve all my problems. Stress, lackluster medical care, and image-related pressures are still prevalent issues. But it sure did inspire a framework to better deal with some of them. Learning to embrace mental health solutions put me on the road to finding personalized solutions that worked for me.

It didn't happen overnight, but over the years, I've witnessed an improvement in how I feel and how my body and mind react. That's worth something.

Wellness, as Goop would rightly say, is a journey. And I can't disagree with that.

Notes

Introduction

1. Rina Raphael, "Namaste En Masse: Can Wellness Festivals Grow as Big as Coachella?," *Fast Company*, Jan. 30, 2017, fastcompany.com/40421458/namaste -en-masse-can-wellness-festivals-grow-as-big-as-coachella.

2. Rina Raphael, "Why This Feminist Weed Camp Isn't Just for White Women," *Fast Company*, Oct. 17, 2017, fastcompany.com/40474705/why-this-feminist -weed-camp-isnt-white-women.

3. Elaine Stone and Sheryl A. Farnan, *The Dynamics of Fashion*, 5th ed. (New York: Fairchild Books, 2018), 180.

4. Lily Harral, "Why Athleisure is Going for Gold in the UK Retail Market During Lockdown," *Savills*, 2020, savills.com/open/fashion/why-athleisure-is- going-for-gold-in-the-uk-retail-market-during-lockdown/

5. "An Inside Look into the 2021 Global Consumer Health and Wellness Revolution," *NielsenIQ*, Oct. 28, 2021, nielseniq.com/global/en/insights/report/2021 /an-inside-look-into-the-2021-global-consumer-health-and-wellness-revolution/.

6. Adi Menayang, "Millennials Are 'the Most Health-Conscious Generation Ever,' Says Report by the Halo Group," *FoodNavigator-USA*, March 27, 2017, foodnavigator-usa.com/Article/2017/03/27/Millennials-scrutinize-health -claims-more-than-other-generations.

Chapter 1: Why the Hell Is the Advice Always Yoga?

1. Erin Donaghue, "New FBI Data Shows Rise in Anti-Semitic Hate Crimes," CBS News, Nov. 13, 2018, cbsnews.com/news/fbi-hate-crimes-up-new-data -shows-rise-in-anti-semitic-hate-crimes/.

2. Rina Raphael, "Is This Workout for Your Feelings What American Women Need Right Now?," *Fast Company*, Sept. 25, 2017, fastcompany.com/40469140 /is-this-workout-for-your-feelings-what-half-of-america-needs-right-now.

3. "2010 Stress in America: Gender and Stress," American Psychological Association, apa.org/news/press/releases/stress/2010/gender-stress.

4. "Women Do 2 More Hours of Housework Daily Than Men," Institute for Women's Policy Research, Jan. 22, 2020, iwpr.org/media/press-hits/women -do-2-more-hours-of-housework-daily-than-men/.

5. Robert Williams, "P&G Campaign Asks for Greater Equality in Household Chores," *Marketing Dive*, Feb. 5, 2021, marketingdive.com/news/pg-campaign -asks-for-greater-equality-in-household-chores/594601/.

6. "3 Out of 4 American Women Are Suffering from Burnout, According to New Harris Poll Commissioned by Meredith Corporation," Dotdash Meredith, meredith.mediaroom.com/2019-10-03-American-Women -Confronting-Burnout-At-Epidemic-Levels-According-To-New-Harris -Poll-Commissioned-By-Meredith-Corporation.

7. Lydia Saad, "The '40-Hour' Workweek Is Actually Longer—by Seven Hours," *Gallup*, May 7, 2021, news.gallup.com/poll/175286/hour-workweek-actually -longer-seven-hours.aspx.

8. John Harrington, "Wouldn't You Like 30 Mandated Days Off? Here Are the Countries with the Most Vacation Days," *USA Today*, July 23, 2019, usatoday .com/story/money/2019/07/23/paid-time-off-countries-with-the-most-vacation -days-brazil-france/39702323/.

9. Rina Raphael, "Almost Half of American Workers Have Cried at Work," *Fast Company*, April 29, 2019, fastcompany.com/90339835/almost-half-of-american -workers-have-cried-at-work.

10. Justin R. Garcia et al., "Sexual Hook-up Culture," *Monitor on Psychology* 44, no. 2 (February 2013): 60, apa.org/monitor/2013/02/ce-corner.

11. Rebecca Dube, "Mom Survey Says: Three Is the Most Stressful Number of Kids," *Today*, May 11, 2021, today.com/parents/mom-survey-says-three-most -stressful-number-kids-t127551.

12. Brigid Schulte, "'The Second Shift' at 25: Q & A with Arlie Hochschild," *Washington Post*, Aug. 6, 2014, washingtonpost.com/blogs/she-the-people/wp /2014/08/06/the-second-shift-at-25-q-a-with-arlie-hochschild/.

13. Caitlin Mullen, "Employed Moms Say Working Is Best Option," *Bizwomen*, Sept. 17, 2019, bizjournals.com/bizwomen/news/latest-news/2019/09/employed -moms-say-working-is-best-option.html.

14. Pallavi Gogoi, "Stuck-at-Home Moms: The Pandemic's Devastating Toll on Women," NPR, Oct. 28, 2020, npr.org/2020/10/28/928253674/stuck-at-home -moms-the-pandemics-devastating-toll-on-women.

15. "New Survey: Black and Latino Americans Face Greater Mental Health, Economic Challenges from COVID-19 Than White Americans," The Commonwealth Fund, Sept. 10, 2020, commonwealthfund.org/press-release/2020/new -survey-black-and-latino-americans-face-greater-mental-health-economic.

16. James F. Fixx, *The Complete Book of Running* (New York: Random House, 1977), 15.

17. Phil Edwards, "When Running for Exercise Was for Weirdos," *Vox*, Aug. 9, 2015, vox.com/2015/8/9/9115981/running-jogging-history.

18. Natalia Mehlman Petrzela (historian and author of *Fit Nation*) in discussion with the author, January 2022.

19. Christopher McDougall, *Born to Run: A Hidden Tribe, Superathletes, and the Greatest Race the World Has Never Seen* (New York: Alfred A. Knopf, 2019), 11.

20. American Friends of Tel Aviv University, "Finding Relief in Ritual: A Healthy Dose of Repetitive Behavior Reduces Anxiety, Says Researcher," *ScienceDaily*, Nov. 2, 2011, sciencedaily.com/releases/2011/09/110922093324.htm.

21. Quoted in Gina Kolata, *Ultimate Fitness: The Quest for Truth About Exercise and Health* (New York: Farrar, Straus and Giroux, 2007), 47.

22. "Highlights from the 2016 Yoga in America Study," Yoga Alliance, yogaalliance .org/Learn/About_Yoga/2016_Yoga_in_America_Study/Highlights.

23. Julie Beck, "'Americanitis': The Disease of Living Too Fast," *The Atlantic*, March 11, 2016, theatlantic.com/health/archive/2016/03/the-history-of-neurasthenia -or-americanitis-health-happiness-and-culture/473253/.

24. Anne Harrington, *The Cure Within: A History of Mind-Body Medicine* (New York: W. W. Norton, 2009), 144.

25. Arielle Tschinkel, "I Have Found Anxiety Relief in an Unlikely Place: SoulCycle," *HelloGiggles*, Oct. 12, 2017, hellogiggles.com/lifestyle/health-fitness /soulcycle-anxiety-relief/.

26. Rina Raphael, "In Jogging Therapy, You Can't Run from Your Feelings," *Fast Company*, Oct. 13, 2017, fastcompany.com/40478128/in-jogging-therapy-you -cant-run-from-your-feelings.

27. Patricia Haefeli, "It Turns Out You Can Run From Your Problems—at Least Temporarily," *Women's Running*, Sept. 15, 2017, womensrunning.com/health/wellness /real-runners-run-away/.

28. Sarah Marsh and Redwan Ahmed, "Workers Making £88 Lululemon Leggings Claim They Are Beaten," *The Guardian*, Oct. 14, 2019, theguardian.com/global-development/2019/oct/14/workers-making-lululemon-leggings-claim-they-are-beaten.

Chapter 2: The House Always Wins

1. Laura Brown, "Drew Barrymore Is Finding the Good News," *InStyle*, July 8, 2020, instyle.com/celebrity/drew-barrymore-august-2020-cover.

2. Jade Scipioni, "Olivia Wilde's Best Career Advice—and the Game-Changer in Her Wellness Routine," *CNBC Make It*, May 20, 2020, cnbc.com/2019/10/18/olivia-wildes-best-career-advice-and-wellness-routine.html.

3. "We Are What We Eat: Healthy Eating Trends Around the World," Nielsen, Jan. 2015, nielsen.com/wp-content/uploads/sites/3/2019/04/Nielsen20Global20Health20and20Wellness20Report20-20January202015-1.pdf.

4. Gwyneth Paltrow, "Sneak Peek: GP Introduces *The Clean Plate*," *Goop*, Jan. 8, 2019, goop.com/wellness/detox/sneak-peek-gp-introduces-the-clean-plate/.

5. Dana James, "5 Mindset Shifts to Make Clean Eating a Habit," *Mindbodygreen*, March 16, 2016, mindbodygreen.com/0-24186/5-mindset-shifts-to-make-clean-eating-a-habit.html.

6. Mary Ellen Snodgrass, *Encyclopedia of Kitchen History* (Abingdon, UK: Fitzroy Dearborn, 2005), 447.

7. Sylvester Graham, *A Treatise on Bread, and Bread-Making* (Boston: Light & Stearns, 1837).

8. S. Margot Finn, *Discriminating Taste: How Class Anxiety Created the American Food Revolution* (New Brunswick, NJ: Rutgers University Press, 2017), 57.

9. "Sylvester Graham, Health Food Nut, Makes Butchers and Bakers Go Crackers," New England Historical Society, April 12, 2021, newenglandhistoricalsociety.com/sylvester-graham-health-food-nut-makes-butchers-bakers-crackers/.

10. Kate Kirby, "Here's What Moon Juice Founder Amanda Chantal Bacon Eats in a Single Day," *Mini*, Nov. 21, 2016, mini-magazine.com/moon-juice-diet/.

11. Rina Raphael, "How Weight Watchers Transformed Itself into a Lifestyle Brand," *Fast Company*, Dec. 4, 2017, www.fastcompany.com/40500280/how-weight-watchers-transformed-itself-into-a-lifestyle-brand.

12. "Why People Diet, Lose Weight and Gain It All Back," Cleveland Clinic, Oct. 1, 2019, health.clevelandclinic.org/why-people-diet-lose-weight-and-gain-it-all-back/.

13. Gwyneth Paltrow, "The Power of Detoxification and Getting Clean," *Goop*, Jan. 6, 2021, goop.com/wellness/detox/clean/.

14. Christine Sismondo, "I Did a Cleanse Promoted by Goop (so You Don't Have to)," *Toronto Star*, Jan. 6, 2020, thestar.com/life/health_wellness/opinion/2020 /01/06/i-did-a-cleanse-promoted-by-goop-so-you-dont-have-to.html.

15. "Weight Loss and Weight Management Diet Market," Allied Market Research, May 2021, alliedmarketresearch.com/weight-loss-management-diet-market.

16. Jordan Younger, "Why I'm Transitioning Away from Veganism," *The Balanced Blonde*, June 23, 2014, thebalancedblonde.com/2014/06/23/why-im -transitioning-away-from-veganism/.

17. Susan Donaldson James, "Blogger Jordan Younger Reveals How Extreme 'Clean Eating' Almost Killed Her," *Today*, Nov. 11, 2015, today.com/health/breaking -vegan-author-jordan-younger-confesses-dirty-secrets-clean-eating-t55086.

18. Jordan Younger, *Breaking Vegan: One Woman's Journey from Veganism, Extreme Dieting, and Orthorexia to a More Balanced Life* (Beverly, MA: Fair Winds Press, 2016), 88. Per her assistant, she says the book no longer "resonates" with her.

19. Jordan Younger, "Some of the Wackiest Things That Have Happened Since 'Coming Out' as a Non-vegan," *The Balanced Blonde*, June 28, 2014, the balancedblonde.com/2014/06/28/some-of-the-wackiest-things-that-have -happened-since-coming-out-as-a-non-vegan/.

20. Jamie McKillop, "What Happened When the Blonde Vegan Wasn't Vegan Anymore," *Well+Good*, July 8, 2014, www.wellandgood.com/what-happened -when-the-blonde-vegan-wasnt-vegan-anymore/.

21. Marie Galmiche et al., "Prevalence of Eating Disorders over the 2000–2018 Period: A Systematic Literature Review, *American Journal of Clinical Nutrition* 109, no. 5 (May 2019): 1402–13, doi:10.1093/ajcn/nqy342.

22. Younger, *Breaking Vegan*, 28.

23. Suman Ambwani et al., "'It's Healthy Because It's Natural.' Perceptions of 'Clean' Eating Among U.S. Adolescents and Emerging Adults," *Nutrients* 12, no. 6 (June 7, 2020): 1708, doi:10.3390/nu12061708.

24. Christy Harrison, "How to Avoid Falling for the Wellness Diet," Christy Harrison, April 9, 2018, christyharrison.com/blog/the-wellness-diet.

25. WW, "How Has James Corden Lost 20 Lbs? The Science Behind WW's (formerly Weight Watchers) Success," April 5, 2021, YouTube video, 5:34, youtube .com/watch?v=eBw3EY4ONUI.

26. Long Ge et al., "Comparison of Dietary Macronutrient Patterns of 14 Popular Named Dietary Programmes for Weight and Cardiovascular Risk Factor Reduction in Adults: Systematic Review and Network Meta-analysis of Ran-

domised Trials," *BMJ (Clinical Research Edition)* 369, m696 (April 1, 2020), doi:10.1136/bmj.m696.

27. Patti Neighmond, "Yo-Yo Dieting May Pose Serious Risks for Heart Patients," *Shots* (blog), NPR, May 1, 2017, accessed Aug. 8, 2021, npr.org/sections/health -shots/2017/05/01/526048767/-yo-yo-dieting-poses-serious-risks-for-heart -patients.

28. Stuart Wolpert, "Dieting Does Not Work, UCLA Researchers Report," UCLA Newsroom, April 3, 2007, newsroom.ucla.edu/releases/Dieting-Does-Not -Work-UCLA-Researchers-7832.

29. Keith Devlin, "Top 10 Reasons Why the BMI Is Bogus," NPR, July 4, 2009, npr.org/templates/story/story.php?storyId=106268439.

30. Tessa E. S. Charlesworth and Mahzarin R. Banaji, "Research: How Americans' Biases Are Changing (or Not) over Time," *Harvard Business Review*, Aug. 14, 2019, hbr.org/2019/08/research-on-many-issues-americans-biases-are -decreasing.

31. Alexandra Owens, "Allure Cover Girl Olivia Wilde's Beauty Secrets," *Allure*, Sept. 18, 2013, allure.com/story/allure-olivia-wilde-beauty-secrets.

Chapter 3: Is My Face Wash Trying to Kill Me?

1. Beautycounter, "Beautycounter in DC 2018," April 1, 2018, YouTube video, 2:47, youtube.com/watch?v=i9URKZvP-MQ.

2. Alix Tunell, "Forget Cadillacs, These Beauty Consultants Want Political Change," *Refinery29*, March 15, 2018, refinery29.com/en-us/beautycounter -political-action.

3. U.S. Food and Drug Administration, "Claire's Stores, Inc., Announces Voluntary Recall of Three Make-up Products," March 11, 2019, fda.gov/safety/recalls -market-withdrawals-safety-alerts/claires-stores-inc-announces-voluntary -recall-three-make-products.

4. David Gelles, "Selling Shampoo, Eye Cream and a Chemical Crackdown," *New York Times*, Oct. 8, 2016, nytimes.com/2016/10/09/business/selling-shampoo -eye-cream-and-a-chemical-crackdown.html.

5. Nancy Tomes, *The Gospel of Germs: Men, Women, and the Microbe in American Life* (Cambridge, MA: Harvard University Press, 2002), 10.

6. "Life Story: Ellen Swallow Richards (1842–1911)," *Women & the American Story*, June 23, 2021, wams.nyhistory.org/modernizing-america/modern-womanhood /ellen-swallow-richards/.

7. Barbara Ehrenreich and Deirdre English, *For Her Own Good: 150 Years of the Experts' Advice to Women* (New York: Doubleday, 1989), 198–99.

8. Sarah Stage and Virginia B. Vincenti, *Rethinking Home Economics: Women and the History of a Profession* (Ithaca, NY: Cornell University Press, 1997), 259–60.

9. "Personal Care Products," Environmental Working Group, ewg.org/areas-focus /personal-care-products.

10. Norah MacKendrick, *Better Safe Than Sorry: How Consumers Navigate Exposure to Everyday Toxics* (Oakland: University of California Press, 2018).

11. The Honest Company, "A Message from Our Founder, Jessica Alba," *Honest* (blog), March 10 2016, www.honest.com/blog/lifestyle/purpose/a-message -from-our-founder-jessica-alba/19793.html.

12. Abbie Boudreau and Aude Soichet, "Jessica Alba Leads Mommy War on Synthetic Chemicals," ABC News, Dec. 3, 2013, abcnews.go.com/US/jessica -alba-leads-mommy-war-synthetic-chemicals/story?id=21084997.

13. Roland Marchand, *Advertising the American Dream: Making Way for Modernity, 1920–1940* (Berkeley: University of California Press, 1985), 66.

14. John Muir, *The Complete Works of John Muir* (Hastings, UK: Delphi Classics, 2017).

15. Rina Raphael, "The Global Beauty Business Goes Au Naturel," *Fast Company*, Sept. 20, 2018, fastcompany.com/90227521/the-global-beauty-business-goes -au-naturel.

16. Rina Raphael, "Herbivore's Moldy Face-Cream Recall at Sephora Underscores an Ugly Issue for Natural Beauty," *Fast Company*, April 12, 2019, fastcompany .com/90334490/herbivores-moldy-face-cream-recall-at-sephora-underscores -an-ugly-issue-for-natural-beauty.

17. Carolyn Crist, "'Clean' Beauty Products Not Always Safe, Dermatologists Say," Reuters, Oct. 2, 2019, reuters.com/article/us-health-cosmetics-clean-safety -idUSKBN1WH2AC.

18. Fred Fedler, *Media Hoaxes* (Ames: Iowa State University Press, 1989), 199.

19. Jessica Bibby et al., "Transitioning to Transparency," Fashion Institute of Technology, 2018, fitnyc.edu/documents/transitioning-to-transperancy.pdf.

20. Douglas Atkin, *The Culting of Brands: Turn Your Customers into True Believers* (New York: Portfolio, 2004), 17.

21. "Lead in Your Lipstick? The Facts on Heavy Metals in Cosmetics," Beauty-counter, Dec. 9, 2016, beautycounter.com/blog/better-beauty/lead-in-your -lipstick-the-facts-on-heavy-metals-in-cosmetics.

22. Tasha Stoiber, "What Are Parabens, and Why Don't They Belong in Cosmetics?," Environmental Working Group, April 9, 2019, ewg.org/what-are-parabens.

23. P. D. Darbre et al., "Concentrations of Parabens in Human Breast Tumours," *Journal of Applied Toxicology* 24, no. 1 (2004): 5–13, doi:10.1002/jat.958.

24. Leigh Krietsch Boerner, "Blue Shift: Why Parabens Shouldn't Scare You," Wirecutter, *New York Times*, Oct. 3, 2016, nytimes.com/wirecutter/blog/why -parabens-shouldnt-scare-you/.

25. Dorota Błędzka et al., "Parabens: From Environmental Studies to Human Health," *Environment International* 67 (2014): 27–42, doi:10.1016/j.envint.2014.02.007.

26. "Antiperspirants/Deodorants and Breast Cancer," National Cancer Institute, cancer.gov/about-cancer/causes-prevention/risk/myths/antiperspirants-fact-sheet.

27. "Do Plastics, Body Care Products or Deodorant Play a Role in Breast Cancer Risk?—Komen Perspectives," *The Komen Blog*, April 1, 2010, blog.komen.org /blog/komen-perspectives-do-plastics-body-care-products-or-deodorant-play-a -role-in-breast-cancer-risk/.

28. "Antiperspirants and Breast Cancer Risk," American Cancer Society, cancer.org /cancer/cancer-causes/antiperspirants-and-breast-cancer-risk.html.

29. "Is Deodorant Harmful for Your Health?" Penn Medicine, June 6, 2019, penn-medicine.org/updates/blogs/health-and-wellness/2019/june/deodorant.

30. "Antiperspirants," American Cancer Society.

31. Anthony F. Fransway et al., "Parabens," *Dermatitis* 30, no. 1 (2019): 3–31, doi:10.1097/der.0000000000000429.

32. "Advocacy for Clean Beauty and a Better Future," Beautycounter, beautycounter .com/advocacy.

33. Scott Faber, "Cosmetics Safety Bill Gains Support from Industry and Advo-cates," Environmental Working Group, July 5, 2017, ewg.org/news-insights /news/cosmetics-safety-bill-gains-support-industry-and-advocates.

34. Katie M. O'Brien et al., "Association of Powder Use in the Genital Area with Risk of Ovarian Cancer," *JAMA* 323, no. 1 (2020): 49–59, doi:10.1001 /jama.2019.20079.

35. Julia Horowitz, "Jessica Alba's The Honest Company Can't Catch a Break," *CNNMoney*, June 12, 2017, money.cnn.com/2017/06/12/news/companies/honest -company-problems/index.html.

36. Thomas C. O'Brien, Ryan Palmer, and Dolores Albarracin, "Misplaced Trust: When Trust in Science Fosters Belief in Pseudoscience and the Benefits of Critical Evaluation," *Journal of Experimental Social Psychology* 96 (2021): 104184, doi:10.1016/j.jesp.2021.104184.

37. Alex Berezow, "Dear EWG, This Is Why Real Scientists Think Poorly of You," American Council on Science and Health, June 1, 2017, acsh.org/news/2017/05 /25/dear-ewg-why-real-scientists-think-poorly-you-11323.

38. Berezow, "Dear EWG."

Chapter 4: Gym as Church

1. Peloton, 30 Min Sundays with Love, Nov. 22, 2020, members.onepeloton.com /profile/workouts/bb7de32e8cca49b1b78679f828360f27.

2. "Sundays with Love," *The Output* (blog), Peloton, Oct. 18, 2020, blog.onepeloton .com/sundays-with-love-peloton/.

3. Jalen Rose, "Peloton Star Ally Love Tells Jalen Rose About Almost Dying at Age 9," *New York Post*, July 1, 2021, nypost.com/2021/07/01/peloton-star-ally -love-tells-jalen-rose-about-almost-dying-at-age-9/.

4. Ally Love, "Peloton's Ally Love Almost Died in a Car Accident at Age 9 and Was Told She'd Never Run Again," *Women's Health*, Oct. 20, 2020, women shealthmag.com/fitness/a34041498/ally-love-peloton-dance/.

5. "Peloton Interactive (PTON) Q4 2021 Earnings Call Transcript" *Motley Fool*, Aug. 27, 2021, fool.com/earnings/call-transcripts/2021/08/27/peloton -interactive-pton-q4-2021-earnings-call-tra/.

6. Recode, "Full Video: John Foley, Founder and CEO of Peloton | Code Commerce," Sept. 15, 2017, YouTube video, 14:45, youtube.com/watch?v=-g5Y-Dp5kDw.

7. Wade Clark Roof, *Spiritual Marketplace: Baby Boomers and the Remaking of American Religion* (Princeton, NJ: Princeton University Press, 2001), 79.

8. "United States Securities and Exchange Commission, Peloton Interactive, Inc.," sec.gov/Archives/edgar/data/1639825/000119312519230923/d738839ds1.htm.

9. Casper ter Kuile and Angie Thurston, "How We Gather (Part 2): SoulCycle as Soul Sanctuary," The On Being Project, July 9, 2016, onbeing.org/blog/how-we -gather-part-2-soulcycle-as-soul-sanctuary/.

10. Kathryn Romeyn, "How an Ex–Talent Manager Co-founded SoulCycle and Sold for $90M," *Hollywood Reporter*, July 3, 2017, hollywoodreporter.com /lifestyle/style/how-an-talent-manager-founded-soulcycle-sold-90m-1015009/.

11. Tim Ferriss, "#372: Julie Rice—Co-founding SoulCycle, Taming Anxiety, and Mastering Difficult Conversations," *The Tim Ferriss Show*, Apple Podcasts, June 5, 2019, podcasts.apple.com/us/podcast/372-julie-rice-co-founding-soulcycle -taming-anxiety/id863897795?i=1000440479706.

12. Sarah Lacy, "Scaling Your Startup . . . with Soul," Startups.com, Aug. 11, 2020, startups.com/library/founder-stories/julie-rice-elizabeth-cutler.

13. TheLeapTV, "Julie & Spencer Rice | SoulCycle | USC Interview," Feb. 28, 2020, YouTube video, 1:25:28, youtube.com/watch?v=lU6vhAq331s, accessed Feb. 7, 2022.

14. Ferriss, "#372: Julie Rice."

15. "Q&A with SoulCycle's Julie Rice: A Local Gym That Helped Spawn an Exercise Craze," *West Side Rag*, March 10, 2013, westsiderag.com/2013/03

/10/qa-with-soulcycles-julie-rice-a-local-spinning-gym-that-helped-spawn-an
-exercise-craze.

16. Lacy, "Scaling Your Startup."

17. Romeyn, "How an Ex–Talent Manager."

18. TheLeapTV, "Julie & Spencer Rice."

19. Ferriss, "#372: Julie Rice."

20. Steven Kotler and Jamie Wheal, *Stealing Fire: How Silicon Valley, the Navy SEALs, and Maverick Scientists Are Revolutionizing the Way We Live and Work* (New York: Dey Street Books, 2018), 141.

21. "Researchers Discover a Completely Legal Performance Enhancer: Friends," University of Oxford, Aug. 31, 2015, ox.ac.uk/news/2015–08–31-researchers -discover-completely-legal-performance-enhancer-friends.

22. Ter Kuile and Thurston, "How We Gather."

23. Aziz Angari, Twitter post, Dec. 13, 2019, 9:43 p.m., twitter.com/AzizAngari /status/1205679604406607872.

24. Wendy Simonds, *Women and Self-Help Culture: Reading Between the Lines* (New Brunswick, NJ: Rutgers University Press, 1992), 42–43.

25. Rina Raphael, "Namaste En Masse: Can Wellness Festivals Grow as Big as Coachella?" *Fast Company*, June 30, 2017, fastcompany.com/40421458 /namaste-en-masse-can-wellness-festivals-grow-as-big-as-coachella.

26. "Your Posture, Right or Wrong, Is Up to You," *Life*, April 12, 1937, 52–56.

27. Karl Toepfer, *Empire of Ecstasy: Nudity and Movement in German Body Culture, 1910–1935* (Berkeley: University of California Press, 1997), 39.

28. Carey Dunne, "The Emperor's New Corsets," *The Baffler* 34, Spring 2017, the baffler.com/salvos/emperors-new-corsets-dunne.

29. Warwick Maloney, "Dr. Bess Mensendieck," *Movement Health*, Dec. 8, 2017, movementhealth.com.au/news/dr-bess-mensendieck/.

30. Dunne, "The Emperor's New Corsets."

31. "Finds Beauty Lies in Muscle Control," *New York Times*, March 9, 1924, times machine.nytimes.com/timesmachine/1924/03/09/101583907.html?pageNumber =63Them.

32. Susan Pinker, *The Village Effect: How Face-to-Face Contact Can Make Us Healthier and Happier* (Toronto: Vintage Canada, 2015), 36.

33. Karen Turner, "Secularism Is on the Rise, but Americans Are Still Finding Community and Purpose in Spirituality," *Vox*, June 11, 2019, vox.com/first -person/2019/6/4/18644764/church-religion-atheism-secularism.

34. "For Mindfulness Programs, 'with Whom' May Be More Important Than 'How,'" Brown University, Feb. 16, 2021, brown.edu/news/2021–02–16 /mindfulness.

35. Nicholas K. Canby et al., "The Contribution of Common and Specific Therapeutic Factors to Mindfulness-Based Intervention Outcomes," *Frontiers in Psychology* (Jan. 14, 2021): 11:603394, doi:10.3389/fpsyg.2020.603394; PMID: 33584439; PMCID: PMC7874060.

36. Michelle Ruiz, "A Conversation with Cody Rigsby, Peloton's 'King of Quarantine,'" *Vogue*, Nov. 25, 2020, vogue.com/article/cody-rigsby-on-becoming -pelotons-king-of-quarantine.

37. Robert D. Putnam, *Bowling Alone: The Collapse and Revival of American Community* (New York: Simon & Schuster Paperbacks, 2000), 184.

38. Ferriss, "#372: Julie Rice."

39. Maxwell Strachan, "SoulCycle Lays Off Long-Time Employees with Zero Severance," *Vice*, May 18, 2020, vice.com/en/article/m7jaqq/soulcycle-lays-off -long-time-employees-with-zero-severance.

40. Alex Abad-Santos, "How SoulCycle Lost Its Soul," *Vox*, Dec. 23, 2020, vox.com /the-goods/22195549/soulcycle-decline-reopening-bullying-bike-explained.

41. Katie Warren, "SoulCycle's Top Instructors Had Sex with Clients, 'Fat-Shamed' Coworkers, and Used Homophobic and Racist Language," *Business Insider*, Nov. 17, 2020, businessinsider.com/soulcycle-instructors-celebrities -misbehavior-2020-11.

42. Catherine Saint Louis, "In New York, a Rivalry Shifts into High Gear," *New York Times*, Oct. 8, 2010, nytimes.com/2010/10/10/fashion/10Spin.html.

43. Warren, "SoulCycle's Top Instructors."

44. Mallory Schlossberg, "I Used to Be Obsessed with SoulCycle—until I realized How Much Is Wrong with the Class," *Business Insider*, April 8, 2016, businessin sider.com.au/why-i-stopped-going-to-soulcycle-2016–4.

45. Saint Louis, "In New York."

46. Abad-Santos, "How SoulCycle Lost Its Soul."

47. Richard P. Feynman, *"Surely You're Joking, Mr. Feynman!"* (New York: W. W. Norton, 1985), 343.

Chapter 5: A Plea to Be Heard

1. Rina Raphael, "Gwyneth Paltrow's Goop Conference Was as Kooky as You Expected It to Be—and That's Exactly What Fans Wanted," *Fast Company*, June 12, 2017, fastcompany.com/40430244/gwyneth-paltrows-goop-conference-was -as-kooky-as-you-expected-it-to-be-and-thats-exactly-what-fans-wanted.

2. Ann Anderson, *Snake Oil, Hustlers and Hambones: The American Medicine Show* (Jefferson, NC: McFarland Publishers, 2004).

3. Jamie Ballard, "Women Are More Likely Than Men to Be Open to Alternative Medicine," YouGov America, Aug. 20, 2018, today.yougov.com/topics/health/articles-reports/2018/08/20/alternative-medicine-men-women.

4. Catherine Thorbecke, Jennifer Pereira, and Eric Jones, "Selma Blair Reveals She Cried with Relief at MS Diagnosis After Being 'Not Taken Seriously' by Doctors," *GMA*, Feb. 26, 2019, goodmorningamerica.com/culture/story/selma-blair-opens-tears-relief-ms-diagnosis-61310469.

5. Julie Miller, "'There's No Tragedy for Me': Selma Blair's Transformation," *Vanity Fair*, March 2019, vanityfair.com/hollywood/2019/02/selma-blairs-transformation.

6. *Nightline*, season 40, episode 41, "Selma Blair Describes the Moment She Received Her Multiple Sclerosis Diagnosis," ABC, Feb. 26, 2019, abc.com/shows/nightline/episode-guide/2019-02/26-022619-selma-blair-describes-the-moment-she-received-her-multiple-sclerosis-diagnosis, accessed Nov. 15, 2021.

7. Pat Anson, "Women in Pain Report Significant Gender Bias" *National Pain Report*, Nov. 8, 2015, nationalpainreport.com/women-in-pain-report-significant-gender-bias-8824696.html.

8. Bernard L. Harlow and Elizabeth Gunther Stewart, "A Population-Based Assessment of Chronic Unexplained Vulvar Pain: Have We Underestimated the Prevalence of Vulvodynia?" *Journal of the American Medical Women's Association* 58, no. 2 (2003): 82–8.

9. Tracy Jarrett, "Endometriosis Increases Risk of Heart Disease in Young Women," NBC News, March 29, 2016, nbcnews.com/health/womens-health/endometriosis-increases-risk-heart-disease-young-women-n547381.

10. Full Frontal with Samantha Bee, "All You Get Is Birth Control | March 21, 2018 Act 2, Part 1 | Full Frontal on TBS," March 22, 2018, YouTube video, 3:53, youtube.com/watch?v=X2FS0s95o_Q.

11. Esther H. Chen et al., "Gender Disparity in Analgesic Treatment of Emergency Department Patients with Acute Abdominal Pain, *Academic Emergency Medicine* 15, no. 5 (May 2008): 414–18, doi:10.1111/j.1553–2712.2008.00100.x, PMID: 18439195.

12. K. L. Calderone, "The Influence of Gender on the Frequency of Pain and Sedative Medication Administered to Postoperative Patients," *Sex Roles* 23 (1990): 713–25, doi.org/10.1007/BF00289259.

13. Sarah Klein, "5 Ways to Make Your Next Ob-Gyn Appointment a Little Less Terrible," *Prevention*, Nov. 4, 2016, prevention.com/health/g20486679/make-your-ob-gyn-visit-less-terrible/.

14. Springer, "Wait, Just a Second, Is Your Doctor Listening?" *ScienceDaily*, July 19, 2018, sciencedaily.com/releases/2018/07/180719112209.htm.

15. Ming Tai-Seale, Thomas G. McGuire, and Weimin Zhang, "Time Allocation in Primary Care Office Visits," *Health Services Research* 42, no. 5 (2007): 1871–94, doi:10.1111/j.1475–6773.2006.00689.x.

16. David Ollier Weber, "How Many Patients Can a Primary Care Physician Treat?" American Association for Physician Leadership, Feb. 11, 2019, phy sicianleaders.org/news/how-many-patients-can-primary-care-physician-treat.

17. Lisa A. Cooper et al., "The Associations of Clinicians' Implicit Attitudes About Race with Medical Visit Communication and Patient Ratings of Interpersonal Care," *American Journal of Public Health* 102, no. 5 (2012): 979–87, doi:10.2105/ ajph.2011.300558.

18. "Discrimination in America: Experiences and Views of African Americans," NPR, Oct. 2017, media.npr.org/assets/img/2017/10/23/discriminationpoll -african-americans.pdf.

19. Nina Martin and Renée Montagne, "Nothing Protects Black Women from Dying in Pregnancy and Childbirth," ProPublica, Dec. 7, 2017, propublica .org/article/nothing-protects-black-women-from-dying-in-pregnancy-and -childbirth.

20. Danielle Ofri, *What Doctors Feel: How Emotions Affect the Practice of Medicine* (Boston: Beacon Press, 2013), 155.

21. Susan Kelly, "Emergency Physicians' Level of Burnout Jumped Last Year," *Healthcare Dive*, Jan. 24, 2022, healthcaredive.com/news/burnout-emergency -physicians-rising/617554/.

22. Elisabeth Rosenthal, *An American Sickness: How Healthcare Became Big Business and How You Can Take It Back* (New York: Penguin Books, 2018), 252.

23. Rina Raphael, "A Shockingly Large Majority of Health News Shared on Facebook Is Fake or Misleading," *Fast Company*, Feb. 4, 2019, fastcompany.com/90301427/a -shockingly-large-majority-of-health-news-shared-on-facebook-is-fake.

24. Paul Bergner, "Lobelia: Legal Considerations in the Samuel Thomson Trial," *Medical Herbalism: Journal for the Clinical Practitioner*, medherb.com/Materia _Medica/Lobelia_-_Legal_considerations_in_the_Samuel_Thomson_trial.htm.

25. Theodore W. Ruger, "The Thomsonian Movement and the Structures of American Health Law," Petrie-Flom Center for Health Law Policy, Biotechnology, and Bioethics at Harvard Law School, Dec. 28, 2009, petrieflom.law.harvard .edu/assets/publications/Ruger_Thomsonian_Movement_and_Structures_of _American_Health_Law.pdf.

26. Samuel Thomson, *A Narrative of the Life and Medical Discoveries of Samuel Thomson* (Columbus, OH: Pike, Platt, 1832), 24.

27. Peter Maisel, Erika Baum, and Norbert Donner-Banzhoff, "Fatigue as the Chief Complaint—Epidemiology, Causes, Diagnosis, and Treatment," *Deutsches Ärzteblatt International* 118, no. 33–34 (2021): 566–76, doi:10.3238/arztebl.m2021.0192.

28. Emily Laurence, "Gwyneth Paltrow Goop Wellness Supplements Line Suffered from Adrenal Fatigue—and It Helped Inspire a New Goop Business," *Well+Good*, March 16, 2017, wellandgood.com/gwyneth-paltrow-goop-wellness-supplements-adrenal-fatigue/.

29. "TINA.org Takes Gwyneth Paltrow's Goop-y Health Claims to Regulators," Truth in Advertising, Aug. 22, 2017, truthinadvertising.org/tina-takes-goop-claims-to-regulators/.

30. Rae Paoletta, "NASA Calls Bullshit on Goop's $120 'Bio-Frequency Healing' Sticker Packs," *Gizmodo*, June 22, 2017, gizmodo.com/nasa-calls-bullshit-on-goops-120-bio-frequency-healing-1796309360.

31. Daniel Morgan, "What the Tests Don't Show," *Washington Post*, Oct. 5, 2018, washingtonpost.com/news/posteverything/wp/2018/10/05/feature/doctors-are-surprisingly-bad-at-reading-lab-results-its-putting-us-all-at-risk/.

32. Erin Blakemore, "1,800 Studies Later, Scientists Conclude Homeopathy Doesn't Work," *Smithsonian Magazine*, March 11, 2015, smithsonianmag.com/smart-news/1800-studies-later-scientists-conclude-homeopathy-doesnt-work-180954534/.

33. Jonathan Jarry (biological scientist and science communicator, McGill Office for Science and Society), in discussion with the author, January 2022.

34. Jonathan Jarry, January 2022.

35. Dr. David Scales (sociologist, physician, and assistant professor of medicine, Weill Cornell Medical College), in discussion with the author, January 2022.

36. The Body of Evidence, "Anecdotes (The Body of Evidence)," July 18, 2016, YouTube video, 7:42, youtube.com/watch?v=QDlPoSSVPuA, accessed Jan. 16, 2022.

37. Klaus Linde et al., "Acupuncture for the Prevention of Tension-Type Headache," *Cochrane Database of Systematic Reviews* 4, no. 4, April 19, 2016, CD007587, doi:10.1002/14651858.CD007587.pub2.

38. Michael Stenger, Nicki Eithz Bauer, and Peter B. Licht, "Is Pneumothorax After Acupuncture So Uncommon?" *Journal of Thoracic Disease* 5, no. 4 (2013): E144–46, doi:10.3978/j.issn.2072–1439.2013.08.18.

39. Skyler B. Johnson et al., "Complementary Medicine, Refusal of Conventional Cancer Therapy, and Survival Among Patients with Curable Cancers," *JAMA Oncology* 4, no. 10 (2018): 1375, doi:10.1001/jamaoncol.2018.2487.

40. Ned Potter, "Steve Jobs Regretted Delaying Cancer Surgery 9 Months, Biographer Says," ABC News, Oct. 20, 2011, abcnews.go.com/Technology/steve-jobs -treatment-biographer-jobs-delayed-surgery-pancreatic/story?id=14781250#.

41. Federal Trade Commission, "In the matter of Easybutter, LLC, a limited liability company, also doing business as Hempme," ftc.gov/system/files/documents /cases/2023047hempmecbdcomplaint.pdf.

42. McGill Office for Science and Society, "Functional Medicine (CS31)," April 13, 2019, YouTube video, 10:44, youtube.com/watch?v=3EDW_upV3ZU.

43. David Gorski, "Dr. Robin Berzin, Functional Medicine Concierge Practices, and the Marketing of Medical Pseudoscience," *Respectful Insolence*, Sept. 5, 2018, respectfulinsolence.com/2018/09/05/robin-berzin-functional-medicine -concierge/.

Chapter 6: Can't Treat What You Don't Know

1. Elisabeth Brooke, *Women Healers: Portraits of Herbalists, Physicians, and Midwives* (Rochester, VT: Healing Arts Press, 1996), 69.

2. Maya Dusenbery, *Doing Harm: The Truth About How Bad Medicine and Lazy Science Leave Women Dismissed, Misdiagnosed, and Sick* (New York: HarperOne, 2019), 7–8.

3. Judith Walzer Leavitt, *Women and Health in America: Historical Readings* (Madison: University of Wisconsin Press, 1999), 53.

4. Patrick Boyle, "Nation's Physician Workforce Evolves: More Women, a Bit Older, and Toward Different Specialties," Association of American Medical Colleges, Feb. 2, 2021, aamc.org/news-insights/nation-s-physician-workforce-evolves -more-women-bit-older-and-toward-different-specialties, accessed Aug. 5, 2021.

5. Mirjam J. Curno et al., "A Systematic Review of the Inclusion (or Exclusion) of Women in HIV Research: From Clinical Studies of Antiretrovirals and Vaccines to Cure Strategies," *Journal of Acquired Immune Deficiency Syndromes* 71, no. 2 (2016): 181–88, doi:10.1097/qai.0000000000000842.

6. "Here's Why Women Are More Likely to Have Chronic Pain," Cleveland Clinic, May 30, 2019, health.clevelandclinic.org/women-are-more-likely-to -have-chronic-pain-heres-why/.

7. Pietro Invernizzi et al., "Female Predominance and X Chromosome Defects in Autoimmune Diseases," *Journal of Autoimmunity* 33, no. 1 (August 2009): 12–16, doi: 10.1016/j.jaut.2009.03.005.

8. Anna Nowogrodzki, "Inequality in Medicine," *Nature*, Oct. 5, 2017, nature .com/articles/550S18a.

9. Chloe E. Bird, "Increased Funding for Research in Women's Health Issues Could Unleash Staggering Returns," *Fortune*, Feb. 11, 2022, fortune.com/2022/02/11/women-health-medical-research-underfunding-equity-rand/.

10. Sergey Feldman et al., "Quantifying Sex Bias in Clinical Studies at Scale with Automated Data Extraction," *JAMA Network Open* 2, no. 7 (2019): e196700, doi:10.1001/jamanetworkopen.2019.6700.

11. Gabrielle Emanuel, "Preterm Birth: Months Early—and a Century Behind," GBH News, wgbh.org/news/preterm-birth-months-early-and-a-century-behind.

12. "Women in Healthcare Leadership 2019," OliverWyman, oliverwyman.com/our-expertise/insights/2019/jan/women-in-healthcare-leadership.html.

13. "Global Female Technology (Femtech) Market: Analysis & Forecast," *Globe-Newswire*, July 29, 2020, globenewswire.com/news-release/2020/07/29/2069355/0/en/Global-Female-Technology-Femtech-Market-Analysis-Forecast.html.

14. Rina Raphael, "Can Silicon Valley Get You Pregnant?" *Fast Company*, Jan. 30, 2018, fastcompany.com/40521525/fertility-tech-is-worth-billions-and-investors-are-finally-paying-attention.

15. Neal Dempsey, "Venture Capital Is Still a 'Boys' Club.' Let's Start to Change That." *Crunchbase News*, August 16, 2021, news.crunchbase.com/news/venture-capital-female-gender-diversity/.

16. Collin West and Gopinath Sundaramurthy, "Women VCs Invest in Up to 2x More Female Founders," *Kauffman Fellows Journal*, March 25, 2020, kauffmanfellows.org/journal_posts/women-vcs-invest-in-up-to-2x-more-female-founders.

17. Laura Lovett, "Femtech Market Has Potential but Struggles to Score Investor Dollars," *MobiHealthNews*, Aug. 28, 2020, mobihealthnews.com/news/femtech-market-has-potential-struggles-score-investor-dollars.

18. Sheila Kaplan and Matthew Goldstein, "F.D.A. Halts U.S. Sales of Pelvic Mesh, Citing Safety Concerns for Women," *New York Times*, April 16, 2019, nytimes.com/2019/04/16/health/vaginal-pelvic-mesh-fda.html#.

19. Susan Berger, "Vaginal Mesh Has Caused Health Problems in Many Women, Even as Some Surgeons Vouch for Its Safety and Efficacy," *Washington Post*, Jan. 20, 2019, washingtonpost.com/national/health-science/vaginal-mesh-has-caused-health-problems-in-many-women-even-as-some-surgeons-vouch-for-its-safety-and-efficacy/2019/01/18/1c4a2332-ff0f-11e8-ad40-cdfd0e0dd65a_story.html.

20. "Transvaginal Mesh Revision Surgeries," *Drugwatch*, drugwatch.com/transvaginal-mesh/revision-surgeries/.

21. Carl Heneghan, "What Next for Transvaginal Mesh?" *BMJ Opinion*, June 5, 2019, blogs.bmj.com/bmj/2019/06/05/carl-heneghan-what-next-for-transvaginal-mesh/.

22. "FDA Takes Action to Protect Women's Health, Orders Manufacturers of Surgical Mesh Intended for Transvaginal Repair of Pelvic Organ Prolapse to Stop Selling All Devices," U.S. Food and Drug Administration, April 16, 2019, fda.gov/news-events/press-announcements/fda-takes-action-protect-womens-health-orders-manufacturers-surgical-mesh-intended-transvaginal.

23. Jonathan Stempel, "Boston Scientific in $189 Million Settlement with U.S. States over Surgical Mesh Devices," Reuters, March 23, 2021, reuters.com/article/us-boston-scientific-settlement/boston-scientific-in-189-million-settlement-with-u-s-states-over-surgical-mesh-devices-idUSKBN2BF29D.

24. Carl J. Heneghan et al., "Trials of Transvaginal Mesh Devices for Pelvic Organ Prolapse: A Systematic Database Review of the US FDA Approval Process," *BMJ Open* 7 (2017): e017125. doi:10.1136/bmjopen-2017-017125.

25. Jonathan Gornall, "How Mesh Became a Four Letter Word," *BMJ* (2018): 363, doi:10.1136/bmj.k4137.

26. "Statement on Agency's Efforts to Increase Transparency in Medical Device Reporting," U.S. Food and Drug Administration, June 21, 2019, fda.gov/news-events/press-announcements/statement-agencys-efforts-increase-transparency-medical-device-reporting.

27. Neil Vargesson, "Thalidomide-Induced Teratogenesis: History and Mechanisms," *Birth Defects Research*, part C, *Embryo Today: Reviews* 105, no. 2 (2015): 140–56, doi:10.1002/bdrc.21096.

28. James Meikle, "Thalidomide 'Caused up to 10,000 Miscarriages and Infant Deaths in UK,'" *The Guardian*, Mar. 6, 2016, theguardian.com/society/2016/mar/06/thalidomide-caused-up-to-10000-miscarriages-infant-deaths-uk.

29. Robert D. McFadden, "Frances Oldham Kelsey, Who Saved U.S. Babies from Thalidomide, Dies at 101," *New York Times*, Aug. 7, 2015, nytimes.com/2015/08/08/science/frances-oldham-kelsey-fda-doctor-who-exposed-danger-of-thalidomide-dies-at-101.html.

30. Ingrid Peritz, "Frances Oldham Kelsey Averted a Thalidomide Tragedy Because She Wouldn't Be Rushed," *Globe and Mail*, Aug. 14, 2015, theglobeandmail.com/life/health-and-fitness/health/frances-oldham-kelsey-averted-a-thalidomide-tragedy-because-she-wouldnt-be-rushed/article25976972/.

31. Leila McNeill, "The Woman Who Stood Between America and a Generation of 'Thalidomide Babies,'" *Smithsonian Magazine*, May 8, 2017, smithsonianmag

.com/science-nature/woman-who-stood-between-america-and-epidemic-birth-defects-180963165/.

32. John Mulliken, "A Woman Doctor Who Would Not Be Hurried," *Life*, Aug. 10, 1962, 28–29.

33. Gardiner Harris, "The Public's Quiet Savior from Harmful Medicines," *New York Times*, Sept. 13, 2010, nytimes.com/2010/09/14/health/14kelsey.html.

34. Emily Olsen, "Femtech Startups Nearly Double Funding Dollars from Last Year, but Still Make up Small Percent of Market," *MobiHealthNews*, Sept. 30, 2021, mobihealthnews.com/news/femtech-startups-nearly-double-funding-dollars-last-year-still-make-small-percent-market.

Chapter 7: Nutritionmania: Why Are We Confused About What We Eat?

1. *Keeping Up with the Kardashians*, season 17, episode 9, "Hard Candy," E!, Nov. 10, 2019.

2. Margaret L. Westwater, Paul C. Fletcher, and Hisham Ziauddeen, "Sugar Addiction: The State of the Science," *European Journal of Nutrition* 55 (2016): 55–69, doi.org/10.1007/s00394-016-1229-6.

3. "Tenfold Increase in Childhood and Adolescent Obesity in Four Decades: New Study by Imperial College London and WHO," World Health Organization, Oct. 11, 2017, who.int/news/item/11–10–2017-tenfold-increase-in-childhood-and-adolescent-obesity-in-four-decades-new-study-by-imperial-college-london-and-who.

4. "Nearly Two-Thirds of Mothers 'Shamed' by Others About Their Parenting Skills," *ScienceDaily*, June 19, 2017, sciencedaily.com/releases/2017/06/170619092158.htm.

5. Ellen Wallwork, "Reese Witherspoon Food Shamed After Sharing Photo of Her Son's Breakfast," *HuffPost UK*, Dec. 3, 2015, huffingtonpost.co.uk/2015/03/12/reese-witherspoon-food-shamed-over-sons-breakfast-photo_n_6855780.html.

6. Janet Forgrieve, "The Growing Acceptance of Veganism," *Forbes*, Nov. 2, 2018, forbes.com/sites/janetforgrieve/2018/11/02/picturing-a-kindler-gentler-world-vegan-month/?sh=30074c722f2b.

7. Sophie M. Balzora, "One-Third of Americans Are Trying to Avoid Gluten–but Is It the Villain We Think It Is?," *NYU Langone Health NewsHub*, nyulangone.org/news/one-third-americans-are-trying-avoid-gluten-it-villain-we-think-it-is.

8. Martha C. White, "Recipe for Success: Cookbook Sales Survive Shift to Digital Media," NBC News, Aug. 14, 2018, nbcnews.com/business/consumer/recipe-success-cookbook-sales-survive-shift-digital-media-n900621.

9. Vani Hari, "Healthy Meal Plans for Looking and Feeling Your Best!," *Food Babe*, Oct. 10, 2017, foodbabe.com/healthy-meal-plans/.

10. Vani Hari, "You'll Never Guess What's in a Starbucks Pumpkin Spice Latte (Hint: You Won't Be Happy)," *Food Babe*, April 6, 2015, foodbabe.com/starbucks-pumpkin -spice-latte/.

11. Nina Teicholz, *The Big Fat Surprise: Why Butter, Meat, and Cheese Belong in a Healthy Diet* (New York: Simon & Schuster, 2015), 43–61.

12. Dustin Moore (registered dietitian and writer) in discussion with the author, April 2022.

13. Centers for Disease Control and Prevention, "Trends in Intake of Energy and Macronutrients—United States, 1971–2000," *Morbidity and Mortality Weekly Report* 53, no. 4 (2004): 80–82.

14. Camila Domonoske, "50 Years Ago, Sugar Industry Quietly Paid Scientists to Point Blame at Fat," NPR, Sept. 13, 2016, npr.org/sections/thetwo-way /2016/09/13/493739074/50-years-ago-sugar-industry-quietly-paid-scientists -to-point-blame-at-fat.

15. "How Much Is Too Much?" SugarScience, University of California, San Francisco, April 27, 2018, sugarscience.ucsf.edu/dispelling-myths-too-much.html# .YYnDStnMLeo.

16. Paul Zane Pilzer, *The Next Trillion: Why the Wellness Industry Will Exceed the $1 Trillion Healthcare (Sickness) Industry in the Next Ten Years* (Lake Dallas, TX: VideoPlus, 2001), 8.

17. Belinda S. Lennerz et al., "Effects of Dietary Glycemic Index on Brain Regions Related to Reward and Craving in Men," *American Journal of Clinical Nutrition* 98, no. 3 (September 2013): 641–47, doi:10.3945/ajcn.113.064113.

18. Wendy Scinta, "The History of Portion Sizes: How They've Changed Over Time," *Your Weight Matters*, April 28, 2016, yourweightmatters.org/portion -sizes-changed-time/.

19. Larissa Galastri Baraldi et al., "Consumption of Ultra-Processed Foods and Associated Sociodemographic Factors in the USA Between 2007 and 2012: Evidence from a Nationally Representative Cross-Sectional Study," *BMJ Open* 8, no. 3 (March 2018), ncbi.nlm.nih.gov/pmc/articles/PMC5855172/.

20. Linda Searing, "The Big Number: Only 7 Percent of Adults Are Consuming the Right Amount of Fiber," *Washington Post*, June 21, 2021, washington post.com/health/fiber-weight-control-heart/2021/06/18/2ff37134-cf7f-11eb -8cd2-4e95230cfac2_story.html.

21. Michael F. Jacobson, "Burying the Snackwell Myth," *Medium*, Dec. 11, 2015, medium.com/@CSPI/burying-the-snackwell-myth-4b6e9dff6d07.

22. "Food Marketing," UConn Rudd Center for Food Policy & Health, April 20, 2020, uconnruddcenter.org/research/food-marketing/#f(1).

23. Warren James Belasco, *Appetite for Change: How the Counterculture Took on the Food Industry* (Ithaca, NY: Cornell University Press, 2007), 28.

24. Marion Nestle, "Food Lobbies, the Food Pyramid, and U.S. Nutrition Policy," *International Journal of Health Services* 23, no. 3 (1993): 483–96, doi:10.2190/32F2–2PFB-MEG7–8HPU. PMID: 8375951.

25. Robert H. Lustig, *Fat Chance: Beating the Odds Against Sugar, Processed Food, Obesity, and Disease* (New York: Plume, 2014), 252.

26. Marion Nestle, *Food Politics: How the Food Industry Influences Nutrition and Health* (Berkeley: University of California Press, 2013), 123.

27. Camila Domonoske, "DNA Tests Find Subway Chicken Only 50 Percent Meat, Canadian News Program Reports," NPR, March 1, 2017, npr.org/sections /thetwo-way/2017/03/01/517920680/dna-tests-find-subway-chicken-only-50 -percent-meat-canadian-media-reports.

28. Ben Quinn, Sarah Butler, and Rebecca Smithers, "Mars Recalls Chocolate Bars in 55 Countries After Plastic Found in Product," *The Guardian*, Feb. 23, 2016, theguardian.com/lifeandstyle/2016/feb/23/mars-chocolate-product-recalls -snickers-milky-way-celebrations-germany-netherlands.

29. "Food Safety in America—Time to Bolster Consumer Confidence," *C.O.nxt*, May 5, 2021, co-nxt.com/blog/food-safety-in-america-time-to-bolster -consumer-confidence/.

30. "We Are What We Eat: Healthy Eating Trends Around the World," Nielsen, January 2015, nielsen.com/wp-content/uploads/sites/3/2019/04/Nielsen20Glob al20Health20and20Wellness20Report20-20January202015-1.pdf.

31. Roland Marchand, *Advertising the American Dream: Making Way for Modernity, 1920–1940* (Berkeley: University of California Press, 1985), 297–98.

32. Catherine Price, *Vitamania: Our Obsessive Quest for Nutritional Perfection* (New York: Penguin Press, 2015), 77.

33. Marchand, *Advertising the American Dream*, 296.

34. Price, *Vitamania*, 71.

35. "2. Americans' Views About and Consumption of Organic Foods," Pew Research Center, Dec. 1, 2016, pewresearch.org/science/2016/12/01/americans -views-about-and-consumption-of-organic-foods/.

36. Benjamin L. Campbell et al., "U.S. and Canadian Consumer Perception of Local and Organic Terminology," *International Food and Agribusiness Management Review* 17, no. 2 (May 2014): 1–20.

37. "EWG's 2021 Shopper's Guide to Pesticides in Produce," EWG, ewg.org /foodnews/summary.php and https://www.healthkick.info/pesticides-in-produce the-clean-15-and-the-dirty-dozen/.

38. Food Science Babe, "Food Science Babe: The Dirty Deception of the 'Dirty Dozen,'" *AgDaily*, March 18, 2021, agdaily.com/insights/dirty-deception-ewg -dirty-dozen/.

39. Food Science Babe, "I really want to bring attention to the deceptive games the EWG plays all in the name of scaring consumers over safe foods to raise money for their organization. This needs to stop. Please share." Facebook photo, March 18, 2021, facebook.com/foodsciencebabe/photos/a.350962359061846 /950422905782452/?type=3.

40. "FY2019 Pesticide Report: Consistent with Trends Over the Past 8 Years, Pesticide Residue Levels Remain Low," U.S. Food and Drug Administration, Oct. 20, 2021, fda.gov/food/cfsan-constituent-updates/fy-2019-pesticide-report -consistent-trends-over-past-8-years-pesticide-residue-levels-remain-low.

41. "Americans' Views," Pew Research Center.

42. Crystal Smith-Spangler et al., "Are Organic Foods Safer or Healthier Than Conventional Alternatives?: A Systematic Review," *Annals of Internal Medicine* 157, no. 5 (2012): 348, doi:10.7326/0003–4819–157–5–201209040–00007.

43. Marcin Barański et al., "Higher Antioxidant and Lower Cadmium Concentrations and Lower Incidence of Pesticide Residues in Organically Grown Crops: A Systematic Literature Review and Meta-analyses," *British Journal of Nutrition* 112, no. 5 (2014): 794–811, doi:10.1017/S0007114514001366.

44. Kenneth Chang, "Study of Organic Crops Finds Fewer Pesticides and More Antioxidants," *New York Times*, July 11, 2014, nytimes.com/2014/07/12/science/earth /study-of-organic-crops-finds-fewer-pesticides-and-more-antioxidants-.html.

45. Peter Whoriskey, "Is Organic Food Safer and Healthier? The Guy in Charge of U.S. Organics Won't Say," *Washington Post*, April 30, 2015, washingtonpost .com/news/wonk/wp/2015/04/30/is-organic-food-safer-and-healthier-the-guy -in-charge-of-u-s-organics-wont-say/.

46. Joanna Schroeder et al., "Organic Marketing Report," *Academics Review* (2016), ww1.prweb.com/prfiles/2014/04/07/11743859/Academics-Review_Organic %20Marketing%20Report.pdf.

47. Michael Pollan, "Naturally," *New York Times*, May 13, 2001, nytimes.com/2001 /05/13/magazine/naturally.html.

48. Vanessa Apaolaza et al., "Eat Organic—Feel Good? The Relationship Between Organic Food Consumption, Health Concern and Subjective Wellbeing," *Food Quality and Preference* 63 (Jan. 2018): 51–62, doi:10.1016/j.foodqual.2017.07.011.

49. "When It Comes to Buying Organic, Science and Beliefs Don't Always Mesh," NPR, Sept. 7, 2012, npr.org/transcripts/160681396.

50. "Individuals May Consider Organic an Important Factor When Defining Healthy Food," Johns Hopkins Bloomberg School of Public Health, public health.jhu.edu/2015/individuals-may-consider-organic-an-important-factor -when-defining-healthy-food.

51. Yancui Huang, Indika Edirisinghe, and Britt M. Burton-Freeman, "Low-Income Shoppers and Fruit and Vegetables: What Do They Think?" *Nutrition Today* 51, no. 5 (2016): 242–50, doi:10.1097/NT.0000000000000176.

52. Cara Rosenbloom, "A Diet Rich in Fruits and Vegetables Outweighs the Risks of Pesticides," *Washington Post*, Jan. 18, 2017, washingtonpost.com /lifestyle/wellness/a-diet-rich-in-fruits-and-vegetables-outweighs-the-risks-of -pesticides/2017/01/13/f68ed4f6-d780-11e6-9a36-1d296534b31e_story.html.

53. Anna Vlasits, "The Growing Diet Divide Between Rich and Poor in America," *STAT*, June 21, 2016, statnews.com/2016/06/21/growing-diet-divide/.

54. James Temple, "Sorry—Organic Farming Is Actually Worse for Climate Change," *MIT Technology Review*, Oct. 22, 2019, technologyreview.com/2019/10/22 /132497/sorryorganic-farming-is-actually-worse-for-climate-change/.

55. Ocean, Inc., "Oceana Report: Plastic Pollution from Amazon Deliveries Grows by 29% in Just One Year," *GlobeNewswire*, Dec. 15, 2021, globenewswire .com/news-release/2021/12/15/2352262/0/en/Oceana-Report-Plastic-Pollution -From-Amazon-Deliveries-Grows-By-29-in-Just-One-Year.html.

56. "2018 Food & Health Survey," International Food Information Council, food insight.org/wp-content/uploads/2018/05/2018-FHS-Report-FINAL.pdf.

57. Meg Greenfield, "Give Me That Old-Time Cholesterol," *Washington Post*, June 20, 1984, washingtonpost.com/archive/politics/1984/06/20/give-me-that-old -time-cholesterol/303be7f3-fd49-4911-ad5b-bb8a9faaa742/.

58. Vani Hari, "Join Me! Investigate Your Food," *Food Babe*, foodbabe.com/about-me/.

59. Susan Donaldson James, "Subway Takes Chemical Out of Sandwich Bread After Protest," ABC News, Feb. 5, 2014, abcnews.go.com/Health/subway -takes-chemical-sandwich-bread-protest/story?id=22373414.

60. Mark Alsip, Kavin Senapathy, and Marc Draco, *The Fear Babe: Shattering Vani Hari's Glass House* (n.p.: Senapath Press, 2015), 28–31.

61. Vani Hari, "Should I Get the Flu Shot?," *Food Babe*, April 16, 2015, foodbabe .com/should-i-get-the-flu-shot/.

62. James Hamblin, "The Food Babe: Enemy of Chemicals," *The Atlantic*, February 11, 2015, theatlantic.com/health/archive/2015/02/the-food-babe-enemy-of -chemicals/385301/.

63. "Dietary Supplement Use Reaches All Time High," Council for Responsible Nutrition, crnusa.org/newsroom/dietary-supplement-use-reaches-all-time-high.

64. David J. A. Jenkins et al., "Supplemental Vitamins and Minerals for CVD Prevention and Treatment," *Journal of the American College of Cardiology* 71, no. 22 (2018): 2570–84, doi:10.1016/j.jacc.2018.04.020.

65. Francis Collins, "Study Finds No Benefit for Dietary Supplements," *Director's Blog,* National Institutes of Health, April 16, 2019, directorsblog.nih.gov/2019 /04/16/study-finds-no-benefit-for-dietary-supplements/.

66. Fan Chen et al., "Association Among Dietary Supplement Use, Nutrient Intake, and Mortality Among U.S. Adults: A Cohort Study," *Annals of Internal Medicine* 170, no. 9 (2019): 604, doi:10.7326/m18–2478.

67. Serena Gordon, "Dietary Supplements Do Nothing for You: Study," *Health-Day*, Consumer Health News, April 8, 2019, consumer.healthday.com/vitamins -and-nutrition-information-27/vitamin-and-mineral-news-698/dietary -supplements-do-nothing-for-you-study-744827.html.

68. Paul Offit, "The Vitamin Myth: Why We Think We Need Supplements," *The Atlantic*, July 19, 2013, theatlantic.com/health/archive/2013/07/the-vitamin -myth-why-we-think-we-need-supplements/277947/.

69. Robert H. Shmerling, MD, "What's in Your Supplements?" *Harvard Health* (blog), Feb. 15, 2019, health.harvard.edu/blog/whats-in-your-supplements -2019021515946.

70. Nikhil Sonnad, "All the 'Wellness' Products Americans Love to Buy Are Sold on Both Infowars and Goop," *Quartz*, qz.com/1010684/all-the-wellness -products-american-love-to-buy-are-sold-on-both-infowars-and-goop/.

71. Andrew Weil, "Cured by Kombucha?," June 20, 2018, drweil.com/health -wellness/balanced-living/healthy-living/cured-by-kombucha/.

72. "Dannon Agrees to Drop Exaggerated Health Claims for Activia Yogurt and DanActive Dairy Drink," Federal Trade Commission, Dec. 15, 2010, ftc.gov /news-events/press-releases/2010/12/dannon-agrees-drop-exaggerated-health -claims-activia-yogurt.

73. "2020 Food & Health Survey," International Food Information Council, foodinsight.org/wp-content/uploads/2020/06/IFIC-Food-and-Health-Survey -2020.pdf.

74. "US Sugar and Alternative Sweeteners Market Report 2020," Mintel, May 25, 2021, store.mintel.com/us-sugar-and-alternative-sweeteners-market-report.

75. Max Knoblauch, "Americans Feel Guilty About Almost a Third of the Food They Eat," *New York Post*, March 13, 2019, nypost.com/2019/03/13/americans -feel-guilty-about-almost-a-third-of-the-food-they-eat/.

Chapter 8: Crystal-Clear Futures: A New Take on New Age Spirituality

1. Thomas G. Plante, "What Do the Spiritual and Religious Traditions Offer the Practicing Psychologist?" *Pastoral Psychology* 56, no. 4 (2008): 429–44, doi:10.1007/s11089–008–0119–0.

2. Claire Gecewicz, "'New Age' Beliefs Common Among Both Religious and Nonreligious Americans," Pew Research Center, Oct. 1, 2018, pewresearch .org/fact-tank/2018/10/01/new-age-beliefs-common-among-both-religious -and-nonreligious-americans/.

3. Anne Harrington, *The Cure Within: A History of Mind-Body Medicine* (New York: W. W. Norton, 2009), 111–12.

4. James C. Whorton, *Nature Cures: The History of Alternative Medicine in America* (New York: Oxford University Press, 2004), 125–30.

5. Anne Harrington, *Cure Within*, 118–19.

6. Marianne Williamson, *A Course in Weight Loss: 21 Spiritual Lessons for Surrendering Your Weight Forever* (Carlsbad, CA: Hay House, 2012), 15–21.

7. Steve Salerno, *SHAM: How the Self-Help Movement Made America Helpless* (New York: Crown, 2005), 248.

8. Rina Raphael, "Is There a Crystal Bubble? Inside the Billion-Dollar 'Healing' Gemstone Industry," *Fast Company*, May 5, 2017, fastcompany.com/40410406 /is-there-a-crystal-bubble-inside-the-billion-dollar-healing-gemstone -industry.

9. Rina Raphael, "Silicon Valley's Quest to Build the Wellness Community of the Future," *Fast Company*, Aug. 9, 2019, fastcompany.com/90387422/how-silicon -valleys-elite-are-trying-to-building-the-wellness-community-of-the-future.

10. Jeane Dixon and Rene Noorbergen, *Jeane Dixon: My Life and Prophecies* (Boston: G. K. Hall, 1971), 12–13.

11. Ruth Montgomery, *A Gift of Prophecy: The Phenomenal Jeane Dixon* (Toronto: Bantam Books, 1965), 13.

12. Michael Isikoff, "Terror Watch: Nixon and Dixon," *Newsweek*, March 22, 2005, newsweek.com/terror-watch-nixon-and-dixon-114707.

13. Montgomery, *Gift of Prophecy*, 34.

14. John Allen Paulos, *Innumeracy: Mathematical Illiteracy and Its Consequences* (New York: Hill and Wang, 2001), 71.

15. Krista Tippett, *Becoming Wise: An Inquiry into the Mystery and Art of Living* (New York: Penguin Books, 2017), 11.

16. Krista Tippett, "My Grandfather's Faith: Contradictions and Mysteries," *The On Being Project*, July 18, 2010, onbeing.org/blog/my-grandfathers-faith -contradictions-and-mysteries/.

17. Tippett, *Becoming Wise*, 170.

18. "In U.S., Decline of Christianity Continues at Rapid Pace," Pew Research Center's Religion and Public Life Project, Oct. 17, 2019, pewforum.org/2019/10/17 /in-u-s-decline-of-christianity-continues-at-rapid-pace/.

19. Chad Day, "Americans Have Shifted Dramatically on What Values Matter Most," *Wall Street Journal*, Aug. 25, 2019, wsj.com/articles/americans-have -shifted-dramatically-on-what-values-matter-most-11566738001.

20. Jeffrey M. Jones, "U.S. Church Membership Falls Below Majority for First Time," Gallup, Mar. 29, 2021, news.gallup.com/poll/341963/church-membership -falls-below-majority-first-time.aspx.

21. Wade Clark Roof, *Spiritual Marketplace: Baby Boomers and the Remaking of American Religion* (Princeton, NJ: Princeton University Press, 1999), 159.

22. Dalia Fahmy, "Key Findings About Americans' Belief in God," Pew Research Center, April 25, 2018, pewresearch.org/fact-tank/2018/04/25/key-findings -about-americans-belief-in-god/.

23. Travis Mitchell, "The Gender Gap in Religion Around the World," Pew Research Center's Religion and Public Life Project, March 22, 2016, pewforum .org/2016/03/22/the-gender-gap-in-religion-around-the-world/.

24. Christian Smith, *Religion: What It Is, How It Works, and Why It Matters* (Princeton, NJ: Princeton University Press, 2019), 200–202.

25. Kathleen J. Sullivan, "A Spiritual Practice Is the Foundation of a Meaningful Life, Oprah Winfrey Tells Stanford Audience," Stanford University, April 21, 2015, news.stanford.edu/news/2015/april/oprah-rathbun-lecture-042115.html.

26. Jamie Ballard, "Exercising More and Saving Money Are the Most Popular 2020 New Year's Resolutions," YouGov America, Jan. 2, 2020, today.yougov.com/topics /lifestyle/articles-reports/2020/01/02/new-years-resolutions-2020-health-finance.

27. Hannah Ewens, "The 'Goop Effect': The Women Who Spend Hundreds Seeking Spirituality," *Vice*, Feb. 18, 2020, vice.com/en/article/jgejj3/spirituality -luxury-upper-class-goop-lab-healing-treatmentss.

28. Robert D. Putnam, *Bowling Alone: The Collapse and Revival of American Community* (New York: Simon & Schuster Paperbacks, 2000), 74–79.

Chapter 9: You're Not Working Hard Enough

1. Rina Raphael, "This Ex-Convict Created New York's New Prison-Themed Fitness Empire," *Fast Company*, Aug. 25, 2017, fastcompany.com/40452499/this -ex-convict-created-new-yorks-new-prison-themed-fitness-empire.

2. Jeff Haden, "Internal Documents Reveal the Marketing Strategy Peloton Used to Become a $1.8 Billion Company," *Inc.*, Mar. 30, 2021, www.inc.com

/jeff-haden/internal-documents-reveal-marketing-strategy-peloton-used-to
-become-a-18-billion-company.html.

3. Rina Raphael, "How Orangetheory Grew to Dominate the Boutique Fitness Industry," *Fast Company*, July 17, 2018, fastcompany.com/90201967/how
-orangetheory-grew-to-dominate-the-boutique-fitness-industry.

4. "The Effectiveness of Activity Trackers and Rewards to Encourage Physical Activity," Duke University, Oct. 5, 2016, duke-nus.edu.sg/allnews/the
-effectiveness-of-activity-trackers-and-rewards-to-encourage-physical-activity.

5. Jordan Etkin, "The Hidden Cost of Personal Quantification," *Journal of Consumer Research* 42, no. 6 (April 2016): 967–84, doi:10.1093/jcr/ucv095.

6. Tara Isabella Burton, "Football Really Is America's Religion," *Vox*, Sept. 27, 2017, vox.com/identities/2017/9/27/16308792/football-america-religion-nfl
-protests-powerful.

7. James F. Fixx, *The Complete Book of Running* (New York: Random House, 1977), 24.

8. Elise Rose Carrotte, Ivanka Prichard, and Megan Su Cheng Lim, "'Fitspiration' on Social Media: A Content Analysis of Gendered Images," *Journal of Medical Internet Research* 19, no. 3 (2017), doi:10.2196/jmir.6368.

9. Angela S. Alberga, Samantha J. Withnell, and Kristin M. von Ranson, "Fitspiration and Thinspiration: A Comparison Across Three Social Networking Sites," *Journal of Eating Disorders* 6, no. 1 (2018), doi:10.1186/s40337–018–0227-x.

10. Denise Prichard, "Trend Report: How You Can Expect Your Workout to Change in 2021," *Mindbody*, Jan. 7 2021, explore.mindbodyonline.com/blog
/fitness/trend-report-how-you-can-expect-your-workout-change-2021.

11. Zoe Weiner, "Is It Time to Phase Out the #FitFluencer Once and for All?," *Well+Good*, Sept. 22, 2021, wellandgood.com/fitness-influencer-fitfluencer
-responsibility/.

12. Stephanie Easton et al., "Young People's Experiences of Viewing the Fitspiration Social Media Trend: Qualitative Study." *Journal of Medical Internet Research* 20, no. 6 (2018), doi:10.2196/jmir.9156.

13. Baine B. Craft, Haley A. Carroll, and M. Kathleen B. Lustyk, "Gender Differences in Exercise Habits and Quality of Life Reports: Assessing the Moderating Effects of Reasons for Exercise," *International Journal of Liberal Arts and Social Science* 2, no. 5 (2014): 65–76.

14. Kim Parker, Juliana Menasce Horowitz, and Renee Stepler, "2. Americans See Different Expectations for Men and Women," Pew Research Center, Social and Demographic Trends Project, Dec. 5, 2017, pewresearch.org/social-trends/2017
/12/05/americans-see-different-expectations-for-men-and-women/.

15. Rina Raphael, "Burned-out Americans Are Helping Wellness Tourism Flourish," *Fast Company*, Oct. 29, 2016, fastcompany.com/3064971/burned-out -americans-are-helping-wellness-tourism-flourish.

16. Rina Raphael, "Travelers Are Abandoning Spas to Join Fitfluencer Retreats," *Fast Company*, Dec. 11, 2017, fastcompany.com/40504343/travelers-are -abandoning-spas-to-join-fitfluencer-retreats.

17. Kasandra Brabaw, "An Eating Disorder Survivor Opened Up About Vacation Weight Gain," *Refinery29*, May 24, 2017, refinery29.com/en-us/2017/05 /156020/vacation-weight-gain-body-positivity.

18. Maggie Lange, "Don't Even Think About Working Out on Vacation," *The Cut*, July 16, 2021, thecut.com/2021/07/dont-work-out-on-vacation.html.

19. Jason Kelly, *Sweat Equity: Inside the New Economy of Mind and Body* (Hoboken, NJ: Bloomberg Press, 2016), 99.

20. "Three out of Four Women Are Suffering from Burnout, According to New Harris Poll Commissioned by Meredith Corporation," Dotdash Meredith, Oct. 3, 2019, meredith.mediaroom.com/2019-10-03-American-Women -Confronting-Burnout-At-Epidemic-Levels-According-To-New-Harris-Poll -Commissioned-By-Meredith-Corporation.

21. Rina Raphael, "Yoga Class While Waiting for Refills? CVS Tests New 'Health Hubs,'" *Fast Company*, May 4, 2019, fastcompany.com/90343800/yoga-class -while-waiting-for-refills-cvs-tests-new-health-hubs.

22. Tamara Lush, "Poll: Americans Are the Unhappiest They've Been in 50 Years," Associated Press, June 16, 2020, apnews.com/article/0f6b9be04fa0 d3194401821a72665a50.

23. David Brancaccio, Chris Farrell, and Daniel Shin, "'The Big Quit' Isn't Going Away Anytime Soon," *Marketplace*, Oct. 27, 2021, marketplace.org/2021/10/27 /the-big-quit-isnt-going-away-anytime-soon/.

24. Katherine Wernet, "Stressed Out in America," *Mindbody*, mindbodyonline .com/business/education/blog/stressed-out-america.

25. Mary Pilon et al., "The Influencers Fighting Instagram's Perfection," *Outside*, Sep. 20, 2017, outsideonline.com/health/wellness/backlash-instagram -influencer-culture/.

26. "'Every Body Yoga' Encourages Self-Love and Everyone to Get on the Mat," *Here & Now*, WBUR, July 13, 2017, wbur.org/hereandnow/2017/07/13/every -body-yoga-jessamyn-stanley.

27. Jen Murphy, "The Hot New Class at Your Gym? Resting," *Wall Street Journal*, Mar. 27, 2022, wsj.com/articles/the-hot-new-class-at-your-gym-resting -11648336639.

28. Rina Raphael, "Stretching Studios Are the Next Big Boutique Fitness Trend," *Fast Company*, Nov. 27, 2018, fastcompany.com/90269526/stretching-studios -are-the-next-big-boutique-fitness-trend.

Chapter 10: Chasing Golden Unicorns: Biohacking the Future

1. Rina Raphael, "Cell Massages to Cryotherapy: Inside the 'Biohacking' Gym of the Future," *Fast Company*, Nov. 16, 2017, fastcompany.com/40492979/cell -massages-to-cryotherapy-inside-the-biohacking-gym-of-the-future.

2. Courtney Rubin, "The Cult of the Bulletproof Coffee Diet," *New York Times*, Dec. 12, 2014, nytimes.com/2014/12/14/style/the-cult-of-the-bulletproof -coffee-diet.html.

3. "Wellness 2030: The New Techniques of Happiness," Global Wellness Institute, June 16, 2021, globalwellnessinstitute.org/industry-research/wellness-2030/.

4. Rachel Monroe, "The Bulletproof Coffee Founder Has Spent $1 Million in His Quest to Live to 180," *Men's Health*, Jan. 23, 2019, menshealth.com/health /a25902826/bulletproof-dave-asprey-biohacking/.

5. Jade Scipioni, "These 2 Habits Can Help You Live Longer, Says Bulletproof Coffee Creator (Who Plans to Live to 180)," *CNBC Make It*, Nov. 20, 2019, cnbc.com/2019/11/20/bulletproof-coffee-founder-dave-asprey-how-to-live -longer.html.

6. Emily Abbate, "The Real-Life Diet of Dave Asprey, Who Thinks Coffee Is a Superfood," *GQ*, Jan. 28, 2021, gq.com/story/real-life-diet-dave-asprey.

7. Tasbeeh Herwees, "I 'Biohacked' My Body—but My Body Hacked Me Back," *Good*, March 7, 2017, good.is/food/bulletproof-diet-biohack.

8. Dave Asprey, *Super Human: The Bulletproof Plan to Age Backward and Maybe Even Live Forever* (New York: Harper Wave, 2019), 170.

9. Judith Rodin and Ellen J. Langer, "Long-Term Effects of a Control-Relevant Intervention with the Institutionalized Aged," *Journal of Personality and Social Psychology* 35, no. 12 (1977): 897–902, doi:10.1037/0022–3514.35.12.897.

10. Tali Sharot, *The Influential Mind: What the Brain Reveals About Our Power to Change Others* (Boston: Little, Brown, 2018), 102.

11. "Why We Believe We Have More Control Over the World Than We Actually Do," The Decision Lab, thedecisionlab.com/biases/illusion-of-control/.

12. Harvey Hartman and David Wright, *Marketing to the New Natural Consumer: Understanding Trends in Wellness* (Bellevue, WA: Hartman Group, 1999), 34–35.

13. Raphael, "Cell Massages to Cryotherapy."

14. Vince Parry (president and chief branding officer, Parry Branding Group), email message to the author, October 2021.

15. Vince Parry, *Identity Crisis: Health Care Branding's Hidden Problems and Proven Strategies to Solve Them* (n.p.: Parry Branding Group, 2017).

16. Vince Parry (president and chief branding officer, Parry Branding Group), in discussion with the author, October 2021.

17. Walter Isaacson, *Steve Jobs* (New York: Simon & Schuster, 2018), 181.

18. Dave Asprey, *Head Strong: The Bulletproof Plan to Activate Untapped Brain Energy to Work Smarter and Think Faster—in Just Two Weeks* (New York: Harper Wave, 2017), introduction.

19. Alex Hannaford, "The Bulletproof Diet: Simplistic, Invalid and Unscientific," *The Telegraph*, Nov. 27, 2014, telegraph.co.uk/books/what-to-read/the -bulletproof-diet-simplistic-invalid-and-unscientific/.

20. Kris Gunnars, "3 Potential Downsides of Bulletproof Coffee," *Healthline*, Feb. 7, 2022, healthline.com/nutrition/3-reasons-why-bulletproof-coffee-is-a-bad -idea#2.-High-in-saturated-fat.

21. James MacDonald, "How Dietary Supplements Can Cause More Harm Than Good," *JSTOR Daily*, Aug. 5, 2019, daily.jstor.org/how-dietary-supplements -can-cause-more-harm-than-good/.

22. Wade Greene, "Guru of the Organic Food Cult," *New York Times*, June 6, 1971, nytimes.com/1971/06/06/archives/guru-of-the-organic-food-cult-guru-of-the -organic-food-cult.html.

23. Joe Schwarcz, "The Right Chemistry: J. I. Rodale Was an Early Opponent of Sugar," *Montreal Gazette*, July 15, 2020, montrealgazette.com/opinion /columnists/the-right-chemistry-j-i-rodale-was-an-early-opponent-of-sugar.

24. Maria McGrath, "The Bizarre Life (and Death) of 'Mr. Organic,'" *New Republic*, Aug. 8, 2014, newrepublic.com/article/119007/bizarre-life-and-death-mr -organic.

25. Rebecca Grant, "How Egg Freezing Got Rebranded as the Ultimate Act of Self-Care," *The Guardian*, Sept. 30, 2020, theguardian.com/us-news/2020/sep /30/egg-freezing-self-care-pregnancy-fertility.

26. Michelle J. Bayefsky, Alan H. DeCherney, and Louise P. King, "Respecting Autonomy—a Call for Truth in Commercial Advertising for Planned Oocyte Cryopreservation," *Fertil Steril* 113, no. 4 (Apr. 2020): 743–44, 10.1016/j.fertnstert .2019.12.039.

27. Kaitlyn Tiffany, "The SoulCycle of Fertility Sells Egg-Freezing and 'Empowerment' to 25-Year-Olds," *The Verge*, Sept. 11, 2018, theverge.com/2018/9/11 /17823810/kindbody-startup-fertility-clinic-egg-freezing-millennials-location.

28. Rina Raphael, "Unable to Afford IVF, Millennials Turn to Hopeful Grandparents," *Fast Company*, July 17, 2019, fastcompany.com/90376652/with-ivf

-too-expensive-millennials-turn-to-a-motivated-source-of-funding-hopeful
-grandparents.

29. Angel Petropanagos et al., "Social Egg Freezing: Risk, Benefits and Other Considerations," *Canadian Medical Association Journal* 187, no. 9 (2015): 666–69, doi:10.1503/cmaj.141605.

30. Romualdo Sciorio et al., "One Follicle, One Egg, One Embryo: A Case-Report of Successful Pregnancy Obtained from a Single Oocyte Collected," *JBRA Assisted Reproduction* 25, no. 2 (April 2021): 314–17, doi:10.5935/151 8–0557.20200087.

31. Ariana Eunjung Cha, "The Struggle to Conceive with Frozen Eggs," *Washington Post*, Jan. 27, 2018, washingtonpost.com/news/national/wp/2018/01/27 /feature/she-championed-the-idea-that-freezing-your-eggs-would-free-your -career-but-things-didnt-quite-work-out/.

32. Claire Cain Miller, "The 10-Year Baby Window That Is the Key to the Women's Pay Gap," *The Upshot* (blog), *New York Times*, April 9, 2018, nytimes.com/2018 /04/09/upshot/the-10-year-baby-window-that-is-the-key-to-the-womens-pay -gap.html.

33. Heather Murphy,"Lots of Successful Women Are Freezing Their Eggs. But It May Not Be about Their Careers," *New York Times*, July 3, 2018, nytimes .com/2018/07/03/health/freezing-eggs-women.html.

34. Emily Jackson, "The Ambiguities of 'Social' Egg Freezing and the Challenges of Informed Consent," *Biosocieties* 13 (2018): 21–40, 10.1057/s41292-017- 0044-5.

35. Lucy van de Wiel, *Freezing Fertility: Oocyte Cryopreservation and the Gender Politics of Aging* (New York: New York University Press, 2020), 51.

36. Ruth La Ferla, "These Companies Really, Really, Really Want to Freeze Your Eggs," *New York Times*, Aug. 29, 2018, nytimes.com/2018/08/29/style /egg-freezing-fertility-millennials.html.

37. Carl Elliott, *Better Than Well: American Medicine Meets the American Dream* (New York: W. W. Norton, 2004), 188.

38. Christopher Barbey, "Evidence of Biased Advertising in the Case of Social Egg Freezing," *New Bioethics* 23, no. 3 (2017): 195–209, doi.org/10.1080/20502877 .2017.1396033.

Chapter 11: Democratizing Wellness: Pushing Back Against 'Wellthness'

1. Rina Raphael, "Inside the $2,000-a-Month, Invite-Only Fitness Clubs," *Elemental*, Jan. 3, 2020, elemental.medium.com/inside-the-2–000-a-month-invite -only-fitness-clubs-b44dc031bf54.

2.   Raphael, "Inside the $2,000-a-Month, Invite-Only, Fitness Clubs."

3.   Tom Corley, "Author Who Studies Millionaires: 240 Minutes a Day
     Separates the Rich from Everyone Else," CNBC, June 22, 2018, cnbc.
     com/2018/06/21/tom-corley-240-minutes-a-day-separates-the-rich-from-ever
     yone-else.html.

4.   Rina Raphael, "Utopic Wellness Communities Are a Multibillion-Dollar Real
     Estate Trend," *Fast Company*, Jan. 24, 2018, fastcompany.com/40512467/utopic
     -wellness-communities-are-a-multibillion-dollar-real-estate-trend.

5.   Rina Raphael, "You Might Get the Best Sleep of Your Life in This House—if
     You Can Afford It," *Fast Company*, Sept. 6, 2019, fastcompany.com/90398249
     /is-this-the-worlds-most-sleep-optimized-home.

6.   Paul Zane Pilzer, *The Next Trillion: Why the Wellness Industry Will Exceed the $1
     Trillion Healthcare (Sickness) Industry in the Next Ten Years* (Lake Dallas, TX:
     VideoPlus, 2001), 50.

7.   Rina Raphael, "Fitter, Healthier, Happier? How Wellness Drinks Took Over
     Instagram," *Fast Company*, Dec. 19, 2018, fastcompany.com/90276523/fitter
     -healthier-happier-how-wellness-drinks-took-over-instagram.

8.   Rina Raphael, "Gwyneth Paltrow Wants to Put Her Goop Inside You," *Fast
     Company*, March 27, 2017, fastcompany.com/3069237/gwyneth-paltrow-wants
     -to-put-her-goop-inside-you.

9.   Douglas Atkin, *The Culting of Brands: Turn Your Customers into True Believers*
     (New York: Portfolio, 2004), 31.

10. "Social Networks Push Runners to Run Further and Faster Than Their Friends,"
     Nature 544, no. 270 (2017), nature.com/articles/544270a.

11. Sarah Stage, *Female Complaints: Lydia Pinkham and the Business of Women's Med-
     icine* (New York: W. W. Norton, 1981), 102.

12. Stage, *Female Complaints*, 108.

13. Stage, *Female Complaints*, 123.

14. Jaclyn Krymowski, "Fitness and Farming—it's No Surprise They Go So Well
     Together," *AgDaily*, July 1, 2020, agdaily.com/features/fitness-and-agriculture
     -a-likely-pair/.

15. Rina Raphael, "Wellness Has a Diversity Issue—These Women Are Changing
     That," *Fast Company*, Feb. 21, 2018, fastcompany.com/40531531/wellness-has
     -a-diversity-issue-these-women-are-changing-that.

16. Rina Raphael, "This Home Comes with Yoga, Sound Baths, Star Energy
     Healing—and 95 Roommates," *Los Angeles Times*, Oct. 24, 2019, latimes.com
     /lifestyle/story/2019–10–24/haven-venice-yoga-sound-baths-95-roommates.

Chapter 12: Guides for the Perplexed

1. Vani Hari, "Food Babe TV: Do You Eat Beaver Butt?," *Food Babe*, Jan. 31, 2018, foodbabe.com/food-babe-tv-do-you-eat-beaver-butt/.

2. Lynzy Coughlin, "Debunking Food Industry Myths with Erin from Food Science Babe," *Motherhood Meets Medicine*, Apple Podcasts, Oct. 6, 2021, podcasts .apple.com/us/podcast/debunking-food-industry-myths-with-erin-from-food /id1553782780?i=1000537708777.

3. Rina Raphael, "'It's Sort of the Wild West': How Instagram Influencers Are Disrupting Healthcare," *Fast Company*, Nov. 20, 2019, fastcompany.com /90427946/as-the-healthcare-industry-increasingly-relies-on-influencers -concerns-mount.

4. Austin Chiang (@austinchiangmd), "Comparing the vaccines #science #learnontiktok #tiktokpartner," TikTok, Nov. 17, 2020, tiktok.com /@austinchiangmd/video/6896305106917149957, accessed Jan. 29, 2022.

5. Food Babe, "New investigation . . . This may be coming to a school near you. We'll likely see disinfectant booths like this in airports, stores, and other public places too," Facebook post, Aug. 12, 2020, facebook.com/permalink.php?story _fbid=3487462847955068&id=132535093447877.

6. Food Babe, "Food Babe Scam: My Response to the Attacks on Me and Our Movement," *Food Babe* (blog), Apr. 16, 2015, foodbabe.com/food-babe-critics/.

7. Holly Whetstone, "Inflation, Pandemic, War Reflect Consumers' Wariness on Grocery Prices," *AgBioResearch*, Apr. 4, 2022, canr.msu.edu/news/inflation -pandemic-war-reflect-consumers-wariness-on-grocery-prices.

8. Douglas Buhler and Sheril Kirshenbaum, "From GMOs to BPA, Why the Wealthy Are More Likely to Fall for Food Pseudoscience," *Genetic Literacy Project*, Sept. 20, 2019, geneticliteracyproject.org/2019/09/20/from-gmos-to -bpa-why-are-the-wealthy-more-likely-to-fall-for-food-pseudoscience/.

Conclusion

1. Arthur J. Barsky, *Worried Sick: Our Troubled Quest for Wellness* (Boston: Little, Brown, 1988), 8.

2. David Foster Wallace, "David Foster Wallace on Life and Work," *Wall Street Journal*, Sept. 19, 2008, wsj.com/articles/SB122178211966454607.

3. Donald B. Ardell, *High-Level Wellness: An Alternative to Doctors, Drugs, and Disease* (Emmaus, PA: Rodale Press, 1977), 3.

Acknowledgments

This book would never have been written had it not been for my patient agent Sarah Fuentes and supportive editor Amy Einhorn. Both were instrumental in getting this project off the ground and steering me in the right direction. Also, the entire team at Henry Holt: Julia Ortiz, Marian Brown, Molly Bloom, Laura Flavin, Christopher Sergio, Omar Chapa, Nicolette Seeback, and everyone else who got this baby out the door.

This book would never have been completed without the guidance, help, and advice of Dedi Felman. Dedi worked with disastrous early drafts and held my hand throughout this process. Not only that, she made working on a research-heavy book . . . fun? I still miss our midday therapy sessions.

So many people devoted their time, expertise, and thoughts: Perry Romanowski, Esther Olu, Bill Sukala, Kelly Dobos, Carl Winter, Jen Novakovich, Steven Loy, Miriam Zoll, Rachel Bloom, Ruthie Schulder, Dr. David Scales, Renée DiResta, Sheril Kirshenbaum, Michelle Wong, Julie Rehmeyer, Don Ardell, Ophelia Yeung, Vincent Parry, Barbara Riegel, and many, many more.

The fact-checking and review process was a team effort. Many thanks to all those who contributed: Dustin Moore, Leah McGrath, Dr. Maude

Carmel, Laury Frieber, Jenny Splitter, Greta Moran, Alison Bernstein, Lea Urpa, Dr. Benjamin Mazer, Dr. Sophie Bracke, Kate Gallagher, Sarah Wassberg Johnson, Bram Berntzen, Dr. Danielle Ofri, Cadence Bambenek, Cody Musselman, Jay Gooch, Kathleen Meehan, Stephen Alain Ko, Mindy Levine, and Tamika Sims.

Plenty of friends got me to this point and helped in various ways. Huge thanks to Tali Malina, Merisa Brod Fink, Beth McGroarty, Rachel Krupa, Dan Gregor, Nick Bilton, Shayndi Raice, and the Mooney Method crew. A special shout-out to Susan Houriet, who gave me some of my first big opportunities in journalism, as well as Anjali Khosla for being such an encouraging and diligent editor at *Fast Company*.

I'm incredibly blessed to have a family that has always been there for me. I'm so very grateful for my Ema (Esther Raphael) and Abba (Dr. David Raphael Z"L), who instilled in me a love of books, science, and debate. I also have amazing, loving siblings: Abraham, Deborah, Nechama, Miriam, and Fred. My in-laws Marion and Dennis Spiegelman were always quick with words of encouragement.

I'm also lucky to have my East Coast family, Gina and Phil Vinick, who looked after me throughout all my years in New York. You treated me like I was your own daughter. I'll never forget that.

Last but not least, I'm forever indebted to my husband Eric Spiegelman, who knows that real wellness is a supportive partner (and a good-looking dog). I'm sorry I was such a nightmare to live with while writing this. I love you. And I promise I'll start getting out of PJs before noon.

Thank you.

A TRAITOR'S HEART

BEN CREED

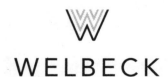

WELBECK

First published in 2022 by Welbeck Fiction Limited, an imprint
of Welbeck Publishing Group based in London and Sydney.
www.welbeckpublishing.com

A CIP catalogue record for this book is available from the British Library

HB ISBN: 978-1-80279-193-8
XTPB ISBN: 978-1-80279-194-5
E ISBN: 978-1-78739-628-9

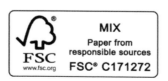

MIX
Paper from
responsible sources
FSC® C171272
FSC
www.fsc.org

Printed and bound by CPI Group (UK) Ltd., Croydon, CR0 4YY

10 9 8 7 6 5 4 3 2 1

'Everyone sees what you appear to be, few experience
what you really are.'
Niccolò Machiavelli, *The Prince*

'Thus men forgot that all deities reside in the
human breast.'
William Blake, *The Marriage of Heaven and Hell*

Prelude

April 12, 1945

So this, thought Oberst Franz Halder, is what Death looks like.

The girl was about twelve years old. She had freckles, strawberry-blonde pigtails and an intelligent, sharp-eyed look. Instead of a black cape, she was dressed in the uniform of the *Bund Deutscher Mädel*, the girls' answer to the Hitler Youth. Instead of a scythe, she was holding out a woven basket containing about thirty polished brass cylinders, each five centimetres long. Each containing a glass vial filled with cyanide.

'*Entschuldigen Sie bitte, mein Herr.* Would you care for one of these?'

Halder waved her away and carried on loitering at the back of the hall. He smoothed the sleeves of his Luftwaffe uniform and kept his eyes peeled for the baron.

Around him, a few hundred candles sputtered. A dozen third-tier Nazis shuffled out of the drizzle and into the draughty Beethoven Salle, the smaller concert venue being used after the Berlin Philharmonic had been bombed out of its home. They were trying not to look hungry, trying to show they didn't care as Germany collapsed about

1

them. Most of all, trying very hard not to think about the moment, any day now, when the Red Army would parade down Unter den Linden while staring at their wives and daughters.

The cold, damp air was beginning to warm with the scent of French perfume, the last dregs that Berlin's high society matrons could coax out of a bottle. In the half-light, a few Waffen-SS and Wehrmacht officers queued to pay homage to Albert Speer, the Third Reich's Minister for Armaments and War Production.

Somewhere, Halder knew, the Gestapo would still be watching.

He glanced at his smudged programme. The final aria of Wagner's opera *Götterdämmerung* – Brünnhilde's last great moment before riding into her beloved's funeral pyre – would open the concert. The playing order had been devised by Speer himself. Halder watched the minister preen before his obsequious guests.

A mournful oboe, tuning the orchestra up for the Wagner, hushed the audience.

There was still no sign of the baron. Halder took his seat and waited for the interval with gnawing impatience. He scratched at the patch of red skin at the base of his neck.

After a minute, a man with a duelling scar, hooded eyes and morose expression sat down beside him.

'Ah ha! You made it, Baron von Möllendorf. I was beginning to worry.'

'I shall miss Wagner,' said the baron, skipping a greeting. 'The master of the leitmotif. Those mystical layers of musical expression that mutually enhance each one's meaning and combine to magnify their power . . .'

2

His voice cracked.

'Are you all right, Baron?' Halder asked.

'Pardon me. I have not eaten for a while.'

'Not many have. To business then. Best be quick before the Lancasters come. You have it?'

Von Möllendorf nodded.

'Here,' he said, handing Halder a soft leather briefcase. 'Your people were most helpful. We completed the task.'

Silence. The soloist, blessed with the physique of a dramatic soprano and the sardonic expression of a cabaret singer, padded onstage to applause. *Götterdämmerung*. The Twilight of the Gods. The burning of Valhalla.

'My dear Oberst Halder, what a pleasure,' said a voice behind him.

Halder turned and looked straight into the genial face of Reichminister Speer.

'A meeting of minds,' said Speer. 'One of our greatest nuclear physicists deep in conference with Hitler's most trusted adjutant. I am glad you have found each other.'

The minister leaned forward.

'Good luck, gentlemen,' he whispered.

The conductor lifted his baton. *Götterdämmerung* began . . .

After the concert, as Halder headed for the exit, the little girl from the *Bund Deutscher Mädel* barred his way again. This time she took one of the shining brass cylinders out of the basket and held it up to him, as if it were a delicious bonbon from Fassbender & Rausch.

'They have asked us to offer them to everyone. In case a swift and honourable end is required, Herr Oberst,' she said.

'Do you know what Goethe said?' he asked her. '"Death will come anyway, whether you are afraid of it or not."'

Oberst Halder sighed and muttered a single word under his breath. His unique battle cry:

'Neubrandenburg.'

He stretched out a hand towards the cylinder.

One never knew . . .

ACT 1
GOLD

1

The corpse had the room to itself. A luxury in Leningrad, where such bourgeois pretensions could attract jealous attention from your neighbours, even accusations of a counter-revolutionary sensibility. The kind of whisper that might elicit a midnight visit from the organs of the state. Luckily for this comrade, thought Major Oleg Nikitin, his brains are already splattered on the wall. Which at least meant that the victim – one Comrade Samosud – was, unlike the rest of the city's one million citizens, beyond the reach of the MGB, the Ministry for State Security.

Even in such a small, mud-caked room crammed full of men perspiring into their uniforms, Major Nikitin did not pass unnoticed. His missing eye – the empty socket encircled by a scaly lava of scars – made sure of that.

Four of those MGB officers in long coats and large caps rimmed with blue bands poked into every grimy corner and examined every surface. They peered at the locks, the window, the exposed light bulb, the gas hob that didn't work because the gas supply didn't work either, at the filthy bucket, at the dust under the sagging bed, and in particular at the dark stain on one wall, new but dried.

Looking on were two officers from the *militsiya*, ordinary street-level police. They were present on the orders of their superior officer but were reluctant to do anything that might get them noticed. Mute witnesses to something or nothing – whatever the MGB best required them to see. Nikitin understood their predicament. He had, after all, once been an MGB officer doing the intimidating.

The men from state security tramped an irritable orbit around the room's centrepiece, which was a slumped body that had been tied to a wooden chair. In the right side of the dead man's head was a neat hole. Beneath it, a second one.

'Comrade Major Nikitin? Oleg, is that you?'

Nikitin ignored the speaker, pulled his own cap lower and shouldered his way to an empty patch of wall in order to regard the corpse from another angle. In the early winter dusk, up here on the fourth floor of this handsome but neglected building, the watery street lamps were no help. And the flickering light bulb was already grating on his nerves.

The corpse wore a grey shirt and a dark-blue padded jacket, both of them open and hanging loose on its stout frame. On the bottom half was a pair of olive-green army-issue trousers and one brown slipper – he couldn't see the other. The dead man looked like he had been in good condition. His pectoral muscles were well defined, the outline of his thighs and calves were visible.

'Oleg?'

Fuck your mother.

Passing unrecognised had been wishful thinking. If his military uniform hadn't made him stand out, the scar tissue that swarmed all over his face always did the trick. It was hard to keep a low profile with a face like his. But, as his bad luck would have it, one of the MGB officers was a comrade of long standing.

'It is you. What do you think you are doing here?'

Nikitin glowered at the speaker. Rumyantsev – an MGB major. Ambitious but not overly blessed with brains. A few months ago, in another life, they had been on civil terms.

'How nice to see you again, Volodya,' said Nikitin. He gestured at the body. 'Looks interesting. What is your conclusion?'

Rumyantsev looked around and barked at his men – who had paused in their endeavours and swivelled their ears towards this conversation – to mind their own business and keep searching for evidence. He turned back to Nikitin.

'I am surprised, Oleg,' he said in a low voice. 'Surprised to see you alive. Alive and in this room, in the uniform of GRU military intelligence, asking me questions. I have heard all sorts of things about you. Should I shoot you now to save time and file my report later?'

Nikitin bared his stained teeth.

'Inadvisable, Volodya. Defence Minister General Pletnev commands me now and he is a man with a long memory. If you want a couple of tanks and an infantry detachment up your arse, of course, then go ahead. And there are other members of the Politburo with a keen interest in my brains remaining inside my head.'

Rumyantsev adjusted his blue cap.

A chill draft blew through a gap where a window should have been. Like last year, the northern winter had come early. Leningrad was already blanketed in snow, which hid some parts of the Sennaya Market area that were improved by invisibility. But the snow could do little to spruce up the area's more basic accommodation: hovels that had been endlessly subdivided, some partitioned by little more than curtains, or a

9

combination of mud-spattered towels and dirty laundry. This one was a notch up. Samosud, whoever he turned out to be, had had no roommates, though there was precious little to adorn his room other than the bed and the useless hob.

'General Pletnev, eh? The Hero of the Seelow Heights. You do have some impressive friends,' said Rumyantsev. 'I'm curious, how did you get here so fast? Was it them?' He nodded at the cops. 'Still got informers in the militia? Letting you know about a mysterious murder?'

That window must have been broken recently, thought Nikitin. No one would have left it with the temperature dropping like it was. Even a couple of pieces of cardboard or plywood and some mud would have been preferable to the late-October wind. And there were shards of glass on the ground that no one had swept up.

Shards of glass on the inside of the room.

'Is he like the other one?' asked Nikitin, pointing at the dead body.

For a split second, Rumyantsev looked furious.

'The other one?'

Yes, I know about the other one . . .

'Well, it has been a pleasure, Major Rumyantsev,' Nikitin said. He marched towards the door.

'Wait!' snapped Rumyantsev.

The two ordinary militia officers didn't move but the MGB agents felt for their pistols.

'In the name of Soviet revolutionary justice, I . . .'

'If you utter the next words, Volodya, they will be your last,' roared Nikitin, whose pistol had materialised from nowhere and was now pointing at Rumyantsev. 'You blue-hats may have power over the life and death of every Soviet citizen, but that power stops with officers of the military's Main Investigative Directorate, where you have power over nothing – not the colour of my piss or the smell of my shit – and if you reach another inch for that Nagant then I shall make you the second corpse in this room and I'll be sure to send Comrade Beria himself a card of condolence.'

Rumyantsev kept still but his gaze never faltered.

'You're dead anyway, Oleg,' he said. 'They say Beria wants you dangling on a hook. With your feet tapping along to "Dark is the Night". Today or another day. He'll get you.'

Nikitin saluted with his pistol, backed out of the room and began to walk down the stairs.

'*In the dark night, I know that you, my love, are sleeping,*' he sang as he went. '*And are furtively wiping a tear by the cradle . . .*'

The lyrics of the song – much loved by Leningraders as part of the soundtrack to Leonid Lukov's wartime film *Two Soldiers* – made him think of Kristina, his wife.

*

Nikitin waited and watched from across the square, cupping his cigarette – a Polish import he didn't much like – in his palm. The MGB officers left, bickering about the next Zenit–CSKA match as they got into their black car.

Moments later the two militia officers appeared, carrying the corpse on a stretcher and struggling with the dead weight. The top half of the body was covered with a coat, while a pair of worker's boots dangled either side of the wooden poles. With each jolt, the left boot gave one of the officers a vengeful kick to the groin. The officers slid their cargo onto the back of a truck: a wartime ZIS with an outsize wooden crate screwed to its fuselage.

People – housewives shopping for supplies, workers who had been let off shift early – were stopping and staring. That was unusual. The Soviet citizen was not meant to come face to face with crime, let alone take an interest in it. But the crowd kept forming until the militia yelled at it to disperse.

The ZIS trundled off and order was restored. Nikitin gave a loud whistle. Spotting him, the militia officers hurried over.

Without a word, one of them felt in his pocket and handed over its contents. A rolled-up piece of paper, about six centimetres long.

'Just as you said, Comrade Major,' said the young militia officer. He was frightened and eager to please. 'At the back of the throat.'

Nikitin smiled.

'Well done. Anyone else still up there?'

'No, Comrade Major.'

'Very well. Give my regards to Captain Lipukhin,' he said. 'Obviously you will now forget about this or . . .'

The two men reddened, nodded, and fled.

Nikitin watched the passage of people to and fro across Sennaya Square for a few minutes before he ventured from his doorway and ascended the creaking wooden staircase back up to the deceased's apartment. He had to move fast.

The stain on the wall was at the same height as the victim's head. He had been shot while trussed to the chair. Nikitin soon found two neat holes amid the red stain on the wall – Rumyantsev and his MGB agents had removed the bullets. Small-calibre pistol rounds.

But he was looking for something else, and within five minutes of groping under cupboards and flicking away spiders and cockroaches, he'd found it. A slightly uneven floorboard under the bed. He lifted the board and his fingers closed on the cold of metal.

A gold medallion, just like the other one. With the same unique stamp.

That made two of them. Two men murdered in the same way, both with scraps of paper in their mouths. Both in possession of the same medallion.

Over the past year, Major Oleg Nikitin had seen friends cross the street to avoid him. Allies had turned to enemies. But his new masters – the GRU – were equally distrustful of him. Even contemptuous. And, for a reason he could not yet understand, impatient.

Nikitin was by training and temperament an interrogator, not an investigator. Now he had more evidence, yet still little idea of how to interpret it.

But – several thousand kilometres away from Leningrad, in the wastelands of the Siberian north – there was one man who could help him.

Provided he was still alive.

2

'Thoughts of love, of home, of women's bodies, a foolish belief in justice . . . None of that will get you through this. You have to find something to hate.'

The old lag who had given Revol Rossel this piece of wisdom on his very first day in Igarka had long since had his throat slit.

The stupid zek hadn't even taken his own advice . . .

Rossel had, though. To the letter.

Something to hate.

Right now, fuck your mother, it was the piece of gravel that had found its way into the toe of his left boot.

The former senior lieutenant in the People's Militia and the five other tethered men strained like a team of carthorses as they tried to move an enormous barrel full of rocks and rubble through the Siberian snow, one painful footstep after another. Three prisoners in front of the barrel, which was shaped like a giant cotton reel, doing the pulling. Three behind. Their eyes ached, their frozen nose hairs pricked them like miniature icicles, their breath broke into a million crystals as soon as it left their mouths. Moving this primitive steamroller, with each pass they flattened the ground another metre for the sleepers and rails that would be laid down from Igarka to Salekhard.

All 1,300 kilometres of it.

Life in a Corrective Labour Camp, under the jurisdiction of the GULAG, or Main Camps Directorate, stripped away the layers of a human being. Left you with almost nothing. As if some mischievous Slavic god was rubbing away at a tiny point on your skull with sandpaper to see what they might discover there. Usually, it was hunger. Because hunger slowly became all that you were.

'Let us say a prayer together,' said Babayan, the thick-bearded priest with messianic, pale-blue eyes, heaving at the barrel to Rossel's right.

'Not another prayer – give us all a fucking break, you Armenian halfwit,' shouted someone.

To his left – shuffling, stick-thin and pale as the permafrost – was Alexander Vustin. A singer, a baritone soloist in Stalingrad's main opera house, a precocious composer of some repute, and now, like many other "politicals" in the camps, an Enemy of the People.

It had been ten long months since Rossel had disappeared into the GULAG system. Two en route to the far north by rail, road and barge. Eight at this colony, so new and remote it was known only as 105th Kilometre, its distance from Igarka. In that time, he had talked about music with Vustin more than he had with anyone in his life. Of the Russians, Shostakovich was good but Prokofiev superior, Vustin proclaimed. Rachmaninov was sometimes kitsch, sometimes great, mostly pleasant. Stravinsky was the genius. Khachaturian could kiss Vustin's arse and anyone else's arse. Rossel was inclined to agree.

'Until Prokofiev lost his nerve and started worrying about what the Party thought of his music,' Vustin had

15

said, shivering so much he could barely find his mouth with his roll-up, 'then he was *dermo*, complete crap, like those simpletons who founded the Russian Association of Proletarian Musicians. Nothing but pompous cantatas for the masses – bombast that signified nothing . . .'

Their conversations had helped to keep Rossel sane. Vustin had not been so lucky. As a boy, Vustin's mother and father had been burned alive in the Nazi bombardment of Stalingrad. Now, as his moods changed, his brittle eyes roamed everywhere, trying not to meet your gaze. Any loud noise would shock the boy. He would throw up his hands to his ears and begin to sing random operatic arias – the Italians, like Verdi or Puccini – as a poetic coping mechanism. Only Rossel's voice would settle him, make him listen, let him see the world again. He could draw Vustin back from the brink of madness into the shared reverie of their musical discourse.

Under their feet was a layer of sand over a layer of ballast, over more sand, over a layer of logs and brushwood. And somewhere in the mix, a layer or two of bones. You either continued laying the line or became part of it. Come the summer, the whole mess would almost certainly sink into the thick, soul-sucking Turukhansky mud.

The haulers, enmeshed in rope, had marginally the worst of it. It was not much fun for the men pushing the barrel behind them, either. Such was its size – almost two metres in diameter – neither group could see the other. They were, however, united in misery. Daily brothers in a bleak despair. Not far away, another group toiled: chopping wood, hauling steel rails. And then another. And another.

Rossel's team staggered as the barrel slipped on the iron-hard ground, dragging them to the left. His knees buckled. The big toe of his left foot ground into the little stone.

Fuck . . .

'Back!'

A guard fifty metres away, one foot on a tree stump, yelled and waved his arm. 'That way, bastards – follow the line, fuck your mother . . .'

The men grunted in unison and bit their lips as they hauled the barrel back on course.

But nothing could stop Babayan praying.

'*Gospodi, Isusye Khristye, syne Bozhii, pomilui menya greshnago* . . . Lord Jesus Christ, Son of God, have mercy on me a sinner . . .'

'Your God had better compensate us for this shit one day soon,' muttered a man from the other side of the barrel. 'Or, as long as he offers me a place by his fire, I'll sin all the Devil likes.'

Babayan spat on the ground, the brown froth turning to ice.

'The Lord already rewards us,' said the Armenian. 'Only yesterday I had a vision of Our Lady of Kazan walking down the track towards us. The good lady and two others. Shadows in the snow, like my mother once saw upon the slopes of Mount Ararat, resting place of the Ark of Noah.'

Babayan's chest rattled. The old priest fell silent for a few paces.

'Little girls, little boys,' said the disgruntled zek. '*Babushki, dyedushki*, cows, pigs, chickens – makes no odds, I'll stick my dick in them all. Anything for a place by that fire.'

17

This far north, high above the Arctic Circle, there were many ways the human spirit could be broken. One was the first moment of real cold. Not just the arrival of snow and frost but the first day it reached minus twenty-five, minus thirty. The realisation that descended upon all the prisoners that it was only going to get colder and darker. It hit them all hard: the politicals sentenced under Article 58; the *Vory*, the Thieves – and their deadly rivals, the *Suki*, or Bitches; and Hitler's orphaned warriors, the clutch of German POWs who had never been sent home.

All of them.

Once the ice crawled into your bones there was no hope of a thaw.

This year, the moment had long since passed. Already, in the first week of November, everyone in the camp was sick with something. Bones ached, chests wheezed, teeth rattled, fingers rotted.

Then, sometime in February, came the unshakeable conviction that winter would never end. Without fail, that was a day for someone to step beyond the wire into the forbidden zone. Become target practice for the guards. The other side of your last breath, some zeks reasoned, had to be a warmer place than here.

'So two other figures followed the Blessed Lady,' Babayan resumed. 'She was as plain to see as you or me but the others were mere spectres. Still, I recognised them – the last Tsar himself, Nicholas, and his poor child, the boy Alexei. God has raised these martyrs to his kingdom. His mercy is infinite.'

As the wind and snow swirled, whiteness danced all around them. Rossel kept his eyes fixed ahead of him on the dirty trail that curved into the taiga. Here was a world of nothing. And they were at its centre.

In another, distant life, he had been a student of the violin at the Leningrad Conservatoire. Despite teenage years wasted in a state orphanage, despite the stigma of his parents' political mortification, he'd still had the talent to force his way in. Enough to dazzle his professors, to excel in his exams, to prompt predictions of an exceptional career.

But he'd been a loose-lipped young man who liked to joke and tell stories.

Too quick with smart remarks. Too candid.

In the Soviet Union, candour could be a fatal flaw.

He had paid for that.

Not just me.

What would Mussorgsky have made of these brittle, jangling flurries? he wondered. How would that great composer have scored this void?

Igarka was a place that made the concept of infinity seem close to hand. Tangible. That of mercy, impossibly remote.

*

Another hour gone, another hour spent listening to the incessant chatter of your own teeth. But Igarka's hourglass was illusory. Sand slipped to the bottom, yes, but it never emptied. And just like the grains in the glass there was no possibility of escape.

To the left and the right, Rossel knew, was thick Siberian forest, though there was a wasteland of fifty or sixty metres,

19

cleared by other prisoners, before you got to the treeline. The railway was due to head west, though no one in 105th Kilometre believed it would ever be completed. Great chunks of it had already sunk into the mire in the summers or simply shattered in the winters. North – maybe two hundred kilometres away, they reckoned – was the edge of Russia and the shore of the Kara Sea. At their backs was the Yenisei River, which if you followed it south would eventually take you to Krasnoyarsk or on to Mongolia.

But to the zeks of 105th Kilometre, these were meaningless, abstract points of context. All they knew was that the railway track stopped about fifty metres behind them and until they had prepared the way it would go no further. And if they stopped moving their human steamroller, the four guards watching them with rifles at the ready would shoot them where they stood.

Gospodi, Isusye Khristye, syne Bozhii . . .

Babayan's daily prayers, Rossel understood, would not be answered. Perhaps the Armenian sensed that, too. For in Igarka, it was the Devil who was omnipotent and omnipresent – in the shape of a guard, an informer, a Thief; in the chill in your bones and the dead weight of hopelessness you felt pressing down on your soul as soon as you opened your eyes each morning.

Rossel stumbled.

Fuck your mother . . .

And sometimes just a stone in your shoe.

Even a slight incline meant trouble. After you'd hauled the steamroller for a couple of kilometres, another centimetre or two felt like you were climbing Mount Elbrus. An upward slope made Rossel's muscles scream; a downward one put all their lives in the hands of the men behind the barrel, heaving back on the wet wooden beams that were fixed like a yoke to its rudimentary axle. And crushing a foot meant not being able to walk back to the camp – a death sentence. No zek would waste one drop of their own precious strength on carrying an injured worker.

At least it had stopped snowing.

Some days it was better not to talk. On other days, talking was what got you through it. Today, Rossel, decided, he would indulge Babayan's babblings.

'What do you see when you look beyond the forest, Revol?' said Babayan. He was certain the old priest wanted to save his soul.

Rossel grimaced as the steamroller veered to the left.

'I see Leningrad. The trams bursting through Theatre Square,' he answered. 'The twinkling chandeliers of the Glazunov Hall in the conservatoire, when I was a student there.'

The barrel let out a banshee wail as it creaked and groaned across the packed ice and snow.

'I see the Anichkov Bridge, and a young fool declaiming the poetry of Mayakovsky through a loudhailer. "Behold what quiet settles on the world. Night wraps the sky in tribute from the stars. In hours like these, one rises to address. The ages, history, and all creation . . ."'

A boy who should have known better.

'Ah, Mayakovsky,' said a man further along the row with a deep sigh. 'Now there was a real *muzhik* – a lover, a drinker, a madman. They say the thought of suicide was like a cancer in him. At first, a whisper. In his last days, a never-ending scream.'

21

Rossel didn't know the speaker but the accent was Baltic. A Lithuanian, perhaps. There were plenty of Balts rotting in the string of camps along the line, all the way to Yermakovo.

Inside his head, Rossel swore. He shouldn't have mentioned being a student at the conservatoire. It was a mistake to reveal anything. Every tiny morsel of someone's soul might be something for the Thieves back at camp to bite into.

If they ever found out that he had been an officer of the Leningrad militia . . .

They would tear him to pieces.

'What else, Revol?' urged Babayan.

'Just pull this fucking thing . . .'

For the next hour they struggled in silence, reserving all strength for their labour. *Shock work is the path to liberation!* declared a ragged banner nailed to the side of the main barracks back in the camp. The camp commander would point to it every time someone was pulled out of roll call, beaten by the guards and sent to the isolating cells.

The sun, which had made only the most reluctant appearance that day, soon retreated again. That meant it was about three o'clock. In another hour, perhaps less, it would be time to return.

'How many years?' said Babayan.

'What?'

Rossel was only half-listening. They had only a few minutes of rest every hour – some zeks had quotas measured in kilograms of coal or fallen logs. Theirs was measured in metres. A tiny shortfall meant less bread, a smaller measure of soup – lukewarm water with a scrap of fish skin in it. He kept his eyes on the treeline.

'How many years is your sentence?' repeated the priest.
Rossel shrugged.

Babayan frowned. 'Everyone counts every day of their
sentence. Everyone knows how long they have served and
how long they have left.'

'Not me. I am here for as long as one man wants me to
be here.'

'Comrade Stalin?'

Rossel found this worth a smile. He shook his head.

The priest grunted. 'I hear it all the time. "If only the
great Stalin knew about this place," the new lads say, "he
would put a stop to it. If only Stalin knew . . ."'

Rossel sighed and forced his shoulders forward in the
yoke.

You have to find something to hate.

Even before arriving in Igarka, even before being sent
out on the long march to the furthest outposts of this
GULAG cluster, long before he and his fellow prisoners
had hauled every tool with them and been forced to build
their own barracks, he had found something to hate.
Someone, at least.

Major Oleg Nikitin.

At first, a whisper . . .

Sometimes, the detective knew, what was true of suicide
could also be true of murder.

3

Up ahead, the distant watchtowers and searchlights of the camp bled a line of light into the darkness. Like phantoms, the column of zeks floated towards it.

Rossel shivered and pulled his ragged scarf tighter around his head. The cold was so intense now it was burning his exposed skin. Raw wind whipped the snow into flurries that stung his face. His gut was growling. Everyone was thinking about one thing. Bread. Except Babayan, whose head was filled with God and the royal family. And Vustin, whose young mind was, as ever, a tangle of musical notes.

'*Gospodi, Isusye Khristye, syne* . . .' chanted the priest.

'Shut it, you dirty Armenian piece of shit. Unless that God of yours is a baker,' shouted a prisoner behind them in the column.

'*Gospodi, Isusye* . . .'

A young guard had drifted closer to the main phalanx of prisoners without them noticing.

'God is dead, Armenian pig,' said the guard. 'Christ is in the sewer. Not another word out of your filthy mouth.'

Do as he says, Rossel thought. He is a zealot, too, every bit as much as you, Babayan. I can tell. I remember them well from my days in the League of the Militant Godless.

'I shall pray for your soul, young man, which shall come to His mercy . . .'

That was a bad . . .

The guard closed the distance to Babayan with unexpected speed and smashed the butt of his rifle into the priest's head. Babayan reeled. He fell into the arms of one of his fellow prisoners, who cursed and pushed him away. He managed to keep on his feet but was no longer walking.

'Don't stop for him,' muttered another zek. 'Don't help the stupid piece of shit. I want to eat.'

'The struggle against religion is the struggle for socialism,' shouted the guard.

It was a slogan Rossel knew well. It was etched on his brain from the endless assemblies of the League of Militant Godless that he had attended as a youth. He had been determined to outdo his comrades in atheist fervour; desperate to wish away God's prying eyes and God's judgment; and – most of all, concerning the fate of his mother and father – to wish away his own judgment, too.

They heard the bolt being drawn back on his rifle. The full stop at the end of Babayan's next sentence would be a bullet from a Tokarev SVT-40.

'Excuse me, comrade. May I interject?'

Rossel felt a twist in his gut. It was Vustin's high-pitched warble. Brought up by his grandfather, a rich landowner – now a hated *kulak* in the eyes of the Soviet state – the boy's naivety was such that even in Igarka he made no attempt to disguise his education and upbringing.

'Who do you think are you, Comrade Interject? The fucking tsar himself?'

The guard shoved his face spit-close to Vustin's. He raised the tip of his rifle and fired into the air.

Vustin blinked twice, put his hand over his ears, and began to sing. A touch of Tchaikovsky. An aria from *The Queen of Spades*.

Now the guard aimed the rifle straight at Vustin.

'Stop singing, *mudak*, or so help me I'll . . .'

But Vustin couldn't stop.

'"*Here come our warriors, our little soldiers, Aren't they smart? Stand aside, there, stand aside! . . .*"'

The guard shoved the rifle into the side of Vustin's head.

'You won't stop, then I'll stop you.'

'"*The foe is wicked, be on your guard! . . . Flee or surrender! Hurrah! Hurrah! . . .*"'

The Tokarev jammed on the first shot, which enraged the guard even more. He ripped out the magazine and yanked at the bolt.

Rossel's throat tightened. He stepped out of line. They were only fifty metres from the fence. The other guards were yelling now, hurrying towards the commotion. A searchlight from one of the watchtowers, drawn by the shot, had picked them out.

'Comrade, please, wait!'

Rossel's voice was muffled. It sounded impotent in the howling wind, the snow and the dark. He raised his hands in surrender and opened his mouth to implore the guard to show mercy.

'The boy is unwell, he does not understand. I can sometimes reason with h—'

The second bullet hit Vustin in the forehead. He went down without another sound.

*

The dead man's tongue lolled out of the side of his mouth.

'It looks, for all the world,' came Babayan's ethereal voice from behind Rossel, 'like the serpent that made its home in Eden.'

A red-faced lieutenant, panting after the exertion of running through the drifts, snapped at the guard who had killed Vustin. 'Idiot! More forms for me to fill in three times over. One less prisoner to push the barrel. You're not fit to guard the shithouse, Dernov.'

Another guard kicked Babayan in the ribs as he knelt over the dead Vustin and ordered him to head for the gates. The Armenian groaned and held his side. Blood was still trickling down his face.

'You can drag him back the rest of the way, blockhead. You,' the guard pointed to Rossel, 'you help him. The rest of you bastards – back to camp, quick.'

Then both he and the lieutenant ran to catch up with the labour brigade, cursing in unison as they went.

Rossel looked down at Vustin. His eyes were open, his expression serene. The hole was neat. In the glare of the camp lights, he could just make out a dark halo spreading around the young composer's head.

Angry at the dressing down he had received, rather than the murder he had just committed, Dernov's face was flushed.

'What are you waiting for?' he shouted.

They took an arm each and began to drag Vustin towards the camp.

'A martyr,' Rossel heard Babayan mutter under his breath. 'The boy has the look of the little tsarevich, Alexei. And the aura of a slaughtered saint . . .'

*

As Rossel and Babayan arrived back in camp, the rest of the brigade was already lined up in the main parade ground. They broke ranks when the composer's corpse was deposited on the snow and the guards made no effort to stop them. In the camp, clothes were priceless.

A fight soon broke out over Vustin's coat.

'What do you want, Rossel?' said Denikin, a professor of Marxist literature from Kursk, as he bent over Vustin's body. 'His socks? His pants?'

Marx's manifesto, Rossel remembered, said Communism could be distilled to a single sentence: the abolition of private property. The professor must have missed that lecture.

As the prisoners tore open Vustin's jacket, a piece of paper flew out. Then another, and another, fluttering and floating over the roll call area, over the camp's inner fence, up among the snowflakes in the searchlight beams and onward into the night. Rossel chased one down and caught it. He looked at it and ran back to the squabbling prisoners, booting them out of the way and joining the mêlée, ignoring the elbows to his face and blows to his ribs. He ripped the coat out of the hands of a burly Ukrainian who thought he had triumphed. Then he reached inside and his rag-covered hands brought out more paper, which he jammed into his own pockets. Rossel looked around but the guards were still too busy watching and laughing at the fight for Vustin's clothes.

Soon the corpse was naked.

He flung the coat at Denikin. 'Here,' he said. 'I think Marx would want you to have it.'

Then Rossel stepped aside and stood still as he watched more of the papers drift over the fence and disappear into the darkness.

They, at least, were free.

Babayan approached, touching Rossel's arm.

'All of a sudden, you seem at peace, my friend,' said the Armenian. 'What was written on Vustin's papers?'

Rossel turned to face the old priest.

'A miracle of sorts, Babayan,' he said. 'One greater than anything in your holy books.'

4

A detachment of German PoWs had come out to the far extremity of the railway work to cart out and lay the sleepers. They were a pitiful sight – hunched, weak, friendless, bullied. They must know how the world regarded them and their fellow countrymen, thought Rossel. And yet, no longer the Wehrmacht's gleaming legionaries, they still looked bemused at how far they had fallen.

It was not the first time the PoWs had been called upon to assist with the railway's construction. They had set to work with only rudimentary directions, measuring the distance between sleepers with lengths of rod and a certain choreography. At rest time they huddled together.

All except one, who leaned on a sloping tree stump a couple of dozen metres away from his *Kameraden*.

Holding up a smoke, Rossel approached. He kept an eye on the guards but they took no notice.

The Fritz was watching him sidelong. Rossel realised that every German in the camp had to make judgments on every Russian, instant assessments of whether they represented danger or indifference.

'Walter,' said the German, extending his hand.

Rossel took it.

'Rossel,' he replied.

Walter frowned. 'Rossel? *Sind Sie Deutscher?*'

Rossel shook his head. 'Russian. But descended from the Volga Germans. *Povolzhskiye nyemtsy.* Volga, Volga. Immigrants. Long time ago – eighteenth century, I think.' He made a looping gesture to indicate the passage of time. Walter seemed to understand. 'My father,' Rossel added. 'Papa. Communist. Bolshevik. Didn't talk about much his ancestors.'

Walter talked on in German, a babble that might have been a commentary on Communism, immigration or the weather. The Fritz took one last heavy drag on the wad of *makhorka* – the roughest of rough tobacco, which Rossel had lent him – and handed it back.

'*Wunderbar. Vielen Dank!*'

The German PoWs numbered around thirty. They had spent seven years in the Soviet Union and found themselves in an Arctic labour camp that didn't even have a proper name. Neither guards nor Russian prisoners mixed with them enough for them to learn more than a few words of Russian. In the eyes of the more rabid camp commanders, fraternization could mean a few more years on the end of your sentence.

But what did that matter to him, he thought, a man who hadn't even been told how long his own sentence was?

Rossel was tempted to get Walter to teach him a few obscenities in German. Just to confuse the guards. But Walter looked a little on the cultured side.

'You like music, Walter? Beethoven, Brahms, Schumann?' Walter nodded.

'Brahms, *da* . . .' The German hummed the last bars of a Brahms lullaby. '"*Morgen früh, wenn Gott will, wirst du wieder geweckt.*" My mother used to sing . . . to me sing it.'

31

'"Tomorrow morning, if God wills, you will wake once again."' Rossel repeated the line in Russian. He smiled. 'Some days in Igarka I have wished God might will the exact opposite . . . I was a musician,' Rossel said, pointing to himself.

'*Musiker?*' Walter approved. 'Mozart, Beethoven, Wagner.' He asked a question Rossel didn't understand but the word 'instrument' was the same in both languages. Rossel mimed playing a violin. Then held up his left hand, pushing down with his right on the glove and rags entwined around it to reveal the absence of two fingers.

'NKVD did this. Or MGB, as they're called now,' he said. Walter thought about it and winced.

'*Physiker,*' he said, tapping his chest. '*Raketen.*' He made the obligatory whooshing sound and pointed at the sky. Then he pointed out a few more of his fellow POWs.

'*Physiker, Chemiker, Physiker,*' he said. '*Ein Kernphysiker,*' he added, jabbing a hand at the tallest, most drooping POW: a man in his late fifties with a long scar across his cheek and a glazed expression in his eyes. The latter had been beaten senseless by the guards shortly after arriving at the main camp in Igarka. Life 105 kilometres further west had not improved his health. He was now no more than a simpleton. But he was a favourite of the Thieves, who made a pet of him at their nightly card games in the camp forge, feeding him scraps and calling him *Tsar Suka*, King Bitch. What the criminals liked, Rossel thought, was how far they sensed the man had fallen. His features were aristocratic but his hunched shoulders, wary eyes and cowering demeanour now gave him the bearing of the humblest servant. His fellow countrymen tried to protect him but they didn't have the will or the numbers to fend off the Thieves.

'Not soldiers?'

Walter shook his head.

'*Nein – ich meine, ja . . . in den letzten Kriegstagen.*'

A whistle blew. Rossel nodded at Walter, who bowed.

Ten years ago the Germans had conquered most of Europe. Now they were grateful for a free puff on a cigarette.

*

It took some dark stars to align for a night like this.

Such nights came when the labour gangs had left a prisoner or two for dead. Not that the other zeks cared much now for lost comrades. But, for a few – once they had chewed on mouldy black bread and drunk rank broth – the emptiness that was left inside was filled with the anger of impotence.

They came when the craziest Thieves from antagonistic clans got off shift at the same time. A challenge to play cards. Insults. Challenge accepted. High stakes – including other men's clothes, tobacco and lives. Such nights came when the stench of one hundred men crammed into one barrack hut mingled with the bittersweet tang of *samogon*: homebrew brewed from pilfered yeast, sugar and leftover grain or potato skin, or diluted industrial alcohol. Mix it all up in the cauldron of the barracks, add a dash of brutal struggle against a ruthless enemy, and you conjured up chaos.

There were two big barracks like these. In one ruled the old-school *Vory*, the Thieves, the ones who adhered to the

BEN CREED

vow never to cooperate with the authorities. In the other ruled the *Suki*, the Bitches – criminals who saw power and opportunity in working, even at arm's length, with the State.

War had broken out between them, war that was vicious and unending.

In both barracks survived the politicals – cowering intellectuals who had written the wrong book or staged the wrong play, or academics, like Denikin, who had proposed the wrong theory. Banished to the coldest corners, wondering if their lives were spinning with the dice at the game of craps taking place in the centre of the wooden building, where there were flickers of light and warmth. To be a political was to live your life as prey. To survive, a man needed to be vigilant. The remotest points of the Soviet justice system, GULAG satellites such as 105th Kilometre were the most lawless places on Earth.

But that didn't mean there weren't rules. And in Igarka, a Thief called Kuba was the one who made them. As a would-be rival was finding out.

Sobol was in a bad way.

On his bunk not far from the centre of the hut, sweating, writhing, clutching his stomach, the thickset thief had repeatedly soiled himself.

'Fuck you, Sobol, it smells like Death's arsehole in here,' said a pug-faced man with a tattoo of Lenin on his neck.

Sobol groaned. He was oblivious to the curses and kicks of the prisoners in the bunks around him, which doubled in vigour with each bout of retching and every involuntary bowel motion. From time to time he would scream out garbled phrases. Once, he cried out for his mother, earning raucous mockery from the barracks at large.

34

Further down the barracks, the tattooist Oblonsky set out his tools. A needle, fashioned from a piece of metal wire that had been heated until it split, threaded through an empty fountain pen. The ink was made from ash or the soot of burnt tyre rubber, mixed with urine. Some camp tattooists claimed to use alcohol to sterilize the mixture, but in 105th Kilometre there was not a drop of alcohol that went undrunk.

'Poisoned,' said Oblonsky, gesturing at Sobol. 'Kuba's orders. Sobol let his guard down.'

Rossel undid the laces of his camp-issue smock.

'*Poganka?*'

Oblonsky nodded.

'Back in the summer,' said the tattooist, squinting at his handiwork, 'somebody picked and hoarded a load of it and slipped a sample into our friend's ration.'

Russia was a nation of forest foragers. The Death Cap mushroom claimed the lives of a few unwary souls each year. It was known to be an agonising way to go.

'He was making a play for Kuba's throne. Normally Kuba gets Medvedev, the Bear, to sort that stuff out. This time he was more . . . subtle.' He nodded at the shitting, shrieking wreck a few bunks away. 'If you can call it that.'

Oblonsky inspected the progress of his handiwork to date – the outline of a large seabird on Rossel's chest – and grunted. 'The other wing today, or most of it. Whatever you can bear. If Ilya Repin had painted on a canvas that squirmed like you do, his daubs would have taken him a lot longer. That's what I tell all my customers.'

The tattooist set to work, puncturing Rossel's skin repeatedly with quick jabs, moving millimetre by millimetre.

Rossel set a piece of old tyre between his teeth and kept as still as he could.

The first buildings of this penal labour camp had been hewn out of timber from the vast northern forests four or five years previously. Intended as just another staging post on a project that consumed prisoners in their hundreds, it had swelled almost to the size of a central camp – the hubs from which expendable workers were sent out to colonise the wastelands above the Arctic Circle.

A speck of grit in the snow to which other specks had clung, and stuck, Rossel thought.

A stocky Georgian with a broken nose appeared at Oblonsky's shoulder. He pointed at the bird on Rossel's chest.

'Hey, you. Albatross. Get ready,' he said. 'Tomorrow night, Kuba wants to hear another one of your stories. Better make it a good one, too. He's not been in the best of moods lately.'

5

In your dreams you could escape. You could walk past the Sphinxes that guarded the Fontanka's elaborate Egyptian bridge. Visit the Hermitage and fall in love with your favourite painting all over again. Stand outside the Kirov Opera, float through its walls and . . . just listen.

But then morning dropped like a guillotine. And you woke up back in 105th Kilometre.

Outside, a luckless Mongolian conscript was sent out to amble around the barracks and hammer two pots together. The perimeter lights were turned on. It was five o'clock.

Inside the barracks the glow from the lights, even amplified by the snow, was muted by the thickening patina of ice on the windows. Every muscle aching from his labours by day and constant shivering at night, Rossel stared up at the misshapen icicles hanging from the rafters. He coughed. The rasping in his chest was something else to worry about. In the camps, if another prisoner didn't steal up behind you and slit your throat, Death – typhus, tuberculosis – hid inside you, waiting.

Some zeks rose immediately. It was the only way to warm up: to get moving, to go rooting for scraps of cloth or anything going spare that might be bartered. Or it might be your turn to take out what Babayan, in a rare attempt at humour, called 'Satan's chalices' – the big pisspots.

With an effort, Rossel got as far as sitting up. He had only one blanket but before winter had arrived he'd had the foresight to stitch pieces of rag into it. Even pieces of cardboard, or scraps of tyre. Anything that might trap and warm some air. In the bigger camps, especially the transit hubs, zeks would bargain anything that wasn't nailed down. In 105th Kilometre, there was nothing spare to bargain. Every scrap was precious.

Take a man's blanket and you took his life.

Stiff and sore, Rossel slipped his own blanket from his torso, felt for his bowl and makeshift fork inside the bag of kindling and sawdust that he'd constructed as a pillow, and slid down from his bunk. Oblonsky was snoring like a bear. He followed a group of three or four zeks out of the barracks, intending to head straight for the canteen.

Over to his left, he saw Babayan, head bowed and making the sign of the cross several times, facing the barracks and crouched over the spot where Vustin's body had been discarded and stripped. As usual, the Armenian was saying a prayer.

'Let those who fear the Lord say his love endures forever . . .'

Babayan heard Rossel's boot crunching in the snow and looked up.

'Vustin was like Venerable Isaac, the hermit of the caves,' he said. 'An innocent, a Fool-in-Christ, as we say.'

He resumed his chanting.

'The Lord is with me, I will not be afraid. What can any man do to me?'

Rossel cast an eye around, partly because it was wise to watch your own back but also because the number of things the powerful could do to the weak out here were limitless.

'Will you not pray for him with me, Rossel?' said Babayan.

Rossel shook his head.

'As I have told you, I was once a member of the League of the Militant Godless,' he said.

Babayan frowned. 'The enemies of Christ,' he said.

Rossel nodded.

'They left their mark. I'm no believer.'

The old priest looked forlorn.

'You're wrong my friend. Our new saint, our great martyr, our Holy Vustin told me he'd never met someone who looked so like he was carrying a great sin inside him.'

'A great sin?'

Babayan smiled.

'That's why the boy liked you, Rossel. All martyrs aspire to carry the Lord's cross. He was jealous of your soul's burden.'

*

A spatter of watery buckwheat gruel did little to stop the ache in his gut. Rossel, eager to find a moment of solitude, rushed it down, stashed his slice of black bread inside his jacket for later, skirted the main parade ground and sat on a log behind the infirmary, by the camp's eastern perimeter fence.

He pulled out the papers he had recovered from Vustin's coat and unfurled them with icy fingers. They were rectangular and yellowing. The typed lettering was beginning to fade but there was no mistaking the nature of the documents.

STATEMENT

'In the interests of Soviet justice and of suppressing all threat of an outbreak of counterrevolutionary activity in the northern administration of correctional labour camps, Bureau XXVI of the regional Ministry for State Security orders the shooting of ARTYOM KERZHAKOV the sentence to be carried out without delay.'

Each document was dated, the earliest from around July 1949 and the latest only three weeks ago, and the names on each were scribbled in block capitals. The signatures were hard to read but Rossel thought he could make out a Major Kirillov. It was a name he had not encountered in 105th Kilometre, or in any of the transit camps through which he had passed, many of which would certainly have been subject to the oversight of the Ministry for State Security, the MGB.

The empty spaces were all filled in by hand. It was a roll call of the dead.

Abramov. Akunin. Alexeev. Astilin. Bogdanov. Braginsky. Vertukhin . . .

Rossel leafed through them. The documents were brief and banal. He tried to picture the faces of the condemned,

wondering if they had ever seen these papers, the bureaucratic imprint of their fate.

Vorilov. Vrasensky. Dolgorukhov. Dmitriyev . . .

He counted to the end. Twenty-four in all.

On the reverse of each was line after line of musical
staves, ruled by a meticulous hand.

Time and key signatures, constellations of notes grouped
in quavers and semiquavers. A composition of unrivalled
ambition. Something only a composer of the calibre of
Stravinsky, or Prokofiev, or Shostakovich would even have
thought of attempting.

It is so precisely written, he thought, printed music looks
amateurish by comparison. Either exposure to the cold or a
poor-quality ink, the brittleness of the paper, or a combination of the three, had caused the notes to fade. But if held
up to the Siberian sky it was all still legible.

There was one that had survived well. The hand was
firmer, the notes rounder, even more confident. Rossel tried
to follow both melody and harmony in his head but the
fugue soon twisted into an impregnable complexity and he
could only follow in outline.

It was the only one with a title:

Fugue 13: The Song of Lost Souls.

Most of Vustin's fugues would challenge the technique of
the most virtuoso pianist, even in a country full of them.
But Fugue 13 was simpler, more lyrical, more heartfelt.

Folding the papers, Rossel tucked them into his jacket. He sat for a few minutes more, until the commotion of roll call.

'Fall in, link arms. If you make so much as a step to the left or the right it will be considered an attempt to escape and the guards will shoot to kill without warning . . .'

If Babayan was right and Vustin was a saint, then the martyred boy had left behind a hymn for all the ages.

6

Captain Verblinksy – pale, thin, pompous and number three in the hierarchy of the camp administration – came to the end of his morning address and raised his head.

The prisoners, almost two hundred of them, were silent, standing in four blocks according to their barracks, contemplating the day before them.

Real cold – minus thirty degrees and worse – came in spells. One had arrived overnight. They had all felt it in their bunks. Rossel glanced along the line of his brigade. The weak would already be feeling weaker. But falling behind on the quota meant smaller rations. Faltering in the fulfilment of your duties meant curses and kicks, being spat on by your comrades.

It was customary for those who had not made it through the night to be dragged out to attend roll call. It made identification of the dead that much easier. But the deceased, whether they had given in to hunger or cold or fallen prey to the attentions of the Thieves, usually had one thing going for them – they were in one piece.

This morning, next to three complete corpses, there was something else.

A severed head.

The captain pointed to it.

'Who the fuck is that? And where is the rest of him?'

An answer was not forthcoming. Verblinsky, eyes wide in outrage, scanned the faces of the punishment brigades but learned little.

A shout came from one of the watchtowers. A guard was pointing at something. Two things, in fact. Two snow-dusted objects: one at the far end of the main parade ground, next to the gates, the other over to the right.

'You,' said Captain Verblinsky, pointing at two zeks. 'And you. Go.'

The two prisoners at the end of the line went to investigate. By the time they were halfway across the parade ground, another guard was pointing in a third direction. Arriving at their first destination, the men bent over to inspect. One recoiled and began to gag. The other, unperturbed, perhaps even relishing his task, picked it up. Then they progressed to the next point, a further fifty metres or so away.

They completed their compass-point tour of the parade ground and returned to Captain Verblinsky, dumping two legs and a torso on the ground before him. The gesture reminded Rossel of newsreel he had once seen. The Victory Parade in Moscow in the summer of 1945. Stalin's armies hurling the standards of the Wehrmacht, Luftwaffe, Kriegsmarine and Waffen-SS at the feet of their great leader.

Poor Sobol.

His agonies had ended in the night.

Captain Verblinsky gulped.

A huge man, a Thief, began to chant through sharpened teeth. It was Medvedev, Kuba's second in command. Known as the Bear, a play on his name.

'In this camp, Kuba, leader of the true Thieves, the Thieves-in-law, rules over every breath taken,' he said. 'North, south, east and west, between the rising and the setting of the sun. *Suki*, this will be your fate too . . .'

The captain glared at him. Not sure how to proceed. Then he ordered the two men who had fetched Sobol's constituent body parts to fall in.

'Band!' Verblinsky shouted. 'Begin!'

The motley prison band struck up 'The Internationale' and Rossel watched the first labour brigade peel off from the far end and shuffle towards the gates, heading to the wastelands. A clear sky was clouding over. His stomach was already growling.

> *Vstavai, proklyatyem zakleimyoniy*
> *Vyes' mir, golodnykh i rabov . . .*

> Arise, you who have been branded with a curse
> A world of the starving and enslaved . . .

The words echoed round his head as Rossel shoved broken hands into his armpits, not for the first time cursing the absence of two fingers on his left and the badly functioning fingers on his right. Playing in the camp band did not spare you from outdoor duties, but it trimmed time spent doing them. And it spared you from joining the vanguard of shock workers who laid the railway tracks.

Two guards, young, surly and suffering in the cold, were summoned to remove the four quarters of the unfortunate Sobol on a stretcher. They scooped up the convict's remains but had not got ten metres before one stumbled, spilling their gruesome load. One of the prisoners started to snigger. Sobol's head had landed under his mangled backside, while his legs pointed in opposite directions.

A moustachioed Chechen in front of Rossel pointed.

'He made my life miserable. Now that bastard can lick his own fucking arse.'

The man next to him collapsed in laughter. Everyone joined in, even the guards. Grinning, the two young guards tried to pick Sobol up again. No luck. This time his head bounced twice and rolled towards a big Ukrainian who picked it up and, dropping into a crouch, made as if he was about to boot it over the perimeter fence.

'Hey, boys, look at me, I'm Lev Yashin,' he said. Yashin was Dynamo Moscow's new young goalkeeper.

Hovering over them, Captain Verblinsky cast loud aspersions on their parentage.

The band wheezed its way to the chorus. In the first weeks of 105th Kilometre's existence, full-throated singing had been obligatory. But it had not been a long-lived tradition. Now only a few politicals made a mocking effort to join in.

Eto yest' nash poslednii
I reshitel'ny boi

This is our final
And decisive battle . . .

A juddering sound came from above. All eyes looked skyward and the laughter died away.

The source was impossible to pinpoint at first but it grew louder until it filled the air. The band was silenced, the labour brigades stilled.

Rossel had only seen a helicopter once before. They were barely used by the Red Army during the war and his only sighting after that had been at an airfield south of Leningrad, not long after he'd been sworn into the militia. He supposed some of the zeks were seeing one for the very first time.

The prisoners gazed towards the clouds, watching the path of the squat, dark-green beetle as it swooped, chattering, towards the ground, zeroing in on a landing spot beyond the camp fence. But the guards pounded a few heads with their rifle butts and the zeks resumed their reluctant marches.

The route taken by Rossel's brigade out to the railway tracks had brought them to within a hundred metres of the helicopter's landing point, close to the camp commandant's living quarters and the MGB barracks. Here, they were beyond the fence and the outer patrol zone.

The helicopter's rotors were still. The whine of its engine had faded.

A small door just behind the rear left wheel was flung open.

A muffled figure emerged from the helicopter's belly, and then another. Now two more. A delegation of uniforms from the camp administration ran up to greet them and the new arrivals pulled down the thick collars of their coats.

Rossel knew the face straightaway. He stopped marching.

The guard alongside him broke step with a curse and hefted the butt of his rifle. Rossel moved his feet again but kept staring at the cluster of figures around the squat fuselage.

Someone to hate.

Major Oleg Nikitin, the MGB officer who had exiled him in this frozen wasteland, was shaking hands with the commandant.

A fifth person emerged from the helicopter. Smaller than the rest. Nikitin turned to welcome them into the group.

As the commandant spoke and gesticulated, the fifth figure looked around to survey the surroundings. The coat they were wearing was too thin for the harsh northern winter.

The brigade marched on but one by one all heads swung towards the new arrival. As though the line were a carnivore that had just picked up a scent.

A woman.

A shout behind them. The brigade halted and a guard, stumbling in thick, badly fitting boots, caught up.

'Prisoner 457, come forward!'

For a moment, he did not understand. It had been so long since anyone in officialdom had addressed him, Rossel had almost forgotten his number.

'You,' said the guard. 'Follow me.'

7

As if he was fanning out a deck of cards before dealing them, Major Nikitin swept a hand over the wooden table, making a sound like sandpaper. The major placed two Manila files on one side of the desk and three packs of cigarettes on the other.

Rossel, slumped in a chair that had uneven legs, looked around this inner sanctum within the main administration building. A couple of logs burned in a small brick fireplace. The flue wasn't up to much and the room, all wood, festooned with red banners – *Forward to Communism, To Freedom with a Clear Conscience* – was smoky and rank. But it was also something almost unimaginable. Hot. As the fire warmed his skin, he felt as privileged as a guest at Leningrad's Hotel Astoria.

Nikitin glanced down at the files. Then back at Rossel.

'You don't look so good, comrade.'

Rossel raised his left hand.

'I apologise,' he said. 'Since you had me sent here, I have not been able to devote as much time to my health as I would wish. The task has been made more difficult, of course, because several years ago an MGB interrogator crushed my hands and removed some of my fingers. As you will doubtless recall, Comrade Major.'

Nikitin sat back.

'And yet, when we last met we parted as –' the major paused – 'I might even say friends.'

Rossel began to shiver and was overtaken by a coughing fit. He wanted to spit in the major's face. If he closed his eyes for a second, he could picture the pleasure of setting about Nikitin's scarred features with a length of pipe. Gouging out his one good eye. Condemning him to darkness. Obliterating that sneer.

Instead, he wiped his mouth.

'You're in a military uniform? Not MGB?'

Nikitin gave a nod.

'Still the detective, I see,' he said. 'A transfer. To the Main Investigative Directorate. GRU. Military intelligence.'

'Comrade Malenkov came through for you, then? Offered you protection?'

It had been a year since Rossel and Nikitin had stood in the moonlit snow on the shores of Lake Ladoga, MGB troops pointing submachine guns at their chests, half a platoon of Soviet special forces pointing automatic rifles at their backs. A few feet away, as if oblivious to the stand-off, two pretenders to the Kremlin's throne, Georgy Malenkov and Lavrentiy Beria, took a moment to decide that a stalemate suited them both. And then retreated. But only to fight another day.

Nikitin had made a fateful choice of his own. He had deserted Beria's side. Not many crossed Beria and lived. Yet here he was.

'He arranged it, yes,' said Nikitin with a scowl. 'They hate me, though. In the GRU, I mean. They think I'm Beria's cuckoo, sitting in General Pletnev's nest.'

'Pletnev? The Hero of the Heights?'

General Pletnev was famed as the officer whose troops had smashed through the last German forces defending Berlin. The Battle of the Seelow Heights. A man who had turned disaster into triumph.

'General Pletnev is defence minister now, Revol,' said Nikitin. 'Stalin moved Marshal Zhukov to the provinces. Early retirement. For the good of his health, if you get me.'

'What had he done?'

'Riding on a white horse at the front of the Victory Parade for the Great Patriotic War? Thousands cheering, people throwing their hats in the air? Stealing the limelight from Stalin like that? A foolish error. Pletnev is smarter. He doesn't like parades. And even if they'd made him ride in one he'd have the good sense to turn up on a donkey, right at the back.'

Rossel pointed at the cigarettes. 'For me? How kind.' Without waiting for a reply he reached out and took all three packs.

The major ruffled his own hair, hard. Flakes of skin flew into the air among the thin blue trails of smoke.

'When I left the MGB, Malenkov and Pletnev had a price for their protection. All the dirt I had on Beria, please. Who was he fucking? How many girls? Any of them underage? Every last smear of shit on his shoes.'

Rossel lit the cigarette. In the camps, at his lowly level in the hierarchy, the best you got was *makhorka* – and even that rough tobacco was cut with dust, dead insects, hair, Christ knew what else. Smoked in newspaper. This was in a different league – actual *papirosi*! *Festivalniye*. A folkloric dancing couple with rosy cheeks adorned the pack. The girl reminded him a little of his missing sister, Galya.

Wherever she is, he thought for what must have been the hundredth time since arriving in Igarka, at least she's not here.

He preferred *Elbrus* but . . .

Rossel sat back and drew in the smoke. He exhaled.

'My father used to say that a warm fire and a good cigarette was as close to Heaven as any man needed to get.'

'One of Beria's girls was my daughter, in case you've forgotten,' muttered Nikitin.

Rossel had not forgotten. Lavrentiy Beria, who had survived and then prospered as head of the Soviet secret police, was still one of Stalin's closest allies. He was also, as Rossel and Nikitin had found out, a monstrous and sadistic sexual predator, among many other vices. Not a good enemy for either of them to have acquired.

'About that, I am truly sorry,' said Rossel.

Nikitin stood and went over to the fire.

Rossel took advantage of the pause to pull another *papirosa* from the pack. He lit it with the first and stashed the pack inside his smock, along with the other two.

Nikitin watched him do it with the familiar grimace that made the patch of scar tissue flow across his cheek. He looked down at his olive-green uniform and touched his epaulettes.

Rossel watched him pace between the desk and the fire. Nikitin was a survivor. As a former MGB interrogator, he was also an expert in human weakness and pain. But he didn't have the guile for Party politics.

They had not seen each other for almost a year. Rossel was surprised to learn that the major was still alive. Not many left the Ministry for State Security of their own volition. Nonetheless, Nikitin seemed to have wound up under the protection of General Pletnev, and the general had succeeded in fending off Beria.

Rossel stared out through the tiny window. Soon he would be back out there, facing his own challenges in a world where the Thieves and Bitches waged constant war with each other, pausing only to victimise the politicals. The prospect weighed on him. A few moments of respite had made him feel only more fatigued.

The *Festivalniye* tasted of everything he had been missing.

He drew too much smoke into his lungs and began to cough again, then recovered.

'Article 58 of the Penal Code, they said at my trial, or what passed for a trial,' said Rossel. 'Charges brought by none other than Oleg Yurievich Nikitin, Major, Ministry for State Security.' He mimicked the judge's high-pitched zealotry. 'Revol Rossel is charged as an Enemy of the People.'

He sat up in his chair.

'As you say, we parted as friends. And yet you are the reason I am here. Now you want something.'

'I hid you in plain sight, Revol,' said Nikitin. 'After we drew attention to Beria's connection to the illicit import-ation of jewellery and his other extracurricular activities – and believe me, his rivals were very interested in what we discovered – you were a marked man. Until now, no one came here to look for you, did they? Beria had put a price on your head. I figured the camps were the safest place to hide you. The last place he'd look other than under the minister's own bed. Would you rather be alive here or dead somewhere else?'

Rossel shrugged.

'That's a question every man here asks himself every single day. The answer he gives mostly depends on the weather, or how long ago he took his last beating from the guards or the Thieves.'

The two of them fell silent. Staring at the face of a man he had once considered an unlikely ally, Rossel looked for any flicker of regret or remorse. But that was the advantage of a face disfigured by an incendiary bomb and a soul that had withered a little with each tortured victim. Nikitin didn't give much away.

Rossel sighed. He was already tired of this game. He pointed at the two Manila files.

'So tell me then, why are you here?'

The major ran the flat of his hand across the tabletop again. Then he picked up the first file.

'Why else would I need you? Someone has been murdered.'

*

It took two more cigarettes for Nikitin to go through everything.

Two bodies in Leningrad, found in the past couple of weeks. Both men. Both showing signs of being beaten and tortured, possibly during an interrogation.

'Whoever did it left them sitting in a chair, with two bullet holes around the right temple,' said Nikitin.

He pushed the two files a couple of centimetres in Rossel's direction.

'The first was a welder by the name of Katz. His body was found on a bench in the wooded area of the Alexandrovsky

Garden, between the statue of the Bronze Horseman and St Isaac's Square. The other was called Samosud. A printer and bookbinder. His corpse was found in his own apartment. In Sennaya Square. But each man had two neat holes in the same place.'

At the mention of familiar Leningrad haunts, Rossel felt the pangs of homesickness.

'During the blockade, I once walked past six corpses as I was strolling down Nevsky Prospect during my regular afternoon constitutional,' Nikitin carried on. 'You'd think Leningraders would be used to dead bodies. But the city is already filled with rumours. They've given a name to the killer – "Koshchei, is here, Koshchei walks among us."'

Rossel sat a little more forward in his chair.

'Koshchei the Immortal? After the monster in the folk tale?'

Nikitin nodded. 'Sorcerer, not monster. Or a bit of both. Newspaper editors have been rebuked for giving the story credence, but not before the stories had been published. Militia officers have been disciplined. Leningrad Party officials have been ordered to get a grip on these foolish rumours. But the name has stuck.'

Rossel thought about this. The folk tale was known to every Russian child. Rimsky-Korsakov had based an opera on it. Koshchei was the villain of Stravinsky's ballet *The Firebird*. He killed for pleasure, abducted the lovers of heroes, and concealed his soul inside animals or objects to protect it, thus keeping himself immortal. Or hidden in an egg, or a needle. Or a needle inside an egg. Rossel's faulty memory of the folk tale had not stopped him from improvising when telling the story to a crowd of Thieves in his barracks. He made no apology. Storytelling had kept him alive – the Thieves adored a good tale.

With a stubby finger, Nikitin nudged the two folders another half centimetre towards Rossel.

'Here's a new twist on the folk tale,' he said. 'Both dead bodies had their tongues cut out and rolled-up pieces of paper placed inside their mouths.'

Rossel stared at Nikitin. Taking revenge on the man he had considered an ally had occupied his thoughts for months. Developing an interest in a couple of murders in Leningrad was the last thing he cared about.

'What was on the pieces of paper?' Rossel asked.

'Katz was left for anyone to discover him, in a place where dozens of people lived or passed by every day,' said Nikitin, ignoring the question. 'But no one saw how he got there or who killed him. No one heard anything – and trust me when I say that the victims would not have endured some of their torments in silence. Samosud was killed in his own apartment. But, likewise, his neighbours heard nothing. The first corpse was found by an old gossip who for her own reasons thought it must have been the work of Koshchei. She told her friend who told her friend and now, well. They say the MGB department that monitors phone calls is astounded by how many people are whispering the name.'

A knock at the door broke the silence.

'Telegram for you, Comrade Major,' said a guard. 'A request for you to call the Yenisei Railway Camp Administration.'

As Nikitin followed the man out of the door, Rossel stared down at the files. But did not open them.

8

On his return several minutes later, the major placed a chipped tin mug next to Rossel.

'Tea?'

Some interrogators would sit still. Say nothing. Wait for their victim to fill the vacuum with incriminating talk. If they were not forthcoming, the interrogator would do his paperwork for a few hours and then leave, making way for the next inquisitor. The victim was given no respite. And so on, for hours. Days with the stubborn ones. They called it the Conveyor Belt.

That had never been Nikitin's style. He had always dealt in fists, boots and clubs. And, occasionally, in sharpened steel. Instant results. Rossel glanced down at his own left hand.

But, today, he had offered him sweet tea.

'Do you know what zeks mean when they talk of the *myaso*?' said Nikitin.

Rossel nodded.

'When someone plans an escape, they go in two or threes,' he said. 'Say two men plan the escape. They invite a third. He's the *myaso*. The meat, the walking larder. He only gets as far as the point where other two decide that they're feeling hungry. The *myaso* gets a chance to sleep by the fire – "rest and warmth, comrade, you've earned it, our

57

turn to take watch." So the fool goes to sleep by the fire. And ends up on it.'

The corners of Nikitin's mouth turned upwards.

'Your old friend Sergeant Grachev has escaped from a camp at Vorkuta. He's taken a young boy called Yenin with him, a political. A student.'

Grachev was a name Rossel had not heard for a while. He would have been happy to keep it that way. A sergeant at Rossel's old police station in Leningrad, Grachev was as crooked as they came – a belligerent barrel of a man who never stopped talking about his exploits in the Great Patriotic War. The Fritzes he had killed, the minefields he had strolled through to get to all the *Frauen* and *Fräuleins* he had violated. The vengeance he had wreaked on the German nation in the name of Mother Russia. More than once, Rossel had encountered Grachev regaling junior officers with these war stories, holding them in thrall, a moment of calm amid the habitual chaos of the police station – a sooty, gloomy mansion on Vosstaniya Street that had once belonged to a merchant. Grachev was a thug with grey teeth and a penchant for spending too much time with any woman in the cells who took his fancy. He had a contempt for authority, a contempt he upgraded to loathing when it came to Rossel, who he regarded as moralistic. And for years, nobody had ever known much more about Grachev than that.

But a man like that made enemies. One of those enemies had found out that Grachev had, as a young man, been on the wrong side in the Civil War. A few well-placed whispers later and Major Nikitin and a detachment of MGB troops had arrested the entire police station, Rossel included. Guilt by association – it was all the MGB needed to put any Soviet citizen on a cattle truck to nowhere.

Some of the militia officers had been released. Many were not. Grachev was given a ten-year term to play his part in that area of the Soviet economy run by the Main Camps Directorate.

Nikitin moved over to the fire, picked up the spike that served as a poker and gave the grate a prod. In spite of himself, Rossel shuffled to the edge of his chair to share the warmth.

Why now? Grachev was many things but not a fool. The chances of surviving an escape attempt like that were either none or slim. It was not something the sergeant would have attempted unless . . .

Two bodies in Leningrad . . .

Grachev escapes.

And now Major Oleg Nikitin travels however many thousands of kilometres just to bring me the news . . .

Nikitin pointed to the tin mug.

'Why not drink some of that tea? And then you could take a little look at those files. If you want any more answers, detective.'

*

Samosud had a long, thin face with hooded eyes and big ears.

The details on him were scarce. Avraam Samosud. Born in Moscow in July 1907. Citizenship: Russian. Ethnicity: Jewish. Discharged from the army in 1947, by which time he had made it to sergeant. Wounded in action twice. The file listed several family members, including his parents.

All were marked as having died in 1941. As Jews, that pointed to one thing – Einsatzgruppen, the Nazi mobile death squads who had followed the Blitzkrieg into western Russia.

Rossel placed the file back on the desk and opened the other document.

Katz. Born in March 1912, in Novosibirsk. A thick black moustache and a high brow. A mournful, pessimistic face. Like the pictures of the exiled Trotsky. The kind of man, Rossel thought, that might greet the bullet that killed him with a 'What took you so long?'

His recorded citizenship and ethnicity were the same as Samosud. The file listed commendations for his participation in agitprop theatre and other forms of cultural enlightenment for his fellow troops. He had also served in a mechanised unit. Katz had fought in Stalingrad, where he had been wounded. Discharged in 1946. His parents' names were listed with no record of any death date. From Siberia, his family would have been well behind the lines.

'There are theories,' said Major Nikitin. 'One, it was an opportunist escape. Grachev saw his moment and grasped it.'

Rossel shook his head.

'That would be rash and suicidal. Grachev is neither. What camp was he in? What were his duties?'

'The main Vorkuta camp. Not one of the colonies but unpleasant enough. In his first week he got into a fight and beat one of Thieves up so badly they spent three weeks in the infirmary. Mostly he was a loner, according to the commandant there. They gave him loner's jobs. Cleaning the place, digging ditches. Some spells in the coal mines. Open pits. But he was surviving.'

Rossel leaned forward.

'That means he was watching and waiting,' said Rossel.

Nikitin smiled. Then nodded.

'Evidently,' said Nikitin. 'And then perhaps he heard of the fate of his former army comrades . . .'

'Excuse me?'

'Ah yes,' said Nikitin. 'You read the files but missed the most interesting part. Look again.'

Rossel fumbled for another cigarette with one hand as he reopened the files with the other.

Katz and Samosud both served in the Red Army. No surprise – most able-bodied men had been called up.

The 8th Guards Army.

The army that Grachev had fought in, as he never tired of reminding people. Because the 8th had made it right across Europe and all the way to Berlin.

Nikitin turned away from the fire and looked straight into Rossel's eyes.

'You see? And not only the 8th but, when the militia dug a little deeper, the same division, the same regiment,' he said. 'So I made it my business to find out where the sergeant had been fulfilling his debt to Soviet society. It took a while but I got there, and I sent some of my new associates to chat to Grachev while I came here to find you.'

Rossel closed the files. 'But now he has disappeared into the forest,' he said.

'Yes.'

Rossel sat back.

'My days as a detective are over, Major. You ended them when you had me sent here.'

Nikitin glanced down at his own jacket and toyed with a button.

'If you help me, Rossel, I can get you out of here. For good.'

Rossel stood.

'I'd like to go back to the barracks now, Major.'

Nikitin shook his head in disappointment and took out a photograph from his wallet.

He placed it on the table between them.

The face in the picture was younger and thinner than the one Rossel knew but was unmistakable.

Vassya.

Rossel picked up the photograph.

'Is she well?'

Nikitin stared at him.

'Why not ask her yourself, detective?'

*

The whole process – Nikitin's swaggering departure, Vassya's reluctant entrance, Rossel's bitter disbelief – was agony. Rossel responded to the appearance of his former lover in the only way he could think of. By pulling out another of Nikitin's cigarettes.

Five minutes or more passed in silence. To his surprise, Vassya broke first, filling the void with words of confession.

'After you were taken, Revol, I tried to find out where you were,' she said. 'I joined the parents and sons and daughters outside The Crosses who throw tins and loaves at the windows with messages tied to them to get word, even a single word, of what has happened to their loved ones.

I even walked past the Bolshoi Dom once in case Nikitin would come out and I could plead with him. Honestly, I flew Polikarpovs into the night sky and the Fascists' flak during the war and I never sweated as much as I did on that day. All for nothing. For six weeks, nothing – no rumours, no contacts. You had disappeared. So, I packed a bag and waited for my own visit from the Chekists. And then I did something very foolish.'

'Which was?'

'I began to hope.'

She sighed.

'Not for you. For myself. Began to hope I had been forgotten.'

After the war, Vassya had resented nothing more than the insult of being forgotten. She had been a Night Witch – one of a group of women pilots who flew mission after mission over German lines in ponderous biplanes, cutting their engines to conceal their presence and position. Gliding at reckless altitude, they dropped bombs from the darkness onto the heads of their enemies.

When peacetime came, they were ordered out of the cockpit and out of the air force.

But she was right. There were times when it was better to be forgotten.

'Six weeks went by,' she said. 'I began to breathe a little easier. Then a certain Captain Karpov of the Ministry for State Security calls at the communal apartment and leaves a message with one of the neighbours. Everyone had pity and fear in their eyes. Everyone wanted to say how sorry they were. No one dared. The message was that I had to go to the Bolshoi Dom.'

For a Leningrad citizen, a summons to the city's MGB headquarters was never good news.

'Captain Karpov has a desk and an office and looks at me as if he cannot wait to kill me himself. He has your file on his desk. He asks questions about us, about you: how long we have known each other, the usual. And after all of fifteen minutes of this he instructs me to go home and pack some essentials and "prepare myself for a long journey." So I prepare myself.'

Vassya reached up and ran a hand through her hair.

'Next morning I come back and Captain Karpov isn't there. I ask for him, and another MGB officer looks over from his desk and says that Captain Karpov was arrested the previous evening and would not be coming back. He advised me to go home and await further communication, with a glimmer of a smile that told me I was the luckiest citizen in the entire Union of Soviet Socialist Republics. So, I did.'

Rossel tapped his right hand on his chest.

'Remember the bird carved on the mantelpiece at Vosstaniya Street station that I used to offer up superstitious entreaties to? These days, I have it inked on my chest. But your story explains why it hasn't brought me any luck. You, Tatiana Ivanovna Vasilyeva, have used up everybody else's.'

Vassya glanced down at the table and did not reply. Once, she would have smiled at that.

Rossel wanted to shout, to accuse her of betrayal. But even in bed, after their lovemaking, they had for the most part stared at each other without speaking. With someone new, you watched what you said in case you ever had to justify it, or repudiate it, at some unknown point in the future. That was instinctive. You loved Stalin, you loved the Party, you loved the Revolution and everything it meant, and that was enough. Apart from the sex, for the most part all they had shared were caresses, kisses, looks and silence.

What does she really owe me?

Perhaps they had not felt for each other as he had thought.

Here and now, part of him despised her. Full-cheeked, full-breasted, sullen, dark, withdrawn.

Just swap places with me for two days, bitch. I'll wait here by the fire.

'I'm sensing you didn't come all this way just to study the architectural magnificence of the GULAG system,' Rossel said.

He looked for a reaction but neither her eyes nor her mouth or anything else revealed the slightest thought. Her voice was dry and matter-of-fact.

'In the air force, if you were a real survivor, you never counted your sorties,' she said. 'You'd go up, drop your bombs, hope that you had killed some Nazis and land again. And the next day the same. And the next . . . In a dogfight, every piece of you has to be focused on today. It's the part that's thinking about tomorrow that ensures you never make it back again. As I said, I had begun to hope. Hope only for myself. That was a foolish mistake. I have a good job now, a very good job – a senior engineer on the new underground system. I'd like to go back to it.'

'And Nikitin has said that will happen if I come back with you?'

Vassya nodded.

'He understands you, Revol. Like I do. He can force you to come back with him. Of course he can. But he knows that won't help him. Because you'll only play along, pretend to play detective but hold back on the insights he really needs. The little things only you notice. He needs you to volunteer. Ready and willing to help. And I am what he thinks will make you do that.'

In the camp's crude but inventive barter economy the remaining *papirosi* would have been gold, but Rossel fumbled inside his jacket with shaking fingers, desperate for a distraction. He dared not look at her any longer. He picked matches off the desk but the bloody things wouldn't keep still and he hurled the half-burned ends onto the floor, hoping they might set fire to the place.

Two deep drags later and he had composed himself. He took a last look at the fire. He would have to make up a story to explain his absence from the labour brigade. But he knew the other zeks would be more interested in a lengthy description of what it felt like to be sat next to a hearth for an hour. If they discovered that he'd sat next to a woman, an actual woman, for a few minutes, they'd go insane.

He glanced through the window again. Already twilight. It must have been more than an hour.

The door opened and Nikitin came back in.

Rossel looked up at Vassya and the major gave them both a bright smile.

'Can I go and get my supper now, Major Nikitin?' he said. 'We might have potatoes tonight. It's a real feast when we do. I find them the perfect accompaniment to the maggots that wriggle in the bread.'

Nikitin's smile vanished.

'In the morning I go to Vorkuta to investigate Grachev's escape,' said the major. 'In a day or so I will be back. When I land, you will give me your answer. If it's no, then you stay here for the next thirty years and I'll make no further attempts to help . . .'

But Rossel was already through the door, pushing past the surprised guard, and out into the cold.

He had trusted the major once before. He wouldn't make that mistake again.

9

Oblonsky's voice was so low Rossel could barely hear it. But he strained his ears – the tattooist was a normally a cheerful man and it took something serious to put him on edge.

'There's a new prisoner here, Revol. A *svodnik*, a pimp. And a bit more.'

He tapped his needle on Rossel's skin without penetrating it.

'A Leningrader. He's been saying things about you.'

Rossel stiffened.

'Not to the Thieves, not yet,' muttered Oblonsky. 'Just sounding us out down here, around the edges.'

'What kind of things?' said Rossel in an undertone. But he knew.

Oblonsky tapped away, not raising his head, concentrating on his subject's flesh.

'That you're a gundog. A militia officer.'

Tap, tap, tap.

'Is it true?'

Rossel pointed at his own chest,

'That line is not quite inked correctly. See there, where the beak of the albatross is.'

Oblonsky dabbed at Rossel's skin, wiping away blood. He scrutinised his handiwork but Rossel knew he wanted more information.

'Listen to yourself, Pasha,' Rossel said. 'Me, a gundog. Here, in Igarka. How does that make any sense? Who is this pimp, anyway?'

'On the other side of the barracks, three bunks down, top bunk. His name is Grishin. He arrived a few days ago. He's trying not to look at us now, but he is.'

Rossel took Grishin in. Not tall but broad-shouldered. A broken nose and a sly, card-sharp's face.

Oblonsky resumed digging under Rossel's skin.

'True or not, if he tells the Thieves – if he tells Kuba and Medvedev. People noticed you were gone today. The wrong sort of people. First, a helicopter arrives, and then you're pulled out of the railway brigade. You're being talked about, Comrade Albatross.'

This time Rossel couldn't help it. A dip of the head, a flutter of the shoulders. To anyone not paying much attention, it was nothing more than the usual flinching when a needle bit too close to bone.

But Oblonsky knew better.

'I hope I get to finish this stupid fucking bird, that's all I'm saying, comrade,' whispered the tattooist, 'otherwise it will be a sorry waste of all my best ash and piss.'

*

Next morning the temperature was thirty below but the sky was clear. Rossel listened to the clatter of the helicopter rising into the air as Nikitin headed towards Vorkutlag, the centre of the GULAG's regional cluster. If he could have found a way of summoning the forces of the earth and skies and bending them in a certain direction, he would have brought the machine down.

He was surprised by the strength of his longing for Nikitin's death.

*

A day hauling the barrel could grind the spirit but Rossel was glad to be clear of the camp. It got him well away from Vassya, for one thing. She must have been confined to the commandant's quarters. He bent his head into a stiff breeze as the brigade tramped out once more into a sombre morning and towards the furthest point of the line, eyes fixed on the ground. Silent. Babayan crossing himself as usual. Each man left alone with his own torment.

By afternoon, the sun's fleeting appearance was masked by thick, low cloud. The huge barrel skidded this way and that. The old priest blasphemed when his ropes got tangled round his neck but the cold took his voice away. Behind them, the Germans swore and squabbled as they tried to get iron stakes in the solid ground to break up whatever lumps and humps the human steamroller had failed to flatten.

The sun disappeared in a hurry and the prisoners fell silent when the guards saw how little progress they had made and cursed them for idle bourgeois bastards who would soon taste Soviet justice. Someone cursed them back, saying the taste of Soviet justice would be better than the taste of the pigswill they got to eat. Each of them, calculating how meagre that evening's ration would be, despaired. Every next step seemed impossible until you took it. Then, somehow, you managed to take one more.

It was a day like any other.

10

No one was watching as Rossel sucked the dregs from his plate and slipped a sharpened utensil, a knife, up his sleeve. He dragged his legs over the bench and headed for the door. Close behind the pimp Grishin.

Rossel had expected Grishin to bear left and head to the barracks but instead he walked straight on. On their right was a row of smaller huts – stores and scrap metal, workshops, fuel cans, tools and machinery that were useless until the ground thawed for a few weeks in what passed for summer. The greenhouses of 105th Kilometre stood at the other end of the camp, slumped in their constituent parts, waiting for someone to care enough to rebuild them.

Grishin walked with the stride of a man not yet reduced to the demands of corrective labour. Someone who was already playing with favours. A man like that, Rossel understood, would have fought more than one fight already during his transportation to Igarka.

He had to be wary.

But the newcomer didn't know the layout of the camp. He would not yet have appreciated the possibilities afforded by the narrow gap between the generator hut and the kiln.

Now was the time.

Rossel picked up his stride, ran through the snow to cover the few metres between them and grabbed Grishin by the collar of his jacket. He shoved him into the gap between the two buildings, blocked at the far end by the roof of the kiln which, derelict, had slumped to the ground. Grishin – straining, wriggling – wheeled his whole arm in surprise. But froze at the feel of sharp, jagged metal at his throat.

Eye to eye, the two of them lurched further out of sight in a vicious embrace.

Even if the thrum of the generator would drown out his screams, it would still have to be quick. Rossel, baring his teeth, placed his right hand over his left for the killing stroke.

Then Grishin lashed out. A big fist slammed into Rossel's stomach. The blow bent him double but one of his flailing hands caught Grishin by the collar.

As the pimp tried to force his way back out to open ground, Rossel kicked, catching his shin. Grishin lost balance and sprawled against the side of the generator hut. Rossel, despite the shooting pain in his abdomen, tackled him.

The two of them went down in the snow.

Grishin was the stronger but not nimble enough. Rossel pinned Grishin's upper arms with his knees. He raised his knife.

Grishin writhed, clutching at Rossel's clothes.

Freed a hand.

Raised a forearm to ward off the blow.

Something fluttered between the pimp's fingers. Sheets of paper, torn from Rossel's coat pocket in the struggle.

'Please, no, I beg you,' shouted Grishin, his face contorted with terror. 'I fucking beg you, I won't say anything, Gundog – I wasn't going to . . .'

73

Grishin struggled some more under Rossel's legs. But then went still.

Holding the knife with one hand, Rossel eased the papers from Grishin's fingers with the other. He stared down at them.

Vustin's compositional hand was immaculate. His clefs, his sharps, flats, rests, bar lines, semiquavers, the dots of his staccato and the sweep of his slurs . . .

These were his scriptures. His psalms.

More pages fluttered and flew away – some pinned against the wall of the storeroom, some vanishing into the shadows.

Rossel rose to his feet.

In the war, yes. But not now. This was different.

On the other side of this he would become somebody else.

Grishin backed away, hands raised.

'I won't let you down,' he said. 'I won't say anything. I promise – not a word. I'll bite my tongue and clench my lips together, tight as a virgin on her first fuck. I won't say anything, Gundog, I promise.'

Grishin walked towards the huts, repeating his vows. Rossel knew they were worthless.

The promise of a criminal was, after all, exactly that.

*

At night, the limits of Soviet authority were demarcated by the lights of the perimeter fence and the watchtowers. In the darkness between, inside the huts and in the shadows they cast, the Thieves and Bitches reigned.

In the gloom of his barracks, Rossel stared up at the ceiling, fighting his exhaustion, trying to stay awake, listening for the approach of Grishin or someone the pimp might have bribed – a 'louse', a lesser thief – to slit his throat. Yet the less rest he got, the worse the following day's hard labour would be.

The *Suki*, the Bitches, ruled the Eastern Barracks. They were willing to work – if it suited them. Since they were rewarded for working with rations and even weapons to use against their rivals, it often did.

The *Suki* also dominated the Northern Barracks but the few veterans of the Great Patriotic War within its walls were disinclined to be as servile as the intellectual weaklings who made up the bulk of the political prisoners. Those who had fought at Stalingrad, at Kursk, at Warsaw, at Berlin, were familiar with violence. The violence within the Northern Barracks had cost seven lives in the past two months alone.

Whether in the dark or the light, the German POWs cowered in Barracks Four, the Southern, never venturing beyond their hut except for labour duties, food and the obligatory scrub and ineffectual delousing once a fortnight. Only then moving together in numbers. Like the musk deer that roamed the taiga at night, ever watchful for the wolves. Some were battle-hardened and able to fight back. But many had only been thrown into the front line at the end of the war when the regular soldiers were either dead or wounded. Fighting was alien to them.

Rossel's bunk was in the Western Barracks. This was where the old-fashioned Thieves, the long-established crime clans, ruled the roost – purists who would rather break an arm than lift a finger for the state. In most camps they were a dwindling force. In 105th Kilometre, rallied into psychopathic fury by Kuba and Medvedev, they were as of old.

At the top were the men of ingrained criminality who lived by the sacred Thieves' Law:

Help other Thieves. Have nothing to do with the authorities. Keep your pledges to other Thieves or pay the price.

Rules and hierarchies stretching back decades. A Thief-within-the-law was to be feared and respected. Never crossed.

Night was a favourite time for the Thieves to settle individual scores with any politicals who had dared display defiance. They prowled the barrack hut, their movements covered by the snores, sobs and growling stomachs of eighty men.

Usually, Rossel did his utmost to put all thoughts of food out of his head. After a night spent dreaming of *syrniki* and *solyanka*, some inmates had been known to step across the perimeter wire in the morning. Preferring death to an almost empty plate.

Tonight, though, he indulged himself. Better to think of that than Grishin. Finally, even though his reveries were filled with *pelmeni* and *pirozhki* and other miracles, he drifted off . . .

*

A hand on his shoulder.

Three men – a *shpana:* a high-ranking Thief-within-the-law, and two henchman – were shaking him awake.

As they filed out of the door, the senior Thief clapped him on the back.

'To the casino, Comrade Albatross,' the Thief said. 'Time for *shobla yobla*.'

Time for the Rabble.

*

After midnight, the *Suki* slipped past the beams of the watchtower searchlights to the factory, while the Thieves and their acolytes sidled into the forge. As they reached it, Rossel crossed into a world of heat and noise. The *shobla yobla* was in full session.

At two tables, a couple of dozen Thieves played cards. They hardly looked up. If his past as a lieutenant in the Leningrad militia was laid bare, Rossel knew their indifference would not last long.

A twist of fear in his gut.

He began to cough again.

In the far corner of the room stood the grinning figure of Grishin.

11

In the centre of the forge, perched on a stool on top of a rickety platform, sat the Emperor of 105th Kilometre. Very short, almost a dwarf, he was a dark-skinned Dargin from the north Caucasus. His swarthiness and love of rum were the reasons he had acquired his nickname: Kuba, after the Caribbean island.

Next to him stood Medvedev, better known as the Bear. It wasn't just a play on his name. The Bear was former weightlifter from Crimea, a giant of a man, adorned from head to foot with tattoos. His bald head and face were completely covered in them, and it was almost impossible to spot even a small patch of white skin. When he grinned, which was often, he bared his pointed yellow teeth, which had been filed into fangs.

At their feet sat their pet creature. Tsar Suka. The hunched, hollowed-eyed, scar-faced German whom Walter had pointed out to Rossel. Among the Thieves, he was indulged, even adored. They were Russians, after all, and so took great pride in keeping a pedigree Aryan as their house mongrel, even one well past his prime.

Rossel was shoved to the near left-hand corner of the room, not far from the door and not close enough to the warmth of the forge. His head was still a blizzard of tiredness and dread. Try as he might, he could not rally his senses.

In this Thieves' court, Kuba and Medvedev, applauded by their imbecile court jester, were infamous for the intricate cruelty of their sentences.

At the tables other Thieves were bickering, pushing and shoving, scratching heads or licking lips as they considered where to place their stakes. The game was *shtoss*, Rossel thought – fast and furious, a magnet for sharps who could count cards or palm them.

Unless they got caught. And if they did, a knife would settle it.

Rossel spotted Misha the Axe in the melee of gamblers – laughing, threatening. *'Pora spat', polnoch, skoro zapoyut petukhi.* Time to go to bed, it's midnight, soon the cocks will be crowing,' shouted Misha in Thieves' slang. 'But I'll ring your neck like a fucking chicken, my good friends, if I find the Ace of Spades hiding in your shoe.'

The rules of *shtoss* were simple enough. The thirteen cards of a single suit were spread out in two rows. Gamblers placed their stakes – coins, buttons, lumps of wax – on whichever card they fancied. Presiding over a separate deck, cards face down, was the dealer.

The top two cards of the deck were turned over. The first was the winning card, the second was the loser. If you'd picked the winner – the matching number or face – you'd doubled your stake. If you'd picked the loser, you kissed your money goodbye.

Rossel saw Kuba whisper into Medvedev's ear and the giant nodded.

'Last round, ladies,' he said.

The clamour intensified. Those on a losing streak wagered everything they had left; those who had kept an eye on what had been discarded and what was still in the deck made fevered calculations.

One last shot!

If Grishin had told them of his past in the militia, Rossel thought, that was all he had.

*

Silence fell upon on the forge.

Kuba clambered down from the stool and stood next to Medvedev. The difference in height between them was so great they looked like a bear and her cub. But it was very clear who was in charge.

Kuba's voice dropped into a plaintive, childlike call. 'Comrade Bobkov, Comrade Bobkov . . . Come out, come out, wherever you are.'

The sweating Bobkov was a political prisoner who had been an entertainer, a comic actor who had strayed from Marxist–Leninist norms. Short and formerly plump, now no longer so, he was shoved into the centre of the room.

'Prosecutor?' demanded Kuba.

A spindly crook with a protruding jaw and a low hairline, standing not too far from Rossel, stepped forward.

'Alexeyev,' he mumbled through his gums.

'Eh? What's that, Arsewipe? Aweks . . . Ayek . . .'

As the crowd hooted and clapped at Kuba's gurning mimicry, the toothless Alexeyev stood still and impotent.

'All right, all right, calm down,' said Kuba, affecting magnanimity but delighted with his court's reaction. 'Speak, Alexeyev.'

'I saw him talking to one of the guards,' said Alexeyev, pointing to Bobkov. 'To a Chekist, not one of the army conscripts. On the far side of the parade ground, behind the coal store.'

The general merriment was instantly replaced by disappointed groans. So what? Informants in a camp were a fact of life. They were treated with contempt but mostly tolerated.

There must be something worse than . . .

'And then Vanya goes into solitary when the guards find his stash of moonshine. They gave him a good battering with their truncheons, too.'

The groans turned to growling. It gathered strength. Bobkov began to tremble.

Kuba raised a hand to quell the Thieves. Rossel watched them lean forward, impatient for the verdict.

Kuba rubbed his hair, short and rough as a ploughed field, and wrinkled his nose.

'They tell me you were a comedian, Comrade Bobkov?' said Kuba.

The defendant nodded.

Kuba raised his hands, palms upturned, and glanced around the room.

'Then make us laugh and we will let you live.'

Bobkov stood still. Lost for words. Petrified.

Medvedev flexed his muscles, which rendered the entertainer even more mute, until a couple of blows round the face brought him out of his trance.

'Right, right, make you chuckle, of course. Young Ivan is . . . Young Ivan is . . .' Bobkov found his voice. He began to gabble at high speed, '. . . in mathematics class and the teacher asks him, "If coal costs one hundred roubles a tonne and your father orders five hundred roubles worth of coal, how much does he get?" Young Ivan replies, "Three and a half tonnes," and the teacher slaps him around the ears, calls him an imbecile. "That is completely wrong!" says the teacher . . .'

Bobkov tried a cheeky grin but didn't pull it off. His voice went into punchline mode. '"I know," says young Ivan. "But my dad says that's what happens at his factory every fucking week, what are you going to do?"'

Bobkov waited for laughter. None came.

Sweat streaming down his brow, he kept digging. He started on a joke about a Soviet expedition of Egyptologists who needed Beria to extract a confession from a mummy to determine its age, but before he got halfway through Medvedev yawned and the comic faltered.

Hell, Rossel thought, is a comedian in a silent room.

Now Bobkov segued into a story about a servant at Stalin's dacha who was fooled by an older, wilier colleague into hoarding the contents of the generalissimo's daily chamber pots in a cupboard 'as if they were pure gold'. Until one day the secret stash of Stalin's shit is discovered.

A couple of titters. Sensing he might be onto a winner, Bobkov raced on.

'Unwilling to declare that Stalin's precious turds were just shit, the political officers are forced to admit that the servant is now the richest man in the Soviet Union.'

Bobkov hesitated. Then he rolled his hand into a fist and raised it upward to signify he was delivering the coup de grâce.

'But to their relief,' he added, 'they realise they are now able to declare him a bourgeois capitalist pig and have him arrested as a hoarder . . .'

Total silence.

Kuba prodded Medvedev. The giant-sized Bobkov up and hit him in the face with an axe handle. The comedian dropped to the floor.

Alexeyev, the prosecutor, bent down and slit Bobkov's throat. As the blood began to flow, Tsar Suka jumped to his feet and began to hum manically – a fragment of a piece of music that Rossel thought he recognised but couldn't quite place. The room collapsed into laughter.

At last, Bobkov was a hit.

*

'Comrade Albatross, we've always liked your stories. But tonight, I'd prefer a song.'

Kuba resumed his elevated position on his stool and pointed at Rossel. A Thief grabbed Rossel's arms and pulled his gloves and rags away.

Tsar Suka stared at Rossel's broken hands, mesmerised. He pointed at Bobkov's body. Kuba grinned, then stepped down from the stool, leaned over and ruffled Bobkov's hair. A couple of the Thieves got to their feet; but no further, uncertain how to proceed.

'His Highness, our noble Tsar, is pointing out that funny bones here has got some fingers he now doesn't need,' said

Kuba. 'A competition, then. If our friend the Albatross does well, he leaves here with some useful spare parts. But if he does badly, we cut off his *khui* and give it to Bobkov. If Hell's everything I'm hoping it's going to be, a spare prick might come in handy.'

Amid general cackling a battered, broken violin was shoved into Rossel's arms. Despite himself he stared at it. The bridge was smashed and the strings ran ragged from the pegs to the tail. Other than his own, which he had left behind in Leningrad and since the war had only ever tucked under his chin to breathe in the memory of playing, it was the first fiddle Rossel had touched in more than a decade. He felt the urge to press it to his lips.

'No, not a fiddle . . .' The instrument was snatched away by Medvedev. 'How about a guitar? Hey, ladies, imagine – Stumpy here playing the guitar!'

The Thieves roared.

Rossel glanced across at the door to the forge. No one was guarding it. If he could get close enough . . .

Another part of his brain said that if you tuned the guitar the right way, all you needed was a thumb and a finger.

What songs did the Thieves like? Rossel thought back to the snatches of Thief life that had reached his ears as a street-level policeman. Glimpses into that world from rare informants.

No, there was no inspiration there.

But then he had it. A song he'd picked up in the transit camp where he had waited for a month before his dispatch northwards.

The story of Kolka the Pickpocket. An all-time criminal favourite.

'A guitar? All right then, Kuba,' Rossel said. 'Get me a guitar and I'll play you something' – he pointed at Tsar Suka – 'even our Tsar can sing along to.'

Kuba nodded. A Thief was sent. After a minute, he returned with another battered instrument with a piece of rough rope as a sling.

It only took one of the remaining two fingers on his left hand to produce four approximate bar chords; and the scarred, broken but still-attached fingers of his right to thrash the thinning strings.

Rossel slipped his right arm through the sling and let the instrument settle under the crook of his arm. He had another ten seconds to finish working out the harmony in his head before plunging in.

> *In Moldavanka they're busy playing music.*
> *With drunken revelry resounding all around . . .*

*

As Rossel played, some of the Thieves beat their fists on the table to the rhythm.

Kolka the Pickpocket was (according to the song) a slave sent to work on the White Sea Canal project, who had turned from the criminal life and embraced the righteousness of the Soviet ideal. Such was the strength of his new conviction, he had even turned his back on a rescue attempt by a clan leader – and had earned himself a death sentence in the process.

> *Tell them, Masha, that he don't thieve no longer.*
> *He's cast it off, that criminal life, for labour . . .*

Rossel fumbled his way from one chord to the next, striking discordant notes, slipping and sliding one-fingered along the fretboard in his quest for the right harmonies.

As he did so, he moved a little further towards the edge of the circle, closer to the door.

He's understood that now he is far stronger

He had to sing like a Thief, with grit in his throat and a snarl in his voice.

That this canal has been his bloody saviour . . .

Thanks to the simple harmony, Rossel settled into the cycle of the chords. He raised his eyes from the instrument and stared back at the front row of gaunt, hungry faces. He'd have to win them over with bravura and some erratic tuning.

He took another stride towards the far edge of the circle.

The song's final verse told of the *pakhan,* the clan boss, giving the order for Kolka the Pickpocket to be taught his lesson. There would be no happily ever after for Kolka, not even after embracing Communist virtues of corrective labour. In the Soviet Union, it was hard to escape your past. Perhaps that's why the criminals loved the song. They saw themselves in it.

Another step.

And another.

One more . . .

But then, shaking his head, Medvedev stepped in front of him and showed his sharpened yellow fangs.

Rossel retreated to the centre of the room. He hurled his knuckles into the final chord and kept his arm aloft as the sound died away.

Instead of the raucous glee that greeted renditions of the song in communal kitchens up and down the Soviet Union, in the forge of a corrective labour camp in northern Siberia it resulted in only silence. Everyone looked to Kuba for his reaction.

But it was Tsar Suka, his ageing court jester, who broke the spell.

Brutally twanging on the battered violin and humming a tune – a falling scale that eventually got too low for his voice – the German circled Rossel.

Heart pounding, understanding that his life depended on the whims of a capricious halfwit and a sadistic dwarf, Rossel was still dimly aware that the melody was prodding a memory in him.

Tsar Suka started again, lips open but yellow teeth clenched, getting louder and slower as the scale descended.

Kuba and Medvedev watched their pet Aryan with glee.

'What's that?' asked Kuba.

The German broke off, bowing his head like a mischievous child, showing his thinning hair.

Not an orthodox scale, the intervals were wrong. And there was that skip to the rhythm at the start . . .

'What's that?' repeated the head Thief, more loudly.

Where had I heard it? Yes, of course . . .

'Wagner,' said Rossel. 'A favourite of Hitler and the Nazis. His operas were based on Nordic myths. Great stories, Kuba, you would like them – heroes and dragons and dwar—'

87

Rossel stopped himself. Medvedev bared his teeth again.

'Dwarves?' said Kuba.

Rossel nodded.

A couple of Thieves sniggered.

Kuba stepped towards him and pulled out a big knife.

'You're a tall man, Comrade Albatross. Handsome, too. At least, you would be with a few more meals inside you. First man I ever killed looked a little like you. I was sitting next to him on a tram in Moscow. A young girl in a red beret, maybe five or six years old, was staring at us both. The little princess glanced at me, then back at the tall glass of water. Then she smiled . . .'

'That's when he knew,' said Medvedev.

Kuba nodded.

'"Mummy, look, there's a funny little man sitting over there, a dwarf" – that's what the little bitch was thinking.'

Kuba used the tip of his knife to prise out some dirt from underneath one of his fingernails. 'So, when he gets off the tram I follow the giraffe into the park. Sneak up behind him. And make him a present of a nice a ruby necklace – slit his throat.'

Rossel's eyes were fixed on the tip of the knife. But his voice sounded calm.

'In the opera,' he said, 'a dwarf called Alberich forges a ring of stolen gold that gives the bearer the power to rule the world. Gods, heroes, villains, all fight over it. But the ring is cursed and everyone who takes possession of it dies, one after the other. Until the rule of the gods ends and the time of men begins. Something from that is, I think, what our friend Tsar Suka was singing.'

Kuba's eyes moved around the room, gauging the mood of his Thieves. In the warmth and heavy smoke, the death of Bobkov, the song of Kolka the Pickpocket, talk of stolen gold, the drawing of the knife . . . all that had hypnotised them. Something caught Kuba's eye. He walked towards the forge before reaching for a small object on a worktable, testing its temperature with quick fingers before deciding it was safe to handle. He picked it up, flattened his hand and slipped the brass washer on his stubby finger.

Kuba had found a ring. Putting his knife away, he threaded his way back to his throne and sat back down.

'They say Stalin sometimes calls himself Koba, after a Georgian king. Me, I think Uncle Joe wants to give himself airs and graces. So, first he mispronounces my name. Then steals it. A ring. A crown. A state. A camp. They always belong to the man who has the balls to reach out and take them.'

Kuba smiled at Rossel. It began as sunshine but ended as ice.

'Grishin here says you used to be a gundog, a militia lieutenant. That's a real shame because I always liked both your singing and your stories.'

Rossel went for the door but was too slow. A thicket of hands, two of them Medvedev's, seized him.

Someone kicked him hard in the back of the knees, dropping him to the floor.

Kuba pointed to Grishin and threw him his knife. 'Start with his prick.'

He then gestured to the dead comedian. 'If Comrade Bobkov here doesn't want it we can feed it to one of the guard dogs.'

The pimp grinned and stepped towards Rossel.

I knew I should have killed you when I had the chance . . .

Rossel closed his eyes.

He tried to retch and could taste bile but, pressed hard into the damp boards by the Thieves, the puke only clogged up his throat. An image of his mother and father, proud Communists until the Party devoured them, rose in his mind. And another – Sofia, a woman he had once loved; her face in quiet repose, turning to him, softly smiling.

He braced his body for the first cut of the knife. Tried to blank his mind.

A pounding at the door to the forge. Then it was smashed open.

He felt the weight lift from his chest and limbs – a short-lived respite as a heavy boot then thumped into his head, followed by a knee thudding into his sternum. A semi-automatic rifle went off close to his ear, deafening him.

Then camp guards were hauling him out into the snow by his hair and the collar of his jacket.

Above the clamour, a familiar voice, berating everyone for their anti-Soviet tendencies and cursing them all for bastards, threatening to have them all slaughtered. Major Nikitin.

And another sound. That of Tsar Suka's rambling, Wagnerian leitmotif.

The camp's fool grinned and shook as he sang his song to the starry Siberian sky.

12

Rossel had been in the air only five times. Days after the Siege of Leningrad had been lifted, he twice went on out-and-back transport missions to pick up rations for the forces defending the city – a Yak-6 so rickety that the Fascists didn't even bother to shoot at it.

The only other time had been a night-time flight in a Polikarpov biplane piloted by Tatiana 'Vassya' Vasilyeva, with Nikitin as the other passenger.

The major, he remembered, had thrown up.

As the rotors of the Mi-4 began to turn, the helicopter spurted dark-grey smoke from the twin exhaust pipes that protruded like stunted horns from its nose. Rossel glanced at Nikitin, who was watching the blades spin with a look of admiration on his face.

Vassya stood to one side, well wrapped up against the cold. As the blades turned even faster, kicking up snow, she lowered her head.

Nikitin clapped him on the back.

'It's only to Salekhard, and then we're on the ground again. After that, a regular plane to Moscow, and another to Leningrad.'

Leningrad.

Just hearing the word spoken out loud made Rossel feel giddy.

The major wrenched open the large hatch at the side of the Mil Mi-4 and levered himself in. Rossel turned to bid farewell to the fences, barbed wire and watchtowers of 105th Kilometre, and to the buildings and people within. Just as he was turning back, he caught sight of the day's labour gangs setting off. Two were heading in the direction of the railway line.

He could just make out the stooped figure of Babayan at the front of the first. At this distance, the old priest looked like he was leading a line of forlorn pilgrims out towards the saints to whom he prayed. Our Lady of Kazan, Blessed Nicholas II, Alexei the Tsarevich, and the newly canonised Vustin.

All his shadows in the snow.

As the dead boy's comrades fell in behind the ghosts who'd marched before them, a fragment of Vustin's gulag hymn came to Rossel. He longed to feel a bow in his hands. Pianissimo, he thought, that's how I'd play it. Almost unbearably gently.

And slow. So slow.

*

Wearing really warm clothes – socks, boots, a thick coat and padded gloves – for the first time in months was enough to distract Rossel from the Mi-4's fumes and noise. The pilots sat above the cabin, the only people with a view. All the passengers were bathed in a harsh red light.

The one thing he could not ignore was sitting opposite him, collar up and fur hat pulled down. Rossel tried to catch Vassya's eye, to read her expression, but she would not turn towards him. Eventually he gave up. He found himself staring all around the cabin, at straps and cables, at the ladder that led up to the cockpit, at metal plates bolted to the floor – all in an effort to ignore her. But occasionally his eyes betrayed him and his stomach churned not only with the fumes but also with his emotions.

It took a while before he realised that Nikitin was trying to shout something at him. Rossel caught only snatches – how Grachev had definitely escaped with another prisoner, a much younger man. 'Probably the *myaso*,' yelled Nikitin. 'But our men closed in on him too fast. They got separated – or, more likely, Grachev left the boy to be caught, while he disappeared.'

The constant roar of the engines was giving Rossel a headache. Vassya was still a statue. Nikitin started to laugh.

'Apparently Grachev kept on boasting to the boy about some tart called Odette. How he was going back to Leningrad to find her.'

That didn't sound like Grachev, thought Rossel. A woman waiting for him by the fire? Not ever likely.

And one called Odette?

Under them the floor shuddered. Nikitin threw out an arm; grabbed Rossel's shoulder to steady himself. Vassya fought for balance. They hovered for a moment more.

Then, at last, they landed at Salekhard.

*

Onwards, further south.

The engines of the rusty Douglas, a wartime present from the Americans, were thrumming.

A hand on his shoulder. Rossel's eyes blinked open.

'I need you to look at something,' said Nikitin.

Rossel had drifted off in pitch darkness. Now the sun, its soft rays rippling along the aircraft's wing, had deepened into red.

'I thought I'd let you rest. But now, here's some homework.'

The major handed him a small piece of paper that had been written on in Roman script. A concise and deliberate hand had been at work. The paper was wide and thin – perhaps fifteen centimetres across, but only three or four in height – and curled at the edges, as if it had been rolled up and then smoothed out. Rossel took it. It was good quality, a little rough. The ink was jet black.

His hand shuddered to the rhythm of the engines and he struggled to decipher the script. As a student at the Leningrad Conservatoire he had been curious enough to translate occasional chunks of operatic libretti. But his Italian was never more than basic.

> O dolce notte, o sante
> Ore notturne e quete
> Ch'i disïosi amanti accompagnate

'I have had it translated,' said Nikitin.

He pulled out a small notebook from within his jacket.

'That means . . . "Oh gentle darkness, oh sacred and sweet nocturnal hours that attend fevered lovers . . ." Or something like that.'

Rossel turned it over. There was nothing on the back except a small patch where the ink had bled through.

'When we found this little ditty,' the major added, 'it had been rolled up and placed in the mouth of a man who had been tortured with pliers, had cigarette burns all over his body, and then finished off with two bullets to the brain.'

Oh gentle darkness, oh sacred and sweet nocturnal hours that attend fevered lovers . . .

As Rossel repeated the phrase out loud, he glanced across at Vassya. She was sleeping.

He sat straighter.

'After or before?'

'After or before what?'

'Did they place the paper in the victim's mouth after or before they killed them?'

Nikitin shrugged.

'After, I think. Does it matter?'

Rossel turned and stared down out of the window at thin blue line that twisted and turned through a grey patchwork of city blocks and the outlines of canals. The Neva River.

He was home.

It is a miracle.

He turned back to face the major.

'To me, no,' he said. 'To our murderer, possibly.'

'In what way?'

Rossel thought for a moment, then sat back in his seat and shrugged.

'Inserting it before killing is an act of inflicting a final humiliation upon the victim. Inserting it after – well, that's sending a message to whoever finds the body. A message to you . . .'

He stared down at the piece of paper in his hand before glancing back up at Nikitin.

'. . . a message to us.'

ACT 2
VALKYRIE

13

Nikitin's black, bug-like GAZ Pobeda drove out of the military airfield on the southern edge of Leningrad and set off to the opposite side of the city. The front and rear lights of cars, trucks and trolleybuses flared in the early morning half-light. Although it was nothing like as cold as the far north, Leningrad was a port city and the winters got under your skin. Snow lay piled up in the gutters while the wet roads gleamed and hissed under the tyres of the hesitant, irritable traffic.

At Moscow Square they turned east, rolling past Lenin striking a dramatic pose – when did he not? – and along Prospect Slavy. *Slava Gorodu-Geroyu! Glory to the Hero City!* proclaimed a huge red banner stretched above the road. Up the ramp, onto the bridge and they were over the dark waters of the Neva, the river flanked by warehouses. Beyond those, new residential buildings were being constructed for the heroes of the Hero City. But like the Siberian railway he had left behind, Leningrad's heroic status was built on bones.

The road bent north and in another twenty minutes they were already as far as the Piskaryovsky area. Nikitin turned off the main road and nosed his way down a series of side streets until he brought them to a halt in front of an impressive greystone apartment block – the kind that was usually reserved for Party officials.

The major took some keys from his coat pocket and handed them to Rossel.

'I still have the odd friend among the blue-hats,' he said.

'This belongs to a member of the MGB?' said Rossel. 'That seems unlikely.'

'Of course not. But I heard it had just become vacant and will only be reallocated in a couple of weeks. It will do for now. Be grateful, comrade – the knowledge and the keys cost me a couple of bottles of Armenian cognac.'

Rossel looked down at the keys.

'Who used to live here?' he said.

'Drugov, Ivan Vitalyevich Drugov. Big Party man. Proud Bolshevik, all the way to his bootstraps. Also the director of the Museum of the Defence of Leningrad. Or rather, former director. He was arrested days ago. Now, I suspect, he's lying on the floor of a cell in the Bolshoi Dom, face down in his own shit.'

Leningrad's citizens were proud of its status as Hero City. But not everyone in Moscow was so enamoured. Particularly Comrade Stalin.

'The place is probably riddled with microphones,' said Nikitin. 'Don't even talk in your sleep. Shout out an old girlfriend's name – Rosa, I love you – and, chances are, next morning at the factory where she works, Rosa doesn't make it in.'

'What did Comrade Drugov do?'

'Section 1A of the idiot's guide to the Penal Code – guilty of understatement.'

'Understatement?'

'The role of Stalin in the defence of Leningrad was insufficiently emphasised in his overall exhibition.'

They looked at each other. Compared to the sacrifices made by close to a million dead soldiers and civilians – not to mention those who somehow survived the starvation, disease and bombardment – Stalin's role had not been significant.

That said, he had made his presence felt. Not least through the offices of Oleg Nikitin, who before the Great Patriotic War had – in his capacity as an interrogator with the People's Commissariat for Internal Affairs, the precursor to the MGB – ended Rossel's promising career as a violinist by separating a couple of fingers from the hand to which they belonged.

Nikitin shook his head. 'Someone is always listening,' he muttered. 'Whatever it is, whether I'm here or not, don't say it. If you get sent back, even I won't be able to get you out again.'

Rossel held up his left hand.

'It's nice to hear you're thinking about my well-being, as always. Especially considering how we first met.'

*

"*It was a time when only the dead smiled, happy in their peace.*"

A line Vustin often repeated from Anna Akhmatova, a Leningrad poet whom the boy revered, came back to Rossel. She was someone else Moscow wasn't keen on: the Party marking Akhmatova out as an artist "in whom fornication and prayer are mingled", her poetry "distant from the people." The last accusation alone was enough to condemn her. But, so far, she had not been arrested.

Vustin, he remembered, would sing fragments of the unpublished poem, trying it out in a major and then a minor key. He had heard the poet read from it in person at a secret recital in Leningrad and instantly memorised them. 'I have based an entire cycle of twenty-four preludes and fugues on her work,' he had once told Rossel as they toiled together in the Igarka snows.

At the time, Rossel had presumed this was another of his fanciful notions.

He placed a hand on the remnant of the music in his pocket. He had been wrong about that.

Dead bodies were waiting for him. Come the next morning, he and Nikitin would review the facts of the case – the method of assassination, the inscriptions on the scrolls of paper inserted into the mouths, the identities of the victims. What linked them? And what had they done to deserve such a baroque demise?

But that was tomorrow.

Rossel yawned.

He went to the window of Comrade Drugov's apartment and drew back the curtain an inch with his crooked left forefinger.

His neighbours, it turned out, were the glorious dead. He could see little besides the pinprick lights of passing vehicles, but out there, behind a screen of young trees, was the Piskaryovskoye Memorial Cemetery. Almost six hundred thousand of those who had perished in the Leningrad siege lay at peace in 180 mass pits. Half the city was there – an army of soldiers, policemen, firemen, nurses, teachers, students, grandparents, mothers, fathers, children . . . For a moment, Rossel felt as if all it might take was one blast of the horn on Judgment Day for them to march en masse towards him.

He was tired, but sleep felt a long way off. He turned around and surveyed his new home. It was, when compared to the conditions of 105th Kilometre, palatial.

But there are ghosts here, too . . .

They stared back at him from silver frames, arranged on top of a Steinway piano. Ivan Drugov and his family. In his position at the Museum of the Defence of Leningrad, Drugov was – or had been until recently – in charge of a large complex near the river, just to the east of the Field of Mars and only a short distance from Rossel's old militia station. The museum featured gas masks and ration cards, photographs of heroic resistance, burnt-out Nazi tanks. It had opened shortly after the end of the war. What would happen now that its director was in chains, he could not tell.

In the main photograph on the piano – surrounded by his wife, young son and daughters – Drugov was dark and thin-faced, with sharp, penetrating eyes. An academic who had done very well for himself, he had about him the purposeful air of a confident Soviet bureaucrat; of someone whose life had taken a turn for the better after the revolution. Now, it seemed, Fate had taken it in a different direction – the most likely destination for the Drugovs would be a cattle train like the one that had taken Rossel to Siberia, months earlier. And then a GULAG facility.

Next to the picture of the Drugov family was one of the older daughter, a girl of perhaps seventeen, holding a violin in one hand and the certificate of her graduation from

Special Music School No 5 in the other. She was pretty, with long dark hair tied in a pigtail and a serious expression – one that suggested intellectual curiosity.

Everything was just as it must have been moments before the family had heard that knock on the door. A half-completed jigsaw of the Battleship Potemkin was lying on a glass coffee table; a book, Gogol's *Dead Souls,* was open and face-down, balancing on the arm of red velvet chaise longue. A copy of *Sovetskaya Zhenshchina* magazine with a picture of the actress Lyubov Orlova on the cover lay on a leather footstool, next to a hand-crocheted white cushion that had tumbled to the floor. On a dining table in the corner of the room, cutlery and plates has been set for five people. On the stove in the kitchen was a congealing pan of *solyanka,* a sour beef stew.

Nikitin had, it seemed, brought him back from the dead only to make him captain of a ghost ship.

The main bedroom was small but comfortable, with a matching oak dresser, chair and bed. On the dresser were more framed family photographs – the Drugovs laughing and smiling on a beach in a Black Sea resort; the boy in front of the Winter Palace in a white shirt and flowing red necktie, the uniform of the Young Pioneers; and the girl, looking less serious this time, stroking a large black cat. There was something about her, in the intensity of her gaze, that reminded him of his sister, Galya. Even though she had been missing for half his life.

Where was the cat?

The thought struck him that, somewhere in the city, an MGB man was coming through the door of his own apartment holding out a new pet. A gift for his excited children.

On the bed was a dark jacket and trousers, chosen by someone who had been told Rossel was tall, and a white shirt, chosen by someone who had been told he was enormous.

Something else, too. A pistol. An ageing Nagant with a cut-down barrel that hinted at past use as an assassination weapon. He assumed it had come from Nikitin and he was disgusted. But he'd rather have it than be unarmed.

Beneath the bed was a scuffed pair of shoes. At least they fitted.

Every night for almost a year, Rossel had slept in his bunk in one camp or another, dreaming of a bed like the one that belonged to the Drugovs. He yawned again, the desire to sleep finally building, and pulled off his grubby coat. As he moved towards the bed, he caught the eye of the Drugovs in another family photograph: father in uniform, fish-scaled with medals, and everyone else in their best clothes. Staring at him, sombre, judgmental and mute.

Rossel went around the room, turning every photograph down on its face, before collapsing onto the bed.

As he closed his eyes, he thought of the message the murderer had left on the body.

'Oh gentle darkness, oh sacred and sweet nocturnal hours . . .'

Koshchei, he suspected, would probably like this place.

14

Rossel had slept until midday – hours of uninterrupted, dreamless sleep for the first time since his arrest – before Nikitin had turned up and started banging on the door. Somehow, it had only made him feel even more exhausted.

'We haven't got much time, comrade. But you look like you need feeding up. I was going to take you to a state-run canteen near the Mining University,' said Nikitin. 'I figured, after the fine dining options available in our glorious corrective labour camp system, even their shitty meat patties would taste like the caviar they serve to the Party bigwigs at the Hotel Astoria. But then I remembered this Georgian place.'

They left Nikitin's car on Kronverkskiy Prospect and walked north, leaving the Peter and Paul Fortress and the Neva River behind them.

This part of the city was just out of his old territory as a militia officer. Like most Leningraders, he had been here dozens of times. After Igarka, returning felt like putting on an old suit. Leningrad could present a face as cold and impersonal as a diamond. Its heart beat in its alleyways, around corners, in secret places you had to know about . . . But, if you knew where to go, you would be seduced. Its outside, however, was prim, respectable.

Whereas the GULAG locked you in, Leningrad shut you out. Unless you were in the know.

Down a side street or three, and Nikitin led them into a courtyard full of well-polished cars. Above an ordinary wooden door was a line of swirling characters: Georgian script, which Rossel couldn't read.

'I know Tamara, the woman who runs this place,' said Nikitin, levering open the door. 'You don't look like one of her regulars and you'll probably scare the other diners but she owes me a favour. Levon, her husband, was a stubborn man. Too stubborn. See that?' He pointed at the letters, stencilled in bright red paint above the door. 'Shemome-chama, it says. Roughly translates as "still eating even when you're full". Which I'm confident you'll be doing shortly, Comrade Rossel.'

The staircase was rickety with a listing steel banister. Nothing hinted at the presence of a restaurant until the second floor, where there were more red Georgian letters on the wall.

'I used to eat here with my wife, sometimes the rest of the family.'

Nikitin's face coloured slightly. The major, Rossel thought, was not by nature one of life's romantic souls. But he was devoted to his wife and children.

'Even my mother would concede defeat when it came to Tamara's cooking,' said Nikitin, resuming his composure. He knocked on the door.

'During the siege, after a year of nothing in their bellies, the neighbours would paint over the sign. They couldn't stand walking past it any more. Levon would paint it back again. They'd paint over, he'd paint it back. Once they take your name, he told Tamara, there's nothing left to take.'

'A man of principle. I like your story,' said Rossel. 'In the camps, men of principle are thin on the ground.'

You'd fit in there well, you *mudak,* he thought.

'And then one day a neighbour broke in and slit his throat,' said the major.

Nikitin's grimace seemed to suggest that Levon's fate was a suitable end for any man stupid enough to stand up for a principle that was not to be found in the works of Marx, Lenin or Stalin.

The door half opened. Tamara was small and plump. She had a grin that suggested it didn't come easily but it materialised for Nikitin. Heat, steam and the aroma of spices rushed out into the cold air and made Rossel's head spin.

'I was still an MGB officer then. So, I found out who the killer was and took him into the Bolshoi Dom,' added Nikitin over his shoulder as the door opened the rest of the way and they walked into a room draped in red velvet. 'Sadly, he expired before he was able to answer all of my questions. Tamara assures me that no one has complained about the sign since.'

*

After months of guarding a mouthful of rotten fish in a bowl of warm water from the skeleton in the next bunk, Shemomechama dazzled.

In comparison to his labour camp, even a proletarian *stolovaya* would have seemed opulent. But *this* establishment – its unexpected majesty; its glittering clientele, all suits and gowns; and its tall thin glasses filled with *Sovetskoye Sham-panskoye* . . .

The restaurant, stuffed full of the elite and their syco-phants, seemed to extend for a hundred metres in every direc-tion. Rossel wasn't sure he could even see the far walls; there was too much food, too much intrigue, too much privilege in the way. He hoped he still had a flea or two, and that the fleas would transfer themselves to others present. And multiply.

Some of the other diners had had the same thought. They were staring at him, a skeleton in a new suit. And, to judge by the looks he was getting, they were contemplating having him thrown out.

But the uniform of the man guiding him to a banquette in the far corner was enough to make even Party members think twice. Military, but with something extra, something unfamiliar. That and the scarred face, boxer's shoulders and Tokarev pistol at his waist.

Tamara fussed around them, placing a bowl of flatbreads on the table and filling two glasses to the brim with Georgian wine. The table was partially hidden by a wooden screen.

'*Lobio* – a big bowl. *Kupati*, I never leave without trying your wondrous spicy *kupati*, Tamara.'

Rossel stopped listening to Nikitin's recitation of Geor-gian culinary splendours and reached for the bread, the two remaining fingers of his left hand closing on their target. He brought it to his nose, brushed it against his lips. The first bite was indescribable. Rossel tore into the remain-der, gnawing at it, turning his head away from the room in embarrassment, but unable to stop.

'You look like the monk who just left the monastery and wandered into a *bardak*,' said Nikitin, laughing.

Rossel gulped down the last morsel and recovered some semblance of self-control.

Nikitin wasn't looking. Instead, he was unscrewing the base of one of two candle-style bulbs attached to the wall. The light went out as he removed the whole fitting. Putting a finger to his lips, the major peered inside. He pulled out a small metal cylinder attached to a wire. A blade appeared in one hand and Nikitin cut the wire, pocketing the cylinder. He repeated the process with the other fitting but found nothing. He met Rossel's gaze.

'Microphones,' he said. 'Every table, broadcasting all their petty intrigues and casual misdemeanours – backhanders, fiddling the quotas, siphoning off factory stores for the black market. Affairs. Jumping the queue for a car or a fridge.'

'Are these customers particularly dumb?' asked Rossel.

'There's always one really stupid one,' said Nikitin, 'boasting to a lover or thanking a business partner for something they got *po blatu*.' *Blat* was the word for getting your hands on something through connections. A Thieves' word, it had infiltrated everyday Soviet life.

Nikitin raised his glass.

'And after half a bottle of vodka everyone else catches up.'

*

Tamara reappeared, laden with steaming dishes.

Rossel peered around the screen and stared at the nearby tables, marvelling at the casual way in which the clientele were consuming the finest caviar, the most succulent smoked fish, the most expensive champagne.

'I was a dead man walking,' said Nikitin.

Rossel looked back at the major, who was using a flat-bread to scoop up a thick, creamy sauce. There was a pause as he manoeuvered it into his jaws.

'Like I told you in the camp,' Nikitin added, still chewing, 'Beria's extra-curricular activities had not gone unnoticed. Especially the girls. Especially the younger ones.'

Rossel leaned forward and lowered his voice.

'Perhaps that's why the minister used to give them flowers afterwards. So he found it easier to live with himself.'

Nikitin shrugged. 'Fuck your mother, this stew is good.'

He dug deeper into the sauce with one hand, fumbling for a napkin with the other.

'After our last little adventure, I was the toast of the entire Politburo,' the major mumbled between mouthfuls.

'Last little adventure' was an understatement. Beria's predilection for girls, some of them very young, was only one of the minister's secrets that Rossel had investigated as a militia officer. Secrets that when uncovered might have been fatal to almost anyone else.

But Beria was indestructible. And vengeful.

'Malenkov's people loved me,' continued Nikitin. 'So did Kaganovich's. And Molotov's. But they were like women – all over me one minute, giving me the cold shoulder the next. From what I hear, right now it's civil war in the Politburo. No one knows who's in favour and who's out in the cold, whose coat is hanging on a rusty nail. Something's even brewing against Beria. Every delegation that came to see me was brandishing a new list of his possible victims. Knives are being sharpened for that bastard. Not before time.'

As Nikitin talked on, Rossel closed his eyes and inhaled. The smell of the spices, the walnut sauce, the melting cheese . . . he thought he might be delirious. The scent of the Georgian wine alone was enough to intoxicate him. Nikitin was piling into it.

'For a month I was the most important person in Minister Malenkov's entire universe. My farts smelled like roses. Then . . .'

'Then?' said Rossel, opening his eyes.

'The job I was promised as Malenkov's personal bodyguard turned out to be a job as a nightwatchman at Hospital 37 down in Kupchino. Kupchino, fuck your mother. I was a sitting duck. Have some *lobio*, it's delicious.'

The major spooned some of the bean stew into Rossel's bowl.

Rossel watched, mesmerised, as Tamara arrived with more dishes and lowered a skewer of lamb onto his plate. Trails of fat glistened amid the nut-brown meat. He had never seen peppers in so many colours, or smelled so many fragrances. There was more meat on that one skewer than a zek would get in three months in Igarka.

He grabbed the skewer.

Nikitin sucked at his fingers.

'One night a couple of Black Ravens roll up at the hospital and half a dozen blue-hats get out.' He smiled. 'Not easy to hide a handsome face like this –' he jabbed a greasy thumb at the scarred side of his face – 'I had to wrap my head in bandages, tape a drip to my arm and climb into a bed in the Burns Unit. In the morning I got out of there. But now I had no job and it was only a matter of time before they hunted me down.'

Yet another course arrived. Nikitin was right about the food, especially the *kupati*.

Wondrous . . .

But the major pushed the plates to the side of the table. 'Enough of eating,' he said. 'Let's talk about murder.'

*

Nikitin stood up and repositioned the screen so their table was almost entirely invisible to the rest of the room.

'Do you remember a film called *The Mandrake*? Before the war – thirty-seven or thirty-eight?'

Rossel nodded.

'A Boris Tarkovsky film. Everyone went to see it,' he said. Tarkovsky was a commanding actor with legions of female admirers. But a supposedly whimsical comedy a few years back had not done his reputation any favours. And, if the rumours were true, vodka had left its mark.

'You're right, everyone did,' said Nikitin. 'They say Stalin himself loved it – perhaps even more than *Volga-Volga*. And it appears that our killer, Koshchei the Immortal, is a fan, too.'

He held the chicken wing between his hands and picked the bits of skin off it with his teeth. He dropped the bones onto a plate and washed his hands in a finger bowl.

'*The Mandrake* – that's where the words in the victims' mouths are from,' the major continued, raising a glistening finger. 'Not our Soviet film. The play by Machiavelli, on which the film was based. That's why they're in Italian.'

'How did you work that out?'

'I asked a woman in the Defence Ministry who was a liaison officer with the Communists in Italy for a few months after the war. Nina recognised it straightaway.

After the film did so well, the New Moscow publishing house brought out an updated version of the play and asked Tarkovsky to write the foreword. Nina swoons over Boris. Buys everything he touches. So . . .'

'If it's no great mystery, then why do you need me?' said Rossel. 'It sounds like the Main Intelligence Department, or whatever you call yourselves . . .'

'Directorate.'

'. . . has it covered. Thanks for the dinner, but . . .'

The two men glared at each other and for a moment, angry though he was, Rossel could remember what it was like to have those dark, half-hooded eyes fixed on you.

But this isn't a cell. I'm not at your mercy now.

Nikitin picked up a napkin and gave his hands and mouth a thorough wipe. He reached into his leather case and took out a set of photographs, pushed some of the empty plates to one side and spread them on the table.

There were six in all. Two featured seated men: both with two neat shots to the right temple, though the other side would be less neat. The next pair of images were close-ups of the jaws of the deceased. Their tongues had been cut out and a rolled-up piece of paper had been inserted part-way into each man's throat. The final photographs were of the strips of paper, unfurled so the writing could be read.

'Two men with their tongues cut out. But each sings a silent song,' said Rossel.

Nikitin nodded.

'Like I told you in the labour camp, we know for certain that both were in the same platoon as Sergeant Grachev, who broke out of his camp. And listen to what the lines in Italian mean . . .'

'I don't get it,' Rossel broke in. 'You don't bring a zek back from those frozen wastelands to help you investigate. Not when you can whistle and have a dozen GRU officers at your command, plus all the Machiavelli scholars in the Soviet Union. You don't need me, so why—'

Nikitin slammed a fist down on the table hard enough to make the cutlery jump.

The major breathed in and out, calming himself.

'You remember I have a wife, a son? And a daughter, Rossel?' he said.

Rossel looked back at him.

'Well, right now I have one person, the Defence Minister, standing between *them* and the cells and interrogators of the Bolshoi Dom. General Pletnev is an impatient man. War heroes are being killed. He wants results in this case, and fast. I have Beria's hand on one shoulder and Pletnev's on the other.'

Nikitin the family man. Isn't that sweet?

'I need your help,' Nikitin said, looking like it hurt to prise the words out of his mouth. 'But I can offer you something in return. I can ensure you never have to go back to Igarka.'

There was a distraction across the restaurant, at the entrance. Unseen by them a militia officer, a youngster, followed Tamara's finger until he spotted Rossel's table and came hurrying over.

'I need an investigator: a proper one, a gundog, someone like you who won't let go,' said Nikitin. 'You did it last time, Rossel. When the only way out was to find the killer, you found the killer. I'm ex-MGB, I'm tainted within the GRU. My new brother officers are going to watch me drown and not lift a finger to help me.'

The young policeman came round the screen and threw an ungainly salute.

'Major Nikitin? I was told I would find you here.'

'Yes.'

He moved closer.

'There's been another one.'

15

All along Kamennoostrovsky Avenue was a line of banners, either flowing from the tops of the lampposts or draped down the fronts of the buildings facing the street. Stalin was the most prominent person to be shown, but he was accompanied by the senior members of his Kremlin court – Beria, Malenkov, Khrushchev, Kaganovich, Voroshilov, Bulganin, Pletnev . . . Beneath them all came the slogans and proclamations: *Leningrad's Rebirth – a new future for the children of the Hero City; All-Soviet Party Congress November 1952; Long Live Our Victorious Nation!; Long Live our Dear Stalin!*

Rossel, Nikitin and the young militia officer halted at the gardens that lay before the neoclassical pillars guarding the entrance to Lenfilm. Along with Mosfilm, it was one of the Soviet Union's major film studios.

A stray dog, sheltering from the wind that was whipping the snow into flurries all along the avenue, had pulled an old boot under a bush and was licking at it. Rossel reached into his pocket. Without Nikitin seeing, he had wrapped some *kupati* inside a napkin and taken it from the restaurant.

Rossel tossed the sausage onto the ground and the animal pounced on it. He reached down and patted its head.

'This way, Rossel,' said Nikitin.

The three men strode up to the grand portico of the studio. Nikitin took off his fur hat as he fumbled for his ID to show to the policeman guarding the door.

'Welcome to the land of make-believe,' he said to Rossel, extending an arm to allow him in.

Rossel looked over his shoulder at the parade of Party leaders and slogans. *All Hail the Triumph of Communism and the Freedom of the Peoples of the World . . .*

'I thought I was already living in it,' he said.

*

Two huge stage lights magnified the dead man's shadow against a white backdrop, creating the impression they were in the presence of a sleeping giant.

The corpse was about thirty years old, his long hair already flecked with grey. A big man, he was propped up in the middle of a medieval-style set on huge golden throne: itself a stage prop for yet another film of Ivan the Terrible's life, this time a musical.

His head lolled backwards, the mouth open. Two bullet holes were clearly visible in the right temple.

A militia captain saw Nikitin and saluted smartly. The major nodded back.

'Has the MGB been here?' he said.

'Not yet, Comrade Major.'

'Good. You did well in sending young Titov here. There will be compensation.'

'Thank you, Comrade Major. But *they* won't be long, they have . . .'

The captain stopped and swallowed. It was wiser not to comment on the activities of the MGB.

Nikitin patted him on the shoulder.

'Then we'd better get a move on.'

This was a cramped corner of the Lenfilm studios. The throne left little room for anything else. Rossel kept still, his shoulder blades pressing into what felt like a flimsy plasterboard screen, while a militia photographer bustled round the corpse. Two other policemen, looking bored, stood to one side, occasionally peering down the twisting corridor that had brought them here. He didn't recognise any of them, including the captain, and was relieved about that. On the other side of the throne, wedged between the stage lights, was smaller and older man – dressed in worker's overalls, fidgeting and looking pale: a props man, who had discovered the body.

The militia captain's thin ginger moustache did not suit him well, though it did distract a little from his bulging eyes and permanent air of anxiety. At least he was doing his job: making notes, ordering the photographer to take certain shots, going over the facts. The Lenfilm props man had found the body not long after filming and other technical work had finished for the day. He had stayed on to fix a problem they'd been having with Ivan's crown – the glue on the costume jewellery kept drying out in the lights and every time the actor moved his head an emerald or a ruby dropped off. Then he had remembered the old props for a long-forgotten film about some tsar or other and come looking for them in the maze of storerooms and mini studios.

'And encountered this jolly scene,' concluded the captain, still flipping through his notebook.

'Do we know who this is?' said Nikitin, poking the corpse with a finger. 'He's a fat bastard – must weigh a hundred kilos.'

The captain nodded. 'The props man, Comrade Petrov here, knew him. Says he has a girlfriend, a bit-part actress who is working on the film. We'll pull his work file from the administrative office but I'm sure his colleague will tell you more.'

'Akimov.' Props man Petrov found his voice. 'Vyacheslav Semyonovich Akimov. Usually an electrician and general odd-jobs man.'

Rossel took out a *papirosa* and lit it.

'Usually?' he said.

He heard Nikitin grunt in satisfaction as he asked the question. A crime scene, Rossel realised, was something the major had known he would not be able to resist.

Petrov grimaced, revealing a top row of crooked teeth. 'They gave him a part in the Ivan the Terrible musical drama. Some sort of nobleman. The actor was ill and they're on a tight schedule. A non-speaking part. All he had to do was march about in fancy clothes and mime one line of a song – and three of the words were *Ivan, Ivan, Ivan* – and then get executed by the tsar. It's that scene they do in every film and play about Ivan. The bit about Boyar Fyodorov. You know – where Ivan has Fyodorov dressed in his own robes before he has him done in. But Akimov was awful. Seventeen takes and he still hadn't done it right. The director was going crazy.'

Rossel moved closer to the corpse and looked into Akimov's wide, staring eyes.

'Looks like take eighteen isn't going too well, either,' he said.

120

'King for a day,' said the captain. 'Poor bastard, not even that.'

Rossel and Nikitin peered into Akimov's mouth.

'There it is,' said Nikitin. He inserted a finger into the dead man's jaw and flicked at the cheek, as if afraid the victim might wake up and bite. At the fourth or fifth attempt, he got what he was after: a tiny roll of paper with words on it.

Nikitin pocketed it.

'The tongue's intact,' said Rossel, straightening. 'Not cut out like the first two.'

'Maybe the killer ran out of time. Heard our man Petrov coming,' Nikitin said.

Rossel took a draw on his cigarette.

'Comrade Petrov,' he said, 'one more thing. Was Comrade Akimov here in the army during the Great Patriotic War?'

Petrov nodded. 'He signed up from the start, made it all the way through. He was proud of it. Wore his medals on Army and Navy Day.'

'All the way to Berlin, correct? With the 8th Guards?'

'Yes.' Petrov looked surprised. 'Did you know him?'

Rossel shook his head.

The two junior militia officers stirred into life like they knew trouble was coming.

'Comrade captain,' one said. 'It's the blue-hats.' MGB officers wore distinctive blue-trimmed caps. 'They're coming.'

Nikitin turned to Rossel.

'Time to go,' he said.

16

Nikitin swore at his car as the ignition rattled and died. On the fourth attempt the engine came to life and they set off, heading north, weaving through the streets until Nikitin turned the steering wheel to the right and came to a halt in a quiet courtyard.

'Koshchei the Immortal,' Nikitin said. 'No one sees him kill, no one sees him come or go, no one sees him dump the bodies of his victims. Leningrad talks of nothing else. Even stranger, the stories are in the papers.'

Rossel looked at him in surprise.

'The papers?'

As far as the Soviet press was concerned, crime did not exist.

'Not any more,' said Nikitin. 'But it was, and for almost a week.'

No wonder Koshchei has everybody's attention.

'As a child,' Rossel said, 'my grandmother would tell me the old tales of Koshchei. How he would hide his heart inside a box, or an egg, or a bird.' He tapped his chest. 'Back then, I sometimes used to wonder if he was hiding inside me.'

The major fumbled in his pocket and pulled out the scrap of paper.

O dolce notte, o sante
ore notturne e quete,
ch'i disïosi amanti accompagnate . . .

'Mean anything to you?'

The hand was precise, each letter the same size as the one before it.

'*O dolce notte* – Oh sweet night – and then something about peaceful nights,' said Rossel.

Nikitin grunted. 'I thought you said you knew Italian?'

'Any classically trained musician knows a little. Though perhaps not enough to translate poetic messages left in the mouths of murder victims.'

'What else can you make out?'

'I don't know – something about lovers.'

'Not much love on display for Comrade Akimov,' said Nikitin.

'What do you know about Machiavelli?' asked Rossel.

Nikitin thought for a moment.

'Not much. He wrote the handbook for plotters and schemers. *The Prince.* You won't find it in the House of Books, but there must be more than a few members of the Central Committee who like to stay up late at night thumbing its pages.'

Survival at the very top of the Party must take more cunning and more emotional energy than I will ever possess, thought Rossel.

'Have you still got the translated copies of the other two?' he asked.

Nikitin reached into his coat and pulled out two pieces of paper. Rossel took them and read:

That ignorance is bliss is widely known;
How bless'd the imbecile is with head of bone!
He thirsts not after gold, nor aches for pow'r,
Believes what he is told, hour after hour.

The second had a similar feel. Trickery, and a certain smugness.

How gentle is deception
When carried to fruition as intended.
For it defies perception.

'How did you get your hands on them?' said Rossel.

'I have kept up my contacts in the militia,' Nikitin replied. 'Every other officer is informing for someone. MGB agents took the scrolls from the first two crime scenes – but not before the militia had photographed them.'

They sat for a few moments in silence.

An educated killer. One who appeared to have a grudge against a very particular group of war veterans. And who enjoyed taunting the authorities and investigating officers with enigmatic references to deception.

'I could spend ten years going back through the records at my old militia station and I still wouldn't pull out anything that would link a man to a crime like this,' said Rossel. 'For a start, the killer's actions seem deranged – and yet his handwriting is very controlled and precise.'

Nikitin started the car again.

'I remember Tarkovsky in the film of *The Mandrake*,' he said. 'He was Callimaco. A slimy toad who kept trying to shag some old bastard's wife. I had no idea it was based on a Machiavelli play, though. Who did?'

Rossel sat back in his seat and closed his eyes.

When he opened them again Nikitin was almost smiling.

'That's what I need to see more of, Gundog,' the major said. 'You, thinking hard. Being a detective.'

17

Akimov lay pale and naked on the slab: the white flesh of his stomach and chest covered with cigarette burns and plier marks; a hole in the middle of his right thigh. Rossel looked away and reached for the tobacco inside his coat pocket. His years as a militia officer had done little to improve his appetite for the still numbing sight of a man who only yesterday had lived and breathed as he did. Now just an inert object lying on an autopsy table.

Besides, most corpses were straightforward cases. Drunken knife fights; crimes of passion; the winter cold claiming another person 'without a defined place of residence'; the loser of a dispute among the Thieves. Most of Leningrad's ordinary dead did not call for much detective work. And it was not worth asking about those who fell prey to the attentions of the MGB. Those inquiries had already been made, the conclusions already drawn.

In his previous career as an officer in the militia, only one set of victims – a quintet of dead bodies left lying in the snow – had called for a prolonged investigation. The victims had been left as bait. Rossel had taken it.

And look where it got me.

'Comrade Senior Lieutenant Rossel, I was hoping I might bump into you again. You look . . .'

Dr Maxim Bondar took a step back.

'Well, I'll be honest, only a touch better than poor Comrade Akimov over there. You need to find a wife quickly, comrade. A nice fat Ukrainian girl who will fill your stomach with *kotletki* and *borshch* and *salo*.'

Dr Bondar was balding, middle-aged, and as thin as his own scalpel. The pathologist's guttural accent gave away his Kievan origins. It was rumoured that Dr Bondar was able to put his access to reliable refrigeration to unintended but lucrative uses. One rumour in particular said that he was considered a good man to store black-market beluga for those who could get it but didn't want to take the risk of storing it on their own premises. The nickname *Ikra*, or Maksim Caviar, had stuck. He didn't seem to mind.

'Not the *salo* you get here – that's dog fat, or horse if you're lucky. You want the real stuff. And a soup cooked by a real Kievan temptress who will put in plenty of marrow bone and then ladle in the cream.'

Dr Bondar's morgue was within The Crosses: a prison Rossel had been in several times as a militia officer and once as an inmate. The latter stay, albeit brief, had not been pleasant. The regime in The Crosses was notorious.

The morgue was concrete almost from floor to ceiling, save for a few white tiles that were clinging on like barnacles. A black hose was coiled in a corner and it was wet underfoot.

Akimov had been moved here during the night from the Lenfilm studios. Now that they got to look at him in detail, they could see that his final moments had not been pleasant ones.

Rossel blew out some smoke.

'It's not currently "lieutenant", Maksim,' said Rossel. 'Comrade will have to do. But it's good to see you.'

'Not lieutenant? I don't . . .'

The pathologist stopped himself. He pursed his lips; looked from Rossel to Nikitin, and back again.

'You have been away, Comrade Rossel?' he said. 'To take a little air, perhaps, or the waters of Mineralnye Vody?'

'That's it, Maksim, exactly right. Lots and lots of bracing fresh air.'

Rossel gestured to Nikitin.

'This is Major Nikitin of the GRU. He's in charge.'

Dr Bondar gave Nikitin a look.

'In charge? Right, I see. It's just that . . .'

'Yes?' said Nikitin.

The pathologist cleared his throat. His eyes darted between his two visitors, hoping for sympathy from at least one of them.

'The MGB have also taken a strong interest in my recent cases. May I assume you are coordinating with them?'

'You can assume what you like, comrade,' barked Nikitin. 'These murders also lie within the provenance of military intelligence. Defence Minister General Pletnev strongly suspects that such depravities could only be the work of enemy agents or their Fifth Columnist allies. Isn't it obvious to you that no Soviet citizen could have committed such terrible crimes without the help of outside collaborators? And this man was a decorated veteran of the glorious Red Army. His fate shames us all.'

Dr Bondar pulled a handkerchief out of his coat pocket, blew his nose, and stood to attention.

'Obvious, yes, Comrade Major. I would be honoured to help General Pletnev in any way I can, no matter how small. As would any citizen who knows the glorious story of The Hero of the Heights. To storm those Fascist positions on the Seelow Heights when all seemed lost was an act of extraordinary bravery. Those who were there say it changed the course of history . . .'

As he walked around the body, Dr Bondar talked on – growing more and more effusive in his praise of the general. Much in the manner, Rossel thought, of a man who is talking to a couple of investigating officers while his mortuary fridges are filled with caviar.

*

Dr Bondar extended a hand towards the body as if introducing it to dinner guests. He was ten minutes into his examination.

'Fairly clearly, our man Akimov has been tortured and then killed with two pistol shots to the head. Let's assume that this is the work of a single killer. The tongue was probably cut after death.'

'Why do you say that?' asked Nikitin.

'Well, this is a big, powerful man and doing so while he was alive would not have been easy.'

'Pair of forceps,' said the major. 'Grab a hold of the bourgeois piece of shit, squeeze the cheeks and there you—'

Rossel cleared his throat.

'You must have such fond memories of the Bolshoi Dom, Comrade Major,' he said.

129

'To be certain,' said Dr Bondar, 'one would have to find the rest of the tongue.'

Rossel nodded. 'Please, continue.'

'Both shots to the temple were fired at point-blank range with a Mauser C96,' said the pathologist.

'A Mauser – a German pistol?' said Rossel.

'Initially, yes. But these days it is a mass-produced weapon that has been used in numerous countries for decades. The weapon could well be of foreign origin, but that does not tell one much about the citizenship of the assassin. It was fitted with a silencer. It fires 7.63 by 25 millimetre bullets – the basis for our own Tokarev 7.62 millimetre rounds, as it happens.'

'How do you know it was a Mauser? Did the militia or the MGB find anything else apart from the bullets?' said Rossel.

Dr Bondar strutted over to a metal cabinet, opened the door and pulled out a large pistol with a long barrel and a bulbous grip. With its large box magazine in front of the trigger, it looked almost too big for a holster.

'This was stuck down Comrade Akimov's trousers,' he said.

Nikitin's face darkened.

'This bastard Koshchei is taking the piss out of us,' he said.

'Leaves the gun but takes the tongue,' said Dr Bondar.

Rossel took a step towards the body. 'Do you know when this one was killed, Maksim?'

'Estimated time of death for this one I have at a little more than twenty-four hours ago. So, given that it is only eight a.m. now, that would be early in the morning yesterday. That is based on both the significant continued degree of rigor, which can indicate that the corpse was moved after death, and loss of temperature of the body.'

Dr Bondar picked up a thermometer as if to emphasise his point. Rossel didn't like to think too hard about where the pathologist had last put it.

Nikitin tapped a finger on the back of a chair with impatience.

'Listen, Comrade Caviar, we haven't got all day. Are the injuries to Akimov here the same as those on the other two? Katz and Samosud? Or not?'

The pathologist coloured a little. Then shook his head.

'Not quite. All three suffered silenced pistol shots to the head. All three were tortured with a knife. But Comrade Akimov here also had a leg wound. Caused by a round fired from long range, which entered his thigh at an angle, made a mess of the femur and ended up embedded in the kneecap, and *that* will have stung. A 7.62 by 54 millimetre round, which indicates a Mosin–Nagant 1891/30. Which, as I'm sure you know, is a sniper's rifle.'

Rossel thought back to the last time he'd seen a Mosin–Nagant fired in anger. It had been by a Russian sniper who had lain for days in a half-dried slick of mud as he picked off Wehrmacht soldiers in the retreat that marked the end of the Volkhov Front, a breakout campaign to lift the Siege of Leningrad. June 1942. A failure. A slaughter. But the sniper had done his best to even up the score.

'A sniper likes a distance kill,' said Rossel. 'This is different. Eye to eye, in their faces.'

'And why not the same wound on the others?' said Nikitin.

Rossel shrugged. 'Akimov needed slowing down?'

Nikitin began to button up his coat.

'Anything else for us, Comrade Dr Bondar?'

The pathologist shook his head and picked up a small saw.

'Not yet, Major. But give me a little time. Comrade Caviar here is never happier than when he's got his nose to the bone, so to speak – elbow-deep in pancreas, liver and kidneys.'

*

On the other side of the road, a small gathering of women huddled together, anonymous in the darkness of the early winter morning. They gazed up at the barred windows of The Crosses: hoping for a wave, a message, a sign of life from loved ones. Not far behind them, ice floes creaked and clattered their way along the Neva.

'Snipers are supposed to be our fucking heroes,' said Nikitin as he strode along the pavement, heading for the Finland Station where he had left his Pobeda.

'They would have to hide it,' said Rossel. 'The rifle, I mean. Wrap it up in something and pass it off as, I don't know, a shovel or a drill or some sort of construction tool. Something like that. A Mosin–Nagant is not a short weapon.'

Nikitin nodded.

'Lenfilm is a mix of wide open spaces and cramped rooms barely bigger than cupboards,' he said. 'A sniper could hide but not get a clear shot, or get a clear shot and be seen by everyone.'

So Akimov had been brought down somewhere else, thought Rossel. Then hidden so that he could be tortured, which he would not have endured in silence. And then moved to Lenfilm and dumped so that his body would be found.

All this in the middle of Leningrad.

No wonder there was talk of a malevolent, supernatural and above all invisible killer on the loose.

18

One of the streetlights in front of the Museum of Atheism and Religion was faulty, blinking on and off as if sending an urgent message in Morse code to some watchful deity. The huge curve of neoclassical pillars that stood in front of what had been Kazan Cathedral, before the Bolsheviks gave the building a new purpose, gaped before them like the jaws of some huge beast.

As they walked past the bronze statues of General Kutuzov and Field Marshal Barclay de Tolly – heroes of Russia's 1812 war with Napoleon – the streetlight buzzed, burned brighter and went out.

Nikitin tutted.

'Perhaps we should say a prayer, Rossel?'

'To whom?'

'Our Lady of Kazan, of course. They say General Kutuzov came here and did the same before he defeated Napoleon.'

'"The struggle against religion is the struggle for socialism." When I was in the League of Militant Godless that was our mantra – the only prayer we knew.'

They stopped in front of the museum's huge bronze doors. A lamp above the door cast the major's scarred face with its missing eye into a thin, blue-tinged light.

'I got the call this morning to say he wanted to see us. Make sure you tell General Pletnev you were in the League, Rossel. Restoring their fortunes to the way things were before the war is his life's work.'

*

The League of Militant Godless had millions of members and thousands of offices all across the Soviet Union. Its aim was simple: to seek out and destroy religious belief in all its manifestations – Russian Orthodoxy, Islam, Judaism – and replace it with a zealous Marxist purity. Churches, mosques and synagogues had been closed; many, like the Kazan Cathedral in the centre of Leningrad, turned into anti-religious museums.

As Nikitin led Rossel into what was now the Museum of Atheism, the major glanced at his watch.

The old nave of the former cathedral was massive. More than fifty pillars lined its aisle and, high above, the dome was modelled on St Peter's in Rome. Rossel craned his neck to look even as Nikitin hurried him along. Presumably, it had been created to evoke the hope of Heaven among the faithful. Instead, he thought, its epic scale suggested a paradise that remained out of reach.

Three enormous portraits of Marx, Lenin and Stalin – a Holy Trinity of Bolshevism – now stood on the altar in place of the some of the main ikons and wall paintings. Under Marx was an inscription from his writings: 'Religion is the sigh of the oppressed creature, the heart of a heartless world, and the soul of soulless conditions.'

135

Like the altar, the interior of the building had been stripped of most of its religious artefacts. Only a few saints remained, painted high up on the walls; mute witnesses to the complete destruction of the ideology that had sanctified them. An empty space marked only by rusted brackets was the place where the ikon of Our Lady of Kazan, to which General Kutuzov had prayed before his ultimate victory over the French, had once looked down upon the faithful. The Holy Virgin had been unable to perform the same miracle for the Legions of the Lord in the face of the forces of Lenin.

It was a working day and most people were at an office, factory or school. Wandering among the pillars and exhibits were a few women with children in tow, two or three groups of respectful pensioners and a chattering line of about thirty children policed by two harassed teachers.

Although meant to detail the triumph of Marxism over the world's great religions, many of the exhibits seemed more suitable for a fairground peepshow. Chief among these was a waxwork displaying figures from the Spanish Inquisition – depraved nuns, sinister monks, swaggering conquistadores. Among them was the figure of Torquemada, the Grand Inquisitor, standing next to a rack upon which a hapless victim was being stretched. A hooded executioner was presenting Torquemada with a selection of torture instruments that included a two-pronged 'Heretics' Fork', which could impale the chin and breastbone simultaneously, prolonging the torment without ending the life of the blasphemer. In another glass case was a full-size effigy of Savonarola, the Florentine friar who had embarked on a campaign of religious zealotry to rid his home city of vice.

Nikitin led the way through a side door and down a dark staircase that was longer than it should have been. Overhead lighting revealed two small wooden chairs near the entrance to the sacristy: formerly the robing room for Orthodox priests, and now the headquarters of the Leningrad division of the League of Militant Godless.

'General Pletnev spends most of his time here,' said Nikitin. 'If not at the General Staff building in Palace Square, this is where you'll find him.'

*

After a few minutes' wait, a young GRU officer appeared out of nowhere, strutted towards them and pointed in the direction of the door to what had been the sacristy.

They entered a room covered in polished rosewood shelves – for storing priestly robes, or these days more likely the by-products of military bureaucracy. Among the heaped files were two pictures in simple wooden frames. One was Lenin. The other was of Marshal Zhukov, Pletnev's commanding officer during the war. It was Zhukov who had reassembled the various shattered components of the Red Army, just as the Motherland teetered on the brink of collapse, and hauled it to its feet; and it was Zhukov who had won the race to the ultimate prize: the capture of Berlin. Pletnev had been one of a select few to have accompanied Zhukov to the signing of the Instrument of Surrender at Karlshorst in May 1945. An honour beyond any medal the Kremlin could have bestowed on him.

But the Hero of the Heights had not become one of Stalin's favourite generals by dint of charm. Like Zhukov,

137

Pletnev had cleared minefields by sending *shtrafnye batal'ony* – punishment battalions – into them as human minesweepers. Like Zhukov, Pletnev had shelled areas of enemy territory that lay between his forces and his objectives, regardless of what stood on that territory. In the Great Patriotic War, life was the currency with which you bought victory. And only victory mattered.

The general watched as Rossel and Nikitin advanced to his desk. His head and face were shaved but not quite smooth, peppered with grey stubble. Pletnev was broad-shouldered and tall but to Rossel he still seemed smaller than he had anticipated. The man's legend was such that you expected to have to look skywards to meet him in the eye.

Grey pupils peered out from thick lids. The general held out a hand.

'Sit, comrades.'

On the desk was a file with Rossel's name on it.

'Where I sit, the archimandrite once did,' General Pletnev began. 'Where you sit, his priestly acolytes used to. In this very room, they conspired to pour poison into the minds of the people. As Marx tells us, man makes religion, religion does not make man. This sacristy was the inner sanctum of the most despicable bourgeois superstition of them all. Their factories did not produce radios or dresses or other such beguiling bourgeois trinkets, but something far more sinister – hope. A fake vision of another world, which prevented the workers from transforming this one.'

Pletnev's voice was soft, even gentle – a beguiling and sonorous tenor – where Rossel had expected a commanding bass. But there was a military precision to his diction.

A practised ability to marshal an argument into something that could not be contested.

'Now, thankfully, the citizens of Leningrad understand, exactly as I do, that Heaven only exists at the end of the next Five-Year Plan.'

The general picked up Rossel's file.

'When I was told you were working with the major, I asked for your file. Are you a superstitious man, Comrade Rossel?'

Rossel's left hand moved towards his chest of its own accord. He let it drop again.

'Not especially, Comrade General,' he said.

Pletnev turned a page.

'And yet. During your time as a senior lieutenant in the militia at Station 17 on Vosstaniya Street, there was the image of a bird? A metal relief on the mantelpiece that you used to touch for luck.'

Rossel nodded, acknowledging Pletnev's eye for the kind of detail that could tell you more about a person's character than a hundred speeches, drunken or otherwise. He wondered who the informants in Station 17 had been. Not that it mattered any more.

'So far, it hasn't brought me much,' Rossel said.

Pletnev closed the file and tossed it back onto the table.

'You think not? Twice arrested by the secret services, twice interrogated in the cells of the Bolshoi Dom, yet still alive. A man who survived the sheer slaughter that was the Volkhov Front. A man who, when not at the front, lived through the Siege of Leningrad. A man to whose continued existence Comrade Beria himself objects, if only he could get hold of him. A man who until recently was an inmate in a corrective labour camp colony north of the Arctic Circle: one that might be considered remote even by the terns that breed there. Not lucky? On the contrary. Had I commanded you at Kursk, or the Seelow Heights, or at any point en route to Berlin, I would have kept you close by, comrade.'

Pletnev clasped his hands and regarded his visitors over the top of them.

'When Death unfurls a crooked finger,' he said, 'some men always find a way to give it the slip. In war, every soldier needs his fair share of that kind of luck. Religious superstition, however, I deplore. Those who long to arrive in a paradise above will never apply themselves to serious business of building one here on Earth.'

The general ran the palm of his right hand across his rough skull. Everything about him was grey – his eyes, his scalp and stubble. Almost as though, Rossel thought, all he needed to do was still himself and he could be set upon a plinth.

'Major Nikitin assures me you are just the man to find this Koshchei, our murderer. He is taking the lives of former Red Army heroes. I want that stopped, and fast. The militia are incompetent, and as for the MGB . . . they have their own agenda. The victims may not be serving soldiers but they are our heroic veterans. I am the Defence Minister and I cannot have people saying I am powerless to defend my men. So, find this Koshchei.'

The voice had changed. Now they were on the battlefield and the general was ordering his officers to attack, regardless of losses.

'I am honoured by Comrade Major Nikitin's faith in me,' said Rossel.

'You should be,' said General Pletnev. 'He has staked a great deal on your abilities.'

*

'Three corpses, all veterans. All in the same section of the army. All tortured in a similar way. All three left with a little Italian ditty stuffed into their mouths.' Nikitin smacked one hand into another as he summed up the similarities.

The major and Rossel had walked away from the Museum of Atheism and into the snowy gardens.

'Yes, but what about the differences?' said Rossel.

'Not many. Two are Jewish, one is not – at any rate, Akimov is not a Jewish name,' Nikitin replied. 'And Comrade Akimov also got a sniper bullet to the leg.'

Rossel nodded.

'Back to similarities. All the bodies were left for someone to find. In Akimov's case, however, anyone in Lenfilm would have heard him screaming. So, he was not killed there – or not tortured there, at any rate.'

'Tortured and then dragged in through a side entrance?' said Nikitin.

'He was a lump,' said Rossel. 'You'd need to be strong to carry him. In fact, a dead body that size? You'd have to be a weightlifter. And where would you hide him while you were stubbing your cigarettes out on his skin? He would likely make a little fuss.'

'In one of the buildings around Lenfilm?' Nikitin looked doubtful. 'It's a busy district.'

'Agreed. Even if you gagged him, you'd have to take the gag off if he was supposed to confess to something,'

BEN CREED

said Rossel. 'Same with Samosud, too. If he was tortured in his apartment, the whole of Sennaya Square would have known about it.'

The major swore, his curses puffing into the winter air.

'How did the killer do it?' he demanded. 'It's as if he had his own MGB basement interrogation cell. And could then make his victims walk in silence to where some idiot investigators would find them, sit down, and be slaughtered like animals.'

They reached the end of the gardens and the edge of Nevsky Prospect. No one paid them any attention. Leningrad was busy – trams trundled down the street; a troop of Young Pioneers marched by, heads held proudly in the air.

'There is one other thing,' said Nikitin. 'Common to the first two dead men, at least.'

He took a gold medallion out of his pocket and showed it to Rossel.

'I found this at Samosud's. Katz had one too. Maybe, it could all just be a squabble among Thieves?'

'They weren't Thieves,' Rossel said. 'No criminal records. No time in the camps. No tattoos.'

Rossel fell silent for a moment.

'You only tell me about this *now*?' he said.

Nikitin shrugged.

'Simple theft I can deal with. Dead men with messages in their mouths, that I need you for. I wanted you fully focused on the scrolls. Besides, I've got a lot on. As you've just seen, General Pletnev is a demanding master.'

Rossel held the major's gaze for a moment. Then took out a *papirosa* and lit it.

'Have you looked at Akimov's residence? Perhaps, he has one, too?' he said.

They had reached the major's car. Nikitin pulled open the driver's door.

'Got people doing that now, while the place is empty,' he said. 'While you and I go and talk to his girlfriend.'

19

A cowboy wearing spurs, leather chaps and a black ten-gallon hat was walking down the corridor. He was chatting to a man in buckskin, a headdress and full war paint.

As Rossel stood aside, he heard the headdress say: 'Get anywhere with little Sveta last night?'

The cowboy shook his head.

'The bitch says she is still in love with her husband. Remember him? The ice hockey goalkeeper who died in that plane crash. "I've got spurs and a ten-gallon hat, Sveta," I said, "I'm Leningrad's very own Billy the Kid!" Still nothing, fuck your mother . . . '

As Rossel and Nikitin turned a corner, a red light above a huge, soundproofed door blinked off. The major pulled at the handle.

Extras in the costumes of the Wild West mingled with the less glamorously dressed members of the Soviet movie industry. Everyone seemed to be shouting. On either side of a raised platform were two huge cameras, with a third in a gantry above and to the back. The set was elaborate and detailed and for the most part almost entirely taken up by the giant prow, paddle and black funnel of a Mississippi steamboat christened the *Red Star*.

It was a surreal sight. St Louis on the Neva.

They had come back to Lenfilm to talk to Akimov's girlfriend. Rossel looked around the room.

'See her?'

Nikitin shook his head.

The set was for a brand-new musical called *Red Dawn-Red Dusk*. Igor Volodin, a wily Lenfilm producer, had decided to combine Stalin's favourite film *Volga-Volga* – the story of a group of amateur actors travelling on a steamboat up the Volga – and the Great Leader's well-known love of Westerns. Looking around at the chaos, Rossel suspected that Volodin was either going to end up as a Hero of the Soviet Union or running a film society in a Siberian corrective labour camp. Depending on how the film turned out.

The frenzy intensified as crew and actors prepared for the next shot. Electricians adjusted cables, make-up girls powdered the noses of extras, the director and his cameramen gathered in a huddle.

Just then, a second stage door opened on the other side of the set and a group of six people came into the room. The new arrivals worked the miracle of sudden and total silence, punctuated by raucous laughter coming from a man at the centre of the group of interlopers. A short, stocky bald man in his mid-fifties was regaling his hangers-on with a story. They hung on his every word.

Rossel caught Nikitin's eye. 'Khrushchev,' the major mouthed at him from across the set.

But Rossel had already recognised him. It was an easy face to remember: like a gargoyle on the side of a medieval cathedral. A study in mischief and pugnacity. As if Khrushchev was so surprised by the power that a miner's son from Kalinovka, like him, had been able to acquire that he was incapable of hiding his glee.

Khrushchev finished his story, something about the terrible fate of a corrupt director of a collective farm in the southern Urals. The acolytes slapped each other on the back to demonstrate how amused they were. This soon became a competition. Khrushchev grinned. Then he spotted something – a broom resting against a wall. He grabbed it and made a couple of vigorous sweeping movements.

'Comrade Stalin calls me the Janitor – did you know that, Orlov?'

Orlov, a thin man with a grey moustache who was still wiping away tears of laughter, shook his head.

'Yes, the Janitor, that's me. Either because I am a dead ringer for Sergei Antimonov who plays Okhapkin, the janitor in *Volga-Volga*. Or . . .' He gave an exaggerated stage wink, 'because I'm the man he brings in to do the really shit jobs no one else wants to do . . .'

As one, the group collapsed in dutiful laughter. But Khrushchev's attention was already wandering. He stopped and surveyed the set, as if noticing it for the first time. Actors, extras and crew – all uncertain as to how to behave in the presence of such a Kremlin heavyweight – remained silent. Khrushchev pursed his lips. His cheeks coloured slightly.

'The Janitor,' he shouted, 'get it? The Janitor . . .'

After an awkward moment, the director, Boris Bamet, broke into a strained chuckle and everyone else except Rossel followed suit.

Khrushchev put a finger to his lips. The laughter stopped. Then he nodded at Bamet, who picked up a loudhailer and shouted for everyone to take their positions. Cast and crew shuffled into place, the overhead lights dimmed. Then Bamet raised his voice again.

'Action!'

Boris Tarkovsky stepped on to the prow of the *Red Star* and began to sing.

The actor was no longer the dashing, handsome 'Comrade Callimaco' who had won the hearts of Soviet womanhood in *The Mandrake*. The midriff was too flabby, the hairline in retreat. But he still had the firm jaw, strong mouth and smouldering eyes that had not only beguiled his audiences but brought comparisons to Yakov Dzhugashvili, Stalin's handsome eldest son.

Which had once been considered a highly useful characteristic for an actor planning his career. Before the war, at least. No one spoke of Yakov now.

Tarkovsky struck a pose that suggested stage lights and cameras had only been invented so that they might one day discover him.

But the microphones were less accommodating.

'Run, river, run, run to the sea, the People's cause runs with you, just as it runs through me . . . *Krasnaya Zvezda! Krasnaya Zvezda! Red Star! Red Star!*'

'"Tarkovsky sings!"' whispered Nikitin. 'I don't think they'll be putting that on the posters.'

*

Take four.

Tarkovsky was still managing to belt out his section of the musical number, but his singing had not improved.

'He's putting everything into it, though, eh?' said Nikitin.

Rossel nodded.

You couldn't fault the actor for effort. Just for tuning, rhythm and any semblance of control. With neither any training as a singer nor any musical talent, Tarkovsky kept missing his cues or losing his place or breaking down in mid-song, clutching at his throat and making frantic signals for more water.

Another break.

Rossel moved closer to the set. Tarkovsky was dressed in a blue uniform and wore a blue peaked cap with gold braid trimmings: a Soviet costume-designer's interpretation of a Mississippi steamboat pilot's uniform. A make-up girl dabbed at his brow, doing her best to stem the sweat dribbling down his cheeks, and fixed his stage-paint.

This close, under the harsh lights, Tarkovsky looked far older than when Rossel had last seen him on screen. He retained the Puckish grin and traces of the outrageous good looks of his youth but his jowls had moved in the opposite direction to his hairline, and some of the gold buttons on his blue pilot's waistcoat looked like they were about to pop.

These days, Rossel thought, he's got more of Stalin about him than the unfortunate Yakov.

'Positions, please,' shouted the director.

A spotty youth with a clapperboard gave the signal for take five.

'Action!'

'Run, river, run, run to the sea, the People's cause
runs with you, just as it runs through me . . .
*Krasnaya Zvezda! Krasnaya Zvezda! Red Star!
Red Star!*'

This time Tarkovsky was better. He kept close enough
to the rhythm for the sound editors to have something to
work with and even hit the top note on 'Red Star! Red
Star!' with some panache.

Bamet was windmilling his arms in the air to give his
star encouragement. But just as the second verse began,
Tarkovsky began to lose control, his voice wobbling and
wheezing like a broken locomotive.

Khrushchev, fingers in his ears and a fresh grin plastered
onto his face, grabbed his broom again and made another
series of exaggerated sweeping motions. His lackeys were
once again unable to contain themselves. Warming to his
role, Khrushchev began dancing beneath the prow of the
Red Star. Everyone was grinning.

'Cut!'

The actors and crew all looked at Tarkovsky. Even beneath
the stage paint it was easy to see the actor's face had reddened.

A puffing Khrushchev bowed to the director, the cameras and to no one in particular.

'I just couldn't stand it any more,' he said.

Tarkovsky recovered himself. He smoothed his uniform,
cleared his throat and took several deep breaths through
his angular nose.

'Your criticism is well justified, Comrade Khrushchev.
I am in your debt. Perhaps if we take a few moments break
I can prepare for an improved performance?'

Khrushchev waved the broom in Tarkovsky's direction as a gesture of mock thanks, took another bow and announced that time and political duties meant he would not be able to stay for it. The actor managed to look disappointed – a piece of acting that Rossel could only admire.

As Khrushchev's delegation departed, Tarkovsky placed a towel over his head and headed for his dressing room.

20

After twenty minutes of asking around, they found Akimov's girlfriend in the canteen.

She seemed to know little, and every time Rossel pressed her she began to sob. She had known about Akimov's military service – he was proud of it – but he had never given any indication that his war record nor any other aspect of his past might either bring surprise benefits or cause his unexpected demise.

She was upset, shocked and disbelieving, but said little to give the impression that Akimov had been the love of her life. 'He was not the sort to hit you, like others. Lived up at Udel'naya, you know, right up in the northern district. We met at a dance and he was lovely, treated me well. He fixed our apartment fusebox and said he knew about that stuff, so when I heard we needed an electrician I brought him in and he got the job. Am I in trouble?'

They had not lived together and had sometimes not seen each other for days. She lived in a communal apartment and therefore had a dozen people who could back up her claim to have been at home ever since leaving work for the day.

They let her go. Nikitin left, saying he had business to attend to. Rossel spent the morning pursuing other standard lines of inquiry. He talked to the film's director and the props man who had discovered Akimov's body but uncovered nothing new. Then he spoke to a lighting technician, who had told the militia he had heard something coming from the direction of the *Ivan the Terrible* set after the sound stage had been switched off for the night. But the man now insisted it had been nothing more than a rat that had found its way into a basket full of costume jewellery.

His head full of unanswered questions, Rossel retraced his steps towards the entrance to the studios.

*

Away from the main sound stage, Lenfilm was a maze of corridors filled with cramped offices – the homes of writers, script editors, make-up girls, minor producers and countless bureaucrats. No one paid Rossel any attention. A runner carrying a tray of herring and a bottle of vodka pushed past him and a few metres further on opened a door.

Beyond that door was darkness, a flickering light and an ill-tempered voice. On a leather chair, surrounded by a dozen empty seats and watching a black-and-white film, sat Boris Tarkovsky.

Without announcing himself, Rossel entered the screening room and closed the door behind him. He took his place four or five seats away; on the same row, roughly in the middle of the room. Engrossed in the film, Tarkovsky did not turn to look at the intruder, not even when Rossel lit up.

The film was one he had seen before. *The Mandrake.* It was Tarkovsky's breakthrough, a pre-war sensation. As far as Rossel could remember, the story was an elaborate farce in which Callimaco, Tarkovsky's role, sought to bed another man's wife.

On the screen was a scene in a convent garden between Callimaco and a corrupt priest, Friar Timoteo.

'But why would the Lord make women so delightful if he did not want man to sin? Why create such delicious pleasures and wish that only foul Beelzebub be allowed to partake of them?' said the friar.

As Callimaco replied, so – seemingly entranced – did Tarkovsky, mouthing the same words.

'But what if God and the Devil are conspirators, noble Friar? What if they both dance together to music no one has – as yet – understood?'

Rossel blew out a ring of smoke that drifted across the screen. He glanced down at the small zinc table that extended from one of the chairs. Tarkovsky, he could see, was onto his third plate of herring and his second bottle of vodka.

At last the actor turned towards him, his face registering no surprise, as if he had all along known he had company. His face was patterned with blotches. Traces of white make-up still adorned his eyes and his cheeks still bore the tracks of his recent humiliation.

'Tell that shit Bamet I'm not coming back,' he said. 'Tell him, Comrade Callimaco says he has quit. Tell him to get some other idiot to bellow barnyard tunes from the prow of that stupid fucking steamboat.'

Rossel offered a cigarette. Tarkovsky took it, saw it was a simple *papirosa*, grimaced and lit it anyway.

'I'm not from the studio, Comrade Tarkovsky,' said Rossel.

The actor appeared not to have heard him. He took another glass of vodka from the tray and downed it in one. Then he stabbed at a small piece of herring before hurling the glass against a picture of Sergei Lukyanov, star of *Cossacks of the Kuban*, which was hanging on the wall. Both the glass and the picture frame shattered.

'They're giving Lukyanov a People's Artist Award. Can you believe that? I only found out this morning. He's already got the Stalin Prize, second class. The planks of wood they used to build the *Red Star* have more emotional range than that prick. And yet here I am. Boris Tarkovsky! Singing "Red Star! Red Star!" off the back of a fucking paddle steamer. And that's supposed to be Soviet culture these days . . .'

Drunks, Rossel thought, required a little patience. But getting them to talk was never a problem.

Tarkovsky grabbed the vodka bottle by the neck and took a mouthful. He swallowed hard and shut his eyes.

'You're not from Bamet?'

Rossel shook his head.

'Then who?'

'I'm an investigator.'

It took several seconds for the words to register. The actor straightened in his seat. For a moment, Rossel expected him to try and make amends, to apologise in abject terms for his many indiscretions. But he was wrong.

'I have friends,' Tarkovsky said. His voice was slurred, his tone defiant rather than aggressive.

'Everybody does.'

'In the Party.'

The two men stared at each other. Before the war, the newsreels had covered the deeds of Yakov Dzhugashvili extensively. But, afterwards, the face of Stalin's elder son was one you were supposed to forget. Something impossible to do once you found yourself face to face with Boris Tarkovsky. Yakov had always worn the uniform of a courageous defender of the Motherland, but could never rid himself of a mournful gaze that hinted at something else lurking beneath his heroic façade.

But with middle-age had come shadows of Yakov's father – shadows that lengthened with Tarkovsky's suspicious look. As he stared at the actor, the hint of a shiver ran through Rossel.

'I would expect nothing else, comrade.' he said. 'You are aware of the recent murder that took place here at Lenfilm?'

'How could I not be?'

'Were you filming that day?'

Tarkovsky did not reply.

On the screen, Harlequins and Pierrots whirled around the dance floor at a masked ball. Callimaco threw passionate looks across the room at the object of his desire: the pure and beautiful Lucrezia.

'Let me assure you that I have no wish to threaten you and nothing to threaten you with,' Rossel said. On instinct, he added: 'Comrade Callimaco.'

Tarkovsky sat forward.

'No one calls me that any more. *Pravda* did. *Izvestia*, too. The name, I am told, was talked of with approval in the Kremlin. But . . .'

'But?'

'Then that idiot Yakov got himself killed in the war.'

It had been assumed that Tarkovsky's spectacular rise, the reason he had got the leading role in *The Mandrake* in the first place, was because of his resemblance to Yakov Dzhugashvili. Doors had been flung open, merely because directors and producers believed that by promoting Tarkovsky they would, by means of a miraculous political osmosis, gain favour with Stalin himself. A process that became even more pronounced once it became known that Stalin loved *The Mandrake* and had conferred on its star the title of 'Comrade Callimaco'.

Then Stalin's elder son had been captured by the Germans only days after the Nazi invasion. Captured, not killed, and thus disgraced.

Two years later, he died in Sachsenhausen concentration camp. His name was forgotten. His fate had tainted Tarkovsky's career.

Tarkovsky reached for the bottle again. Rossel stretched out his hand and, taking the actor by the wrist, stopped him.

'The murder, Comrade Tarkovsky, of your colleague Akimov. Were you here? Did you see anything?'

The actor glanced down at his wrist.

'I am on the Party committee here, comrade,' he said. 'I took my examinations in Dialectical and Historical Materialism two weeks ago. And passed them.'

You can't touch me.

Rossel let it go.

'The Party committee is lucky to have you, Comrade Tarkovsky. Your vigilance is an example to us all,' he said.

He stood, getting in the way of the projector and casting his silhouette over the screen.

The actor looked up.

'I wasn't on that day,' he said. 'There had been a problem with the set. They couldn't get that stupid funnel to stand up straight. They brought in carpenters to take a look. I spent the morning with an old friend before visiting the stage orphanage at Kirovsk. I used to be a pupil there. They ask me back from time to time, *pour*, with apologies to Voltaire, *encourager les orphelins*.'

Rossel stopped at the door.

'I went to a state orphanage, too,' he said. 'In Kostroma. Along with my sister. It had high walls and small windows. We didn't like it much.'

They had been sent there after the arrest of his mother and father. As children of 'enemies of the people', he and Galya were themselves suspect.

Tarkovsky had relocated the vodka.

'Then you will understand better than most how far I had to climb to become Comrade Callimaco.' He poured and raised his glass. 'Long live the world revolution.'

He turned back to the screen. Callimaco, who was on the point of bedding the innocent Lucrezia, was removing his black mask.

'Why, child, from our very selves we hide – even from his own mirror the wise man remains a mystery . . .'

As before, Tarkovsky repeated the words exactly as Callimaco said them.

21

Rossel had hoped to slip away, to take time to reacquaint himself with Leningrad. To get some of its grime under his fingernails, put some miles under his feet.

But Nikitin was waiting for him at the studio exit.

'We must report to the general,' he said.

'Why? We've only just seen him and we haven't got anything to tell him.'

Nikitin smiled.

'Yes we do. Take a look at this.'

*

General Pletnev adjusted the pictures of Lenin and Marshal Zhukov behind him so they were straight. He sat back down at his desk in Kazan's old sacristy and fixed Rossel and Nikitin with a stare.

'I have many things to occupy my mind. As a native of Leningrad I have been given the honour of organising the city's Party assembly in a few weeks' time.'

The assembly was the main preparatory meeting before the following year's All-Union Conference. A very important event.

'Stalin himself will attend,' said the general. 'So, be brief. What have you got?'

Something interesting, Comrade General. Let's see how you react.

'The third victim's name was Akimov,' said Rossel. 'He was also a veteran of the 8th Guards Corps during the war. I instructed the militia to go through the war records of all three of the deceased, since all three were in possession of one of these.'

He took a large gold medallion about ten centimetres in diameter from his pocket and dropped it onto the table.

The militia had found it in Akimov's room, under a floorboard. In normal circumstances they might not have taken such a thorough look, but Nikitin had told them what to search for, and they had found it.

General Pletnev stared at it. On the face of the medallion an eagle, its wings spread, carried a swastika in its talons. Around the rim in capital letters was engraved a single word: Neubrandenburg.

The general picked it up.

'That is the Luftwaffe insignia,' he said. 'Loot, perhaps? Something these soldiers stole while rifling through a bomber pilot's attic in Germany?'

Rossel watched him.

'Possibly.'

'And the others. You say they had medallions like this, too?'

'Correct,' said Rossel. 'The first man to die – the welder, Katz – tried to sell his to a Jew who has a stall out near Malaya Okhta, according to the militia. The next day Katz failed to turn up to work, and the day after. He was a serial absentee but his boss was annoyed enough to send round a comrade to drag him out of bed to the factory. That comrade instead found him dead – dead in an intriguing fashion. The militia arrived and found the gold medallion on the floor.'

'Comrade Katz miscalculated,' said Nikitin. 'The Jew may have had links to the Thieves but he was also an MGB informant. He knew a swastika spelled trouble. So, he told the MGB blue-hats.'

'Wait a moment,' said Pletnev. 'The killer and the MGB knew about the existence of a large gold medallion in the possession of this welder, and yet it was left for the militia to recover?'

'It is interesting,' said Rossel, who had been wrestling with the same problem without coming up with an explanation. A killer who left Italian verses inserted in the throats of his victims, but who ignored a lump of gold in each corpse's possession.

Pletnev ran a finger over the lettering around the rim of the medallion.

'And what, or where, is Neubrandenburg?' he asked.

'An eastern German city,' said Nikitin. 'Our boys took it at the end of the war. Pretty much burnt it to the ground.'

The general grunted. 'I do not remember it,' he said. 'And yet . . .'

He stood, placing his fingers on his brow as if trying hard to remember something. Rossel looked at Pletnev for every twitch of every facial muscle. The general exuded power, absolute confidence in his ability to handle every situation.

A moment later, Pletnev straightened his shoulders and nodded. He marched over to a row of filing cabinets and without hesitating pulled open a drawer and removed a file.

He tossed it on the desk.

'Open it,' he said.

Rossel did. Inside was a photograph of what looked like an enormous, low-ceilinged cellar. Two men in US army uniforms, clutching notebooks, were surveying row after row of crates and sacks.

'That is the bottom of a mineshaft in a village called Merkers in Germany. Summer of 1945,' said the general. 'In those crates and bags, and in many others, was more than one hundred tonnes of gold. Bars, rings, jewellery, gold fillings. And thick wads of Reichsmarks. Our intelligence concluded that there were other such caches. Places the Fascists had hidden their spoils of war with aim of returning to it one day.'

Rossel pointed to the medallion.

'You'd need a lot of these to add up to one hundred tonnes,' he said.

Pletnev nodded. 'You would. But there are stories.'

'Stories?' said Nikitin.

'Stories of buried treasure. Hidden under Himmler's *schloss*. Or was it Göring's? Or in the cellar of the mansion of a murdered Jewish banker? Or in a bunker near the hunting lodge of a high-ranking SS officer? And so on.'

Rossel looked at the only other sheet in the file. It was a typed inventory, in English, of the contents of the mineshaft at Merkers. The list continued over the page.

The general laced his fingers behind his back and set off pacing at the slow march.

'At the time Beria said it was all nonsense, but then it emerged he'd been questioning high-ranking Fascist prisoners about it. The MGB are rumoured to have interrogated a few suspects down the years. None of them confessed to anything – well, anything useful.'

Rossel closed the file. He was beginning to see what the general was driving at.

'But now this turns up,' he said.

'And now this turns up,' agreed Pletnev. 'And there was one other story I haven't mentioned. A rumour of a small band of Red Army soldiers who went astray for a few days at the end of the war. Who discovered the location of one of the troves and took the secret with them back to Russia. Hoping one day to return. A rumour, I might add, that has been remarkably slow to die.'

Pletnev resumed his seat and looked straight at Rossel.

'Hidden Nazi gold. Seven years of fruitless searching and then this. Imagine the reaction when the MGB found out.'

'They must have got themselves a little overexcited,' said Nikitin.

The general leaned back.

'If these murders are linked to this wartime treasure hunt, whatever the truth of the matter, I will need you to redouble your efforts,' he said. 'This hoard would be of considerable interest to the Soviet state. We need currency and gold. Every single day, the Americans outspend us.'

So it's not just Beria who has gold fever . . .

'You are aware of the ritual aspect of the three murders, Comrade General?' asked Rossel. 'The torture, the double shot to the head . . .'

'Yes.'

'And the scrolls in the throat?'

Pletnev raised his eyebrows.

'Scrolls?' he said.

'Pieces of paper on which someone has written lines from a play by Machiavelli, *The Mandrake*, and placed in the victims' throats.'

The general ran his hand over the downy stubble that pockmarked his pate. For a moment, he seemed lost in thought.

'"Confuse the enemy, disguise your true intentions, make them concentrate their forces in the wrong place",' he said eventually. 'This must be a diversionary tactic, a ruse. Military commanders use them constantly. I suggest that you do not fall for it.'

Pletnev nodded at them as if to say their time was up. Rossel got to his feet, picked up the medallion and pocketed it.

He and Nikitin headed for the door.

*

As Rossel and Nikitin walked back to the major's car, trams, buses and cars were fighting their way through the icy wind that blew down Nevsky Prospect.

'If you wanted to get the secret location of a hoard of gold out of someone, why do all that – the lyrics, the tongue, the mutilation?' Rossel said. 'Surely you would just put a gun to Katz's head and ask him in a very direct manner – "Where did you get this bar of gold from, Comrade Katz?" Or Comrade Samosud, Comrade whoever . . .

I mean it wouldn't be any more complicated than that, would it?'

Nikitin shrugged.

'Unless all that is just to throw us off the trail – make it seem as though we are looking for a Koshchei, a phantom, a maniac. When in fact it's just a treasure hunter.'

Rossel took a *papirosa* from his pocket and lit it.

A tram passed by on the other side of the street. A pretty girl dressed in the uniform of an Oktyabrina, the youth group for girls dedicated to Lenin, had her face pressed against a partially misted window. She half-smiled at Rossel just as the tram disappeared around a corner.

Rossel blew a stream of smoke after the tram.

'But is the gold the real treasure?'

22

The temperature was falling again; the kind of cold that made factory smoke and exhaust fumes hang in the evening air. The car stopped a street away from the Drugovs' former home.

Rossel made a move to get out. Then sat back down again.

'Has she joined the Party?' he said.

Nikitin looked straight ahead.

'Has who joined the Party?'

'Vassya.'

Just saying her name, the soft familiarity of his own intonation, made him realise how much he had missed her. In Igarka, the memory of their time together had been something to block out. Their brief happiness too painful to recall. A way to weaken his spirit.

But ever since Nikitin had brought her to the camp, he couldn't stop thinking about her.

The major still didn't look at him.

'Tatiana Vasilyeva is doing well,' said Nikitin. 'One of the senior engineers on the new metropolitan railway system. She has a new apartment in the centre of town. A telephone. A prosperous Soviet life in the proletarian paradise we are all building together. A would-be Party member.

A romantic dalliance with someone like you would only set her career back.'

Everyone who wanted to make progress in Soviet society had to join the Party. Rossel reflected on how little he really knew about Vassya's life. Had she been in the Komsomol? Had she done well in her Marxism–Leninism studies? Had she spent summers picking fruit on a collective farm?

All they had ever really spoken about was the war. They were both loners, both survivors.

That instinct, he thought – survival – was why she would try and join the Party. But she would have needed a helping hand.

'A boyfriend?'

'Why don't you ask her yourself, investigator?'

The major pulled out a piece of paper from the inside breast pocket of his coat and held it up. On the paper was written an address in a very respectable part of town, and a number.

'She didn't look too delighted to see me last time, Major.'

Nikitin sniffed.

'I don't understand my wife. But she understands me. As far as wisdom goes that's the only real gold-plated insight I have ever possessed, comrade. And yet, when I asked her out the first time and she said no, I was wise enough to ask her again.'

Rossel took the paper, got out of the car and breathed in a lungful of cold air.

Leningrad's air, Leningrad's lamplight, Leningrad's snow. Leningrad's stillness . . .

In that, for him at least, there had always been wisdom.

*

The manuscript for Vustin's prelude and fugue thirteen in E minor was complete. Rossel sat at Ivan Drugov's grand piano, on which he had placed a notepad and pencil and a brass ashtray that was now full. But he neither smoked nor wrote a word as he picked out the winding, interlocking themes of the fugue as best he could with his right hand and the two fingers of his left.

The fugue had a title, which was unusual. Neither Bach nor Shostakovich, in his most recent masterpiece, had given names to any of the component parts of their complete cycles of twenty-four preludes and fugues. But Vustin had. 'The Song of Lost Souls.'

The Steinway was a shade out of tune but its tone was warm and beguiling. An arpeggio, followed by ornamentation around the fifth note, teetering there like a gymnast at the top of her routine on the double bars before falling to the minor third . . . then the preparation for modulating to the dominant. The second statement of the theme, this time in the tenor register.

Without the requisite fingers, he had to hum the bass notes as best he could. The process took him back to the torturous score-reading exercises he had to do as student at the Leningrad Conservatoire. His first love had always been the violin. But he had been an enthusiastic if indifferent pianist. Nevertheless, he managed to get to the end of Vustin's fugue. It was slow, ingeniously constructed, exquisite. Six pages of eerie melancholy – Igarka and its desolate colonies at night, captured in sound.

The gulag's collective sigh . . .

He listened to the final notes fade away.

Then turned his attention back to the notepad.

The three bodies of Katz, Samosud and Akimov: each with a Machiavellian lyric placed in the throat their tongues cut out, the two executional shots to the right temple.

The killer seemed to be accusing Katz of gullibility. *'That ignorance is bliss is widely known . . .'*

Samosud, the opposite. *'How gentle is deception . . .'*

Nikitin had put his Italian translator to work on an accurate Russian rendition of the Akimov scroll.

'Oh gentle darkness, oh holy and sweet nocturnal hours / That soothe the burning pain of love's desires . . .'

Was it a love letter? Dispatching Akimov with such brutality was an odd way to show infatuation. Unless it was a revenge attack on an unfaithful lover.

Or a way of denying the victim to a rival?

But it still didn't make sense. The three sentiments – naivety, deception, love – were all in *The Mandrake,* but the film had been released before the war and hardly seemed relevant to three murders committed several years later.

The victims' shared past, their time in the 8th Guards, still seemed the most salient connection. And the one of which Nikitin was most convinced.

A killer who was invisible, yet eager to leave messages to those investigating the crimes. And who seemed indifferent to the possessions of his victims, even if they included a large, solid-gold medallion.

Rossel stood up and sighed. He stepped away from the piano and sat down in what, he assumed, had been Ivan Drugov's favourite armchair. It was squat, functional and covered in brown leather – a mass-produced item out of keeping with some of the luxury imported items that a member of the Party could get their hands on. But it had an antimacassar with a deep discolouration, which also gave off a whiff of hair oil, suggesting it been well used.

The stain was, he thought, now all that probably remained of the unfortunate Drugov.

He stared at the black telephone, on a small table, just out of reach.

In the silence, he could feel the eyes of the teenage Drugova on him, staring out from one of the picture frames with her fiddle on her shoulder.

He looked down at the paper Nikitin had given him and lifted the receiver. He half-expected the line to have been cut off, but the tone told him otherwise.

Rossel dialled Vassya's number. Waited. Nothing. As he let the receiver drop onto the cradle he thought he heard one of the tones cut short and the sound of someone's voice. But it was too late.

Silence.

His hand moved towards the phone again.

It rang.

For a split second, he had the surreal feeling one of the Drugovs might be on the other end of the line – the daughter ringing to ask for Vustin's number.

He picked up the phone.

It was Nikitin.

'He's killed someone else,' the major said.

23

Lieutenant Yelchin – a lifelong militiaman in his fifties, with mousy hair and a hacking cough – met Rossel and Nikitin on the street with a wave to slow them down. He followed it with a stiff salute, then led them into the building site covered with wooden scaffolding and tarpaulin, and guided them to the lift. They descended to the cavern that would, he said, one day be the main platform of Vladimirskaya Metro Station.

'It's so deep because everything here is built on a swamp, as you know, Comrade Major,' Yelchin said as they stood on a simple platform with a filthy floor. He was nervous, casting looks at Nikitin as if inviting his approval for the tip-off he'd given him. 'That makes the ground unstable.'

The lift stopped and he pulled back the gate. 'Also, it's being built to withstand one of those atomic bombs the capitalists have.' Aware he might have implied a technological advantage on the part of the enemy, Yelchin quickly added: 'Imperialist criminals.'

Nikitin took no notice and strode forward, Yelchin half-running to catch up. Rossel looked around the vast, grey tunnel. The metro project had been started in the 1930s but the war had interrupted. Progress in recent years had been slow.

The air was dank and smelled of wet concrete and plaster. Pillar after pillar, thick and squat, ran along the concourse. Rossel looked over the edge of the platform, but there was only more concrete and a few sacks.

He caught up with Nikitin.

The major was in a foul mood. He had grumbled all the way to the scene of the crime – 'This stupid piece of shit gets his brains blown out just as I was sitting down to a decent bowl of *solyanka*' – but Rossel knew it was more than that.

He would have to report again to General Pletnev in the morning. And they had nothing. Instead of finding answers they had only found another dead body – and if this one was another veteran . . .

The militia officers who had been summoned to the scene at this late hour kept a wary distance, unsure of Nikitin's uniform. Not MGB, not standard military, not militia. Rossel scanned them for familiar faces but to his relief found none. They looked harder-nosed than the militia cops who had been at the film studios, though. This was a tougher area. The big employer in the neighbourhood was the Kirov Factory, which had kept going even during the blockade with a skeleton crew and any equipment that had not been stripped and reassembled in the Urals.

The body was tied to a plastic seat, next to a wheelbarrow and a couple of open bags of cement. It had been left in the middle of the platform. The officers had found two huge lights, meant for penetrating the darkest corners of the Leningrad Metropolitan's tunnels, to train on the latest victim. It was an inadvertent recreation of the Akimov murder scene at Lenfilm.

Nikitin looked at Rossel, who nodded. The two men approached the body.

'There it is,' said Nikitin.

A tiny piece of rolled-up paper. Rossel took a pen from his inside pocket, slipped the end of it under the fold, lifted it out and unravelled it.

> . . . *tu, col tuo gran valore,*
> *nel far beato altrui fai ricco, Amore;*
> *tu vinci, sol co' tuoi consigli santi,*
> *pietre, veneni e incanti.*

'Understand it?' said Nikitin.

'No. Something about courage, love, sanctity. We'll need your friend. One other thing.' Rossel pointed at the man's right temple. 'Two shots again. And everything else is the same – the chair, the bindings, the position of the body. How was this one found?'

Nikitin summoned Yelchin. Two security guards had heard screams and then a shot, then another shot. It took them another few seconds to reach the bottom and, being unarmed, they took only the briefest look around before taking the lift back up.

'As soon as they were at the surface they called us. And I called you, Comrade Major.'

'Good lad,' said Nikitin.

On the other side of the corpse, two tunnels led into the murk.

Rossel turned towards Lieutenant Yelchin, who eyed him back with wariness. Rossel knew the type from his own days as a militia lieutenant. If you didn't ask the wrong questions, you didn't get the wrong answers. And the best way to make that happen was not to ask many questions at all. Keep your nose clean by not sticking it into the wrong places. He wondered what Nikitin had on him.

'You said the guards heard the commotion at around 19.00, correct?' Rossel said.

Yelchin took out a handkerchief and coughed into it, making a noise like a pneumatic drill as the phlegm rattled around his throat. He nodded.

'Yes, and we got the call at around 19.15. I don't think they saw much more than I just described.'

'And do we know who he is?' Rossel said, gesturing with a thumb to the body.

Yelchin took a notepad from his pocket and read from it. 'Glaskov. A cook, from Repino. We are checking as you requested, Comrade Major, for his wartime . . .'

The militia lieutenant's voice trailed off. He stopped and put his notebook away. Then stood to attention. As one, his men did the same.

Rossel looked back along the platform, at the group who had just pulled back the safety bar of the lift and stepped out from it. Four men wearing the distinctive blue-rimmed caps of the Ministry for State Security service were walking towards them.

'MGB,' said Nikitin. 'This should be interesting.'

*

The MGB colonel introduced himself as Colonel Belsky of the Fifth Directorate. The Fifth was responsible for monitoring and repressing dissent within the Party apparatus and the wider Soviet Union.

'GRU, you say?' Belsky looked from Rossel to Nikitin and back again. He was short and stocky, with a pasty complexion and large bags under his eyes. 'This isn't a military intelligence matter. Besides, I have orders from the highest authority that my men and I should take over this case.'

'I have orders too, Colonel. From General Pletnev, Defence Minister. Perhaps you have heard of . . .'

'A great war hero.' Belsky spoke over the jibe. 'I shall be sure to mention the general's name to Comrade Beria.'

Beria's name was Colonel Belsky's trump card. A single word that had the ability to unlock any door, cast aside any barrier, stifle any objection. But when you go to work every day as a blue-hat, Rossel thought, in every street you're a tsar riding in a procession. Everyone defers to you. Until, one day, you bump into a Nikitin. Running into someone like the major, who didn't back down, had unnerved Belsky's officers, who were looking at their boss for cues.

'I thought it was Comrade Ignatyev who led the MGB now,' said Nikitin.

'Oh, please, please,' laughed Colonel Belsky. 'I think we are all aware of the reality.'

Nikitin set his jaw and shoved his face close to the colonel.

'Of course,' he said, 'Ignatyev sits on Beria's knee, while Beria grabs him by the balls. And squeezes.'

The MGB colonel and his men moved their hands towards their pistols.

Nikitin did the same.

Rossel heard a dog bark. All eyes swivelled to the tunnel on the right. Two militia officers, one holding an excited Alsatian on a leash, had emerged, and were shouting to Yelchin to come quick.

'We have him! We have Koshchei cornered.'

As one, officers, MGB agents, Nikitin and Rossel headed for the mouth of the tunnel, dropping off the edge of the platform and running into the dark.

*

We're close now, we have to be . . .

Footsteps echoed around the tunnel walls, creating a mesmerising percussive effect – the sense of pursuers both behind and ahead. Beams from half a dozen flashlights made dancing patterns in the air and on the walls, while the stench of the new paint being used on the tunnel caught in the back of Rossel's throat.

The two officers with the growling Alsatian led the way, with Rossel close behind. Temporary lights dangled from the roof, not all of them lit. Both Rossel and the dog handler had already smacked their faces on a couple of them as they ran forward.

'Which way?'

Rossel didn't know who had spoken, but the reason was clear. They had covered about 500 metres and now the tunnel split into two.

'That's the main line,' said one of the officers. 'That's just a service tunnel – look, it stops there.'

The handler dropped to one knee, patted the dog, whispered in its ear.

'Which way, Annika? Which way, girl?'

Everyone took a moment, panting and gasping. Both Rossel's lungs and legs were giving out. Hands on his knees and his brow dripping with sweat, he glanced behind him, but half a dozen torches made it impossible to make anything out.

In front of him, the Alsatian growled. The militia officer unclipped the leash and the animal shot off, taking the left-hand fork; its handler running after it. Rossel, forcing his tired limbs to obey, followed.

He chased after the light up ahead as best he could but the distance between it and him widened. The heavy breathing behind faded.

He was alone.

How many paces?

No more than two hundred covered, he thought.

After that he'd lost count.

The tunnel curved. For a few seconds he was in total darkness. He followed the bend, one hand on the wall, and caught up with the dog handler.

The handler was crouched behind a wagon filled with spades, buckets and an enormous drill. Perhaps fifty metres ahead stood a rail carriage, its outline clearly visible thanks to a dim light swinging from the ceiling – a bulb slung over a hook.

Beyond it, a dead end.

Lieutenant Yelchin ran up behind them.

'I think we have him, Comrade Lieutenant,' the handler said as his superior tried to catch his breath. 'This looks like a siding or some sort of service tunnel. If I know anything about my Annika she'll already have that bastard by the—'

A loud bang. Everyone dived for the floor.

'Who was that?' shouted Yelchin. 'Kozlov, you fucking idiot.'

'Sorry, Comrade Lieutenant – I saw him, I swear,' said the underling.

Rossel's cheek was pressed to the cold metal of the rail track. He could see under the carriage. There was a shaft of light at or near the end of the service tunnel.

Annika was lying on her stomach beneath it. She was still.

Rossel clambered to his feet. So did the dog handler.

'Koshchei is not here,' said Rossel. 'The dog wouldn't just lie there like that if he was.'

Rossel stepped forward, squeezing down the right-hand side of the carriage towards the animal. He paused at the end, using it as cover, looking up to find the light source. Steel rungs embedded in the concrete showed him where the escape route was. A metallic scrape far above told him the rest. He darted past the dog, which snarled and jumped to its feet. A hunk of meat dangled from Annika's jaws.

Clambering up the same pile of boards the fugitive must have used, Rossel made sure his pistol was easy to reach, pushing it into a jacket pocket, and began to climb.

Heaving a manhole cover off, Rossel waited at the top, listening.

A few cars. A tram going past.

Three times he stuck his head up and down, before daring a longer look. Grunting with the effort, his arms screaming for him to stop, he hauled himself out into the silent road and the biting wind. A few flakes of snow were twirling round the chimneys of the Kirov Factory, which rose above a forbidding brick wall a couple of hundred metres away.

Koshchei had vanished.

*

Nikitin kicked at a workman's bucket. It somersaulted a couple of times and then splashed black paint across the wall.

'Shit. We lost him.'

Rossel sat on the steps of the rail carriage, recovering his breath, as a procession of militia and MGB officers went up and down the exit shaft.

'This explains it,' said one of the officers from inside the carriage. 'A mattress, blankets, some milk, a tin of *tushy-onka*, and the rest of the nice chop he threw the dog.'

Rossel entered the compartment. A military-issue mat, a thick sleeping bag, rough blankets. Tea, sugar and a small stove.

On the floor, catching the torchlight, he saw something glinting amid the grey cement dust. He bent to pick it up. Holding it in his left hand, he held it to the light and stared at it – a small silver locket with a scratched glass cover, containing a lock of hair. On the back was inscribed a number: 1500.

He showed it to Nikitin.

'Odd,' said the major. 'What do you think it means?'

Rossel shook his head.

'I don't know. A factory batch number, perhaps?'

Nikitin took it.

'And some hair. How romantic.' He thrust it into a pocket. 'I'll add it to Dr Bondar's list. Though my feeling is he'll just give us more questions and no bloody answers.'

178

24

Rossel sat at the Drugovs' piano; a full ashtray in front of him, as well as a half-bottle of cognac he'd found in a kitchen cupboard. He took a pull on his *papirosa* and a drink from the bottle, and looked again at the little gold calling-card that had been left on his doormat.

Dear Comrade Detective,
I called, you were out. Feverishly detecting, no doubt. I am having a small gathering this evening. Orphans come free. Your presence would honour and delight me.
With respect,
Comrade Callimaco.

On the back was a celebrated address. The Yusupov Palace.

Rossel's first instinct had been to ignore it. But another evening surrounded by the shades of the Drugov family was becoming less inviting with each glass. He stubbed out his cigarette, stood up, walked into the hall and adjusted his coat in front of the mirror. As he pulled his gloves over his broken fingers, the last line from *The Mandrake* he'd heard Tarkovsky mouth along to at the film studios came back to him:

Why, child, from our very selves we hide – even from his own mirror the wise man remains a mystery . . .

Ivan Drugov's luxurious sable *ushanka* was hanging on a coat stand. Inwardly promising to return it, Rossel slipped it on. After all, he thought, it wasn't every day a man received an invitation to the Yusupov.

*

Tarkovsky's apartment was, indeed, palatial. The drapes, chandeliers and rug – a rich blue one with the Yusupov coat of arms: two oddly malnourished lions holding up an ornate shield – looked almost new, as if the room had only been recently decorated in anticipation of the arrival of the last Romanov tsar and his family. It was said the Romanovs had even been Russia's second-wealthiest aristocrats – after the Yusupovs.

Everything was polished, ornate, priceless. By day, most of the palace was a museum, including an exhibition of the notorious death with which it was forever associated: the murder of Rasputin. By night, Tarkovsky – whose private rooms were in the furthest recesses of the palace – sometimes walked the corridors alone.

A grand piano occupied the centre of the room. Beyond it, windows led onto a balcony overlooking the Moika. Scattered about were dozens of bottles of Soviet champagne: enough to suggest the party had taken up the entire evening and much of the afternoon as well. But the mood among the twenty or so guests – most in what looked like costumes borrowed from Lenfilm – was languid.

Everyone seemed to have eaten and drunk their fill. In his rough suit and cracked leather shoes, Rossel could only hope that the throng would assume he had come dressed as an archetypal apparatchik down on his luck.

Only Tarkovsky, who was in his element, and a gaggle of mostly female hangers-on fought off the ennui. The actor was playing the master of ceremonies, regaling the company with tales of rapacious aristocratic cavorting at the palace. He was ringed by a ballerina, a squaw, a couple of Marlene Dietrich lookalikes and a very pretty redhead called Dasha, who was barely out of her teens. A sailor and what could have been Ivan the Terrible completed the crowd around the piano.

Holding an almost empty glass, a tall, thin man with long grey hair and the demeanour of a hungry crow circling a battlefield stood a little apart from Rossel. He was listening to the chatter with his head inclined slightly away from the revellers; like a priest behind a confessional screen, mulling over the necessary level of a penance. On Rossel's arrival, Tarkovsky had introduced him as Alexander Fadeyev, the Head of the Writers' Union.

Next to Fadeyev, at the other end of a green and gold chaise longue, was a woman in her late twenties. She had dark hair tied in a bow, wore a simple red dress and was smoking a cigarette of black paper. Her pose was relaxed and carefree, but also disdainful. Her soft smile sometimes curled into something resembling a sneer as her face moved in and out of the light. Tarkovsky had presented her with mock awe. 'Beautiful Natalia. Natalia Ivaskova.'

Rossel took refuge behind a *papirosa* as the party went on around him.

At first, he'd wished he hadn't come. But the chatter and the laughter were both bewildering and invigorating. After life in Igarka, the carefree atmosphere was addictive.

Natalia tipped her head in his direction and spoke over Fadeyev's long grey hair.

'Is it true? Are you a real detective, like Boris says?' Her voice was soft, quite low. 'Or are you just playing one on screen in some cheap Lenfilm potboiler?'

'As it happens, I'm not a detective. Not any more. But I'm not an actor either. What about you?'

'I am an actress. Learning to be one, at any rate. A career change.' She pointed at her left ankle. 'I was a dancer at the Kirov. A good prospect, some said. But then I shattered the end of my fibula. In a rehearsal of *The Nutcracker*, of all things. Brittle bones, the doctors say. And now . . . I am not a dancer any more.'

'A detective who isn't a detective and dancer who can't dance,' he said. 'We have something in common. Where are you from? Not Leningrad, I think, with that accent.'

Her face darkened. She glanced at Fadeyev, but he was still scowling at the group around the piano. Rossel wondered if they were together.

'So you *are* a detective, of sorts,' she said, recovering her smile. 'Well, I'm from a city that no longer exists, near a lake that has no name.'

Rossel shook his head. 'There are many of those,' he said. The authorities were closing off more and more towns and cities to the outside world to keep their military secrets away from spies. Only residents with permits were allowed to come and go. And the MGB, of course . . . Many of the closed cities were in the Urals. Natalia's accent had that lilt – not quite Siberian, but heading in that direction.

'I'd say Sverdlovsk, or Chelyabinsk,' he said. 'I'd need another clue to be sure.'

She put her hands together in mock applause. 'Very good, comrade. Not quite a bullseye, but close enough.'

She held out her empty glass.

'Get me another?'

*

A raucous rendition of a song from a musical Rossel didn't know came to an end. A ripple of applause went around the room as the other guests came back to life.

Various toasts drifted across the smoky air – to friendship, to love, to happiness . . .

Tarkovsky, teetering slightly, took a long drink from the neck of a bottle of champagne and cried out, 'To success!' Instantly, it was agreed that this was the perfect salutation for such an evening. Shouts of 'To success!' echoed around the room.

The host grabbed one of the two girls dressed as Marlene Dietrich around the waist. He turned her towards him and then kissed her.

'And so, as I was saying,' he said, breaking off the kiss and breathing hard, 'before I was so rudely interrupted . . .' Now he did the same thing to the other Dietrich. Then he continued his speech. 'You may have heard, and who am I to persuade you otherwise, some say . . . and by some I mean those in the very *highest* echelons . . .' Boris paused here and looked around the room, which went quiet, '. . . that, in my youth, I bore more than a passing resemblance to a certain Comrade Yakov . . .'

Boris pointed to his own face so no one could possibly miss his point.

The actor picked up a box of cigars that he claimed were a gift from the Soviet ambassador to Havana. 'One of them, the ambassador assures me, contains a secret microfilm of President Truman doing unspeakable things to a two-dollar whore dressed as a hotdog,' he proclaimed. 'Let's see which of you gets the lucky cigar!'

Fadeyev snorted in disgust and moved off to another part of the room. Rossel looked at Natalia.

'Alexander is a big man in the world of Soviet culture,' she said with a shrug. 'A devotee of Socialist Realism: the only artistic principle with any validity, so he claims.'

'I can't imagine a Lenfilm production of a musical Western sits too well with that particular aesthetic,' said Rossel.

'He is not happy. And his mood has not been improved by this evening. It is not what he was expecting.'

'Just what was he expecting from Tarkovsky?' Rossel said.

She was about to answer but their host was demanding more attention, this time apparently in response to a challenge to his own Marxist–Leninist purity.

'I tell you I am becoming a leading authority on Marx and Lenin,' he said, 'as befits someone blessed with this face.' He adopted the classic pose of Lenin himself, arm in the air at the Finland Station. '"While the miser is merely a capitalist gone mad, the capitalist is a rational miser"!' he said, declaiming Marx.

The woman dressed in a tutu untangled herself from the arms of the sailor and drunkenly saluted Tarkovsky. Encouraged, Boris tried again. '"Capital is dead labour, which, vampire-like, lives only by sucking living labour . . ."'

Ivan the Terrible jumped to his feet, belched with vigour and joined in enthusiastically. 'These bourgeois vampires will not taste one single drop of my blood!' he said, laughing.

As the room burst into mock applause, Tarkovsky shouted out a passage Rossel remembered well: '"Perseus wore a magic cap that the monsters he hunted down might not see him . . ."'

At this, Dasha, the pretty redhead, ran to the pile of coats and hats stacked on a sofa near the door and grabbed an outsize *ushanka*. She returned and reached up to place it on Tarkovsky's head, pulling it down so it covered his eyes. 'Now you are Perseus, Borya,' she said, smiling.

Tarkovsky began to move around the room, going from person to person, embracing them blindly while shouting, 'I see no monsters!'

'Here,' the guests were shouting, 'Borya, this way – I am a monster!' Some he groped, others he kissed or licked or nibbled, all the while shouting out the mantras of Bolshevism, most of which were drowned out by howls of laughter.

Tarkovsky arrived at a sitting figure. The actor moved his hands across the man's hair and face, shouting out names at random. Then he slapped his victim a couple of times on the face. This time there were no matching shouts and cheers of 'I see no monsters!'

Natalia got off the sofa, walked forward, and removed Boris's hat.

The actor found himself staring into the face of the Head of the Writers' Union.

'Alexander Sergeyevich, I do beg your pardon,' said Tarkovsky.

Fadeyev smoothed his long hair back into place, taking his time about it.

'You didn't finish Marx's quotation,' he said.

'I didn't?'

'You said, "Perseus wore a magic cap that the monsters he hunted down might not see him." But do you know the other half?'

Tarkovsky gulped. 'Yes, Alexander Sergeyevich. *Wir ziehen die Nebelkappe tief über Aug' und Ohr, um die Existenz der Ungeheuer wegleugnen zu können,*' he said.

Rossel's impromptu German lessons in the labour camp had left him with only a basic grasp of the language. But he could tell Tarkovsky knew it well.

'Which means?' said Fadeyev.

'It means, "we draw the magic cap down over our eyes and ears as a make-believe that there are no monsters" . . .'

'Quite so,' said Fadeyev. 'It was Marx's condemnation of the wilful blindness of the bourgeoisie to the evils of their own capitalist system.' He looked around. 'All this frivolity. It suggests to me that you yourself are blind to your own Marxist duties. This spectacle compares poorly to the sobriety of the Soviet leadership and the iron will of our great leader, Comrade Stalin.'

Fadeyev walked to the end of the room, picked up his coat, flung open the door and slammed it behind him.

'Poor darling Boris,' whispered Natalia returning to Rossel. 'Leningrad is a minefield. And almost every day he finds a new way to step on something explosive. I hear that Khrushchev has invited him to declaim and sing for Stalin himself at the Anichkov Palace in a few weeks' time. A big Party gathering – a rarity for Leningrad, and an honour. Boris is petrified.'

She touched him on the arm.

'The snow has stopped. Will you walk me home?'

*

At this hour, they seemed to have Leningrad to themselves. But even if the streets and embankments had been filled with cheering hordes on a May Day celebration, Rossel wasn't sure he would have noticed.

Heaven knew how long they had been walking before they arrived at her building, or even where it was. She leaned forward to kiss him on the cheek and lingered close to him.

He breathed in her perfume.

The scent reminded him of Sofia; a girl he had been in love with when he was a student at the conservatoire.

A relationship that had not ended well.

Natalia looked at him and touched his face.

'Call again,' she said.

She turned and disappeared inside. Rossel listened to her shoes clicking on the stone steps all the way up.

25

In the unexpected winter sunshine, a woman and her two children, a girl and a boy, were throwing snowballs at each other in front of a newly built statue of Rimsky-Korsakov.

The great composer was absorbed in one of his own scores. His right arm was raised a couple of inches above the metallic manuscript, as if surprised to have found a mistake – a false note amid the harmonies of his own operatic rendition of the story of Koshchei the Immortal.

Rossel looked past the statue at the building of the Leningrad Conservatoire, where he had honed his talents as violinist. His mind was a whirl of bittersweet memories – of pieces he had played, concerts he had given, people he had known. People he had loved.

With his right hand, Rossel shielded his eyes from the sun. The thumb of his left tapped at the stubs of its missing little and ring fingers, an occasional nervous habit.

He had been nearing the end of his studies – winning prizes, getting top marks in his recital examinations – when it had all ended. First, an arrest – a denunciation and a midnight knock on the door – and an interrogation from which a violinist could not recover.

Then the Siege of Leningrad. He had been freed from the dungeons of the secret police to be thrown into the city's frantic defence. A reprieve that was meant to be brief.

But he had survived.

In a city of ghosts, this was where his own past was buried. But he seemed fated to return. Not for the first time, he was hoping that someone inside could shed some light on his current mysteries.

*

Professor Belova was a musicologist and an expert on the history of Italian opera. She was short, plump and on the wrong side of sixty. Her grey hair was tied up in a bun, as it always had been, and her wireframe glasses had not moved from the end of her nose in the twelve years since Rossel had last sat in one of her classes. They gave the professor the air of an intellectual purist; someone for whom the mechanics of music were all that mattered, while to actually play it was an indulgence.

Violin and piano teachers got the best rooms at the conservatoire. So Belova had led a nomadic existence as a professor, shunted around the building from lecture to lecture. Today she had led him to a sparse side room containing a few chairs, a small wooden table and a jumble of discarded instrument cases and music stands lining the walls.

'A detective? I am surprised,' she said.

'Me, too.'

'But then, the blockade changed many things.'

'Yes.'

The professor waited for further explanation.

189

'You said you have something to show me,' she said, giving up.

Rossel took copies of the verses taken from the mouths of the victims out of his pocket and laid them on the table.

The ode to Katz:

> *That ignorance is bliss is widely known;*
> *How bless'd the imbecile is with head of bone!*
> *He thirsts not after gold, nor aches for pow'r,*
> *Believes what he is told, hour after hour.*

To Samosud:

> *How gentle is deception*
> *When carried to fruition as intended.*
> *For it defies perception.*

To Akimov:

> *Oh gentle darkness, oh holy and sweet nocturnal hours*
> *That soothe the burning pain of love's desires . . .*

Finally, the GRU's translation of the scroll found in the mouth of Glaskov, the latest victim:

> *Our hearts are racked with hope and then with terror;*
> *For thou strik'st fear into the very marrow*
> *Of gods and mortals with thy bow and arrow.*

Belova straightened her glasses and stared down at them.

'Is there anything significant about these particular lyrics, professor?' Rossel said. 'Why would someone select these pieces and put them together? Why *The Mandrake* – what might its significance be?'

She reread the four verses, mouthing the words.

'They are very different, are they not?' Rossel added.

'Yes and no,' said Belova, looking up. 'Yes, in that they appear to express very different sentiments. But no, in that they have one thing very clearly in common.'

She read them once again.

'Every student who listens to me for the first time thinks how odd it is that I talk about Machiavelli, but he really was a pioneer,' Belova said, almost to herself. 'He wrote *The Mandrake* around 1518. By then he was in exile from the political life of Florence following a return to Medici rule. Indeed, some scholars read the play as an overt critique of the Medici.'

For a moment she fell silent.

'I occasionally lecture on the phenomenon of *canti carnivaleschi,* carnival songs.'

'Carnival songs?'

'Yes. They celebrated the carnival season in sixteenth-century Florence. They were usually satirical and often obscene. But Machiavelli did something completely new with them. He put them in his plays. Mostly because he was infatuated with a woman called Barbera Salutati – a singer, a courtesan, a muse . . . He wrote a series of them for her to perform between the acts of the play. This was decades before Monteverdi, who is popularly regarded as the inventor of opera, had so much as hummed a nursery rhyme.'

'And these verses,' Rossel said. 'They are all from those songs?'

'Yes. Not the play itself but from the songs between the acts. His gift to Salutati, in the hope that she would, shall we say, look favourably upon him.'

Belova turned up her palms in apology. 'That is about all I can tell you.'

'Thank you, Professor,' he replied. 'You have been most useful. I am sorry to drag you away from your duties, I hope they are not too onerous?'

'A lecture on the early work of that inimitable composer, Maestro Vronsky. I met him once. Charming man . . .'

Rossel glanced at his watch.

'Incidentally, what do you think of *The Mandrake*?' he asked.

Belova pushed her glasses a little further up the bridge of her nose.

'In academic circles, where rational argument is often taken to the level of a bloodsport, its meaning is of course disputed. But I, for one, have always sided with Voltaire's interpretation.'

'Voltaire's?'

She nodded.

'He held it was a play that "mocks the religion which Europe preaches". Especially the Pope.'

'*The Mandrake* is an anti-religious work?'

Belova shrugged.

'Well, Voltaire believed it was, and vehemently so. But then he would. And so, I suspect, does the Party and Comrade Stalin himself. Hence the commissioning of that film before the war starring that beautiful man. What was his name? The actor who played Callimaco . . .'

Belova picked up the piece of paper with lyrics on it.

'This one reminds me of a line from *The Prince,* for which Machiavelli is far more famous.'

She pointed at the lyrics that had been found in Samosud's mouth, which began: 'How gentle is deception . . .'

'Can you remember it?' he asked her.

'Yes. "Everyone sees what you appear to be, few experience what you really are."'

'A wise man, Comrade Machiavelli,' said Rossel.

'Other academics assert that *The Mandrake* holds a mirror to his politics. That it expresses, albeit in a frivolous manner, the deep cynicism of his more renowned and lasting political work.'

Belova waved the paper in front of Rossel before placing it back in his hand. She glanced at his missing fingers but made no comment.

Rossel was about to leave when Belova took a breath as if about to speak. She hesitated.

'What is it, professor?'

'You don't think . . . no, I'm being foolish.' She shook her head.

'Think what?'

'Machiavelli wrote those lyrics into the play to win over a woman. Perhaps they might mean the same thing to the murderer as they did to him. Could they, in fact, be a declaration of love?'

26

He was a small man. A big coat, yes – expensive material, well cut. But the wiry frame within it was decidedly small. Nikitin was certain he could reach across the table, put a hand around his scrawny white throat and – a sharp twist would be all it would take – break the man's neck.

And yet . . .

This forgettable Party bureaucrat – nothing more than a clerk – wearing his best coat so he could pretend to be at home in the luxurious surroundings of the Hotel Astoria; right now, this pompous idiot was his best chance.

His whole world.

The room in which they were meeting was of modest size but well appointed. Between them sat a low, polished table, upon which were laid three photographs.

'Kristina is your wife, yes?' said the man. 'Dima, your son. The girl, Svetlana, your daughter.'

Nikitin stared back at him.

'They are, as you correctly suspected, on a list,' the man added. 'I do not need to tell you what that means.'

'But?'

'My minister is still confident that he can intervene and . . .'

'Yes?'

The major heard the note of fear in his own voice. He reached up and touched the scar tissue on his cheek.

How can a man with a face like mine be so afraid?

The clerk sat back.

'They sell lapel pins in the lobby here with pictures of Lenin on them,' he said. 'I'm going to buy some and take them home to my own boy in Moscow. He is a great collector of *znachki*.'

He would have to play along.

'Dima, he collects things, too,' said Nikitin. 'He likes football. Zenit is all he talks about. He has a little book of players' autographs.'

The clerk took a sip of coffee from a gold-rimmed porcelain cup.

'Minister Beria has a little book,' he said. 'You have met him, you know some of his habits. You can imagine the kind of things that get jotted down in it.'

Nikitin leaned forward and picked up the picture of his son.

'I have brought Dima up in a very down-to-earth fashion,' he said. 'I have not encouraged him to think for himself. A simple man does not make life complicated, I tell him. Even though he is too young to understand what I mean. The child thinks only of Grandpa Lenin, of Comrade Stalin, of the Party. My wife and daughter are blameless, too. They do not deserve to be on any list.'

The clerk put down his cup.

'Names go on lists. Names come off them. As I have told you before, my minister assures me he is in a position . . .'

'Enough of the games,' said Nikitin. 'Ask me.'

'Ask you what?'

In the dark night, I know that you, my love, are sleeping . . .

'Whatever it is you need me to do to save my family.'

27

Oleg Novikov, Deputy Chief Engineer of the *Leningradsky Metropoliten*, had the sallow skin of a man who hadn't seen daylight in some time. Once winter was in full swing, he said, he went to work in the dark and went home in the dark, spending the hours in between either in this concrete block just south of the Fontanka or installing signalling in the tunnels.

Aged about sixty, his face was so pockmarked he looked like it had been rolled in gravel. His clothes were grey and functional, and the forefinger and middle finger of his right hand so yellow with nicotine it was as if he had dipped them in paint.

He was also very loud. Listening to him, Rossel felt like he was being hit over the head with a hammer. Novikov spread the large blueprints of the new metro out on the trestle table in his office.

'When my men have built this beauty, the workers of Leningrad will travel to their jobs like they were the fucking Romanovs. You too, Comrade Rossel,' he said. 'You'll feel like your balls have been dipped in caviar and your arse is being transported to Heaven on a feather bed. Eight stations connecting the Moscow railway station in the centre with Avtovo.'

The engineer tapped at the plans.

'We're here, at Tekhnologichesky Institut. And that will just be the start. There are already shaft and service tunnels running directly north, almost up to the top of Nevsky. Eventually, there are even plans to tunnel under the river. Can you imagine that? Peter the Great built this whole city on a swamp but even he didn't have the *khui* on him to tunnel under the Neva.'

Novikov took the cigarette that seemed permanently stuck to his bottom lip out of his mouth and began coughing, bringing up an industrial amount of phlegm. He spat out a dark brown gobbet into an empty metal wastepaper bin, which made a loud pinging sound. Then he slapped his chest twice in an attempt to regain control of himself and pointed at the blueprints again.

'These tunnels will be the death of me, comrade,' he said.

'I do hope not. But sadly, they have been exactly that to Comrade Glaskov.'

'That the name of the poor bastard they found last night?'

You'll never guess what, Nikitin had said. Glaskov was in the same platoon as Katz and his comrades. Isn't that a surprise?

'That is why I wanted to look at these plans,' said Rossel. 'The line from here to Uprising Square and the Moscow Station cannot be the only tunnel, correct? You need sidings, ventilation shafts, storage . . .'

'Yes,' agreed Novikov. 'And like I said, we have already started the excavation for more lines. This one, for example, from here running south to Park Pobedy, is well underway. The tunnels have been carved out as far as Moskovskiye Vorota in the south. Some of the stations, too – or at least where the stations will be once we get round to it. The signalling, though – it's always the bastard, signalling, especially in this damp.'

'But you said service tunnels were running north,' asked Rossel. 'Can a man fit in them?'

'Easily. But they are half-flooded in some areas, they need pumping out. There, look – up to Nevsky. And after Uprising Square, almost up to the river. It's the Neva that's the barrier. We've not cracked it. Yet.'

Rossel looked closer at the map. Up to the river in two directions there were shafts all over the place: for access, ventilation, pumping . . .

'Easy to get in and out?' he said.

'Not until recently. The covers are heavy; metal set in concrete, which sits on a lip inside the shaft. Then you can lock the cover into place, if you have the right key. And it's a long way up and down, fuck your mother. But now we have the lifts working. And enough open tunnels to connect to most of the city centre.'

'Lifts?'

'Service lifts, the builders use them to take down bricks, cement, scaffolding . . .'

'Big enough to transport a body?'

Novikov gave him a stare. 'If you wanted to.'

The wall of Novikov's office was half metal, half glass. On the other side three people – two men and one woman – were in a meeting, all jabbing fingers at a clipboard. The woman seemed to be having the final word. She stuck a pen back in her top pocket and strode off. Rossel watched her go.

'Our senior engineer, Tatiana Vasilyeva, can be ferocious in argument,' Novikov said, winking at him, 'but I am still happy to introduce you, Comrade Detective?'

Rossel shook his head. 'You mistake my—'

An office boy with a pudding-bowl haircut and carrying a Manila file under his arm knocked at the door. Novikov waved him in and took the file.

He pointed at the boy. 'Young Yura here, like all our city's youngsters, has had his head filled with tales of Koshchei the Immortal and other childish rubbish. Even so, it's dark and deserted down there, fuck your mother. Even the parts where we've made the most progress are a long way from being ready. You might not be looking for Koshchei – just a hairy-arsed builder with a map.'

*

After a day of clear skies and only a few flurries, heavy snow was falling from a bleak evening sky.

Ploughing your way along the wide main roads such as Zagorodny in this weather was energy sapping, but, on the quieter side streets like this one, the snow restored to Leningrad its faded beauty.

As he watched the flakes descend, his grandmother's words came to him.

The Lord is all around us, Revol. Even in the snow that falls from the sky . . .

Something she would not have said in front of his mother, a music teacher, and his father, a naval officer, who had been a zealous Marxists – volunteering for collective farms in the summer and teaching literacy and numeracy classes in far-flung regions in winter. Both had even been delegates to Party congresses in Moscow.

Though that had not saved them. They had been arrested as Stalin tightened his grip and eliminated the Old Bolsheviks: those who had been the first footsoldiers of the Revolution. Rossel and his sister, Galya, were branded 'family members of enemies of the people' and placed in an orphanage.

'Your mother, your father, they are traitors to the Soviet Union. So you will not have any difficulty in denouncing them.'

He could still feel the NKVD investigator's question hanging in the air.

Rossel's cheeks reddened.

I didn't have to answer it.

He turned his head skywards, stuck out the tip of his tongue, let a flake fall upon it.

Yes, all around us. Can't you see? Each tiny snowflake is a communion host . . .

'You must forget your mother now, boy,' the investigator had said. 'Just like you, *she* has a traitor's heart . . .'

*

A woman wrapped in a black fur pushed her way out of the metro offices. She was carrying a bunch of roses wrapped in newspaper, holding them close to her chest to protect them from the snow and wind.

Rossel crossed the street.

Vassya saw him move. She slowed and then turned towards him.

'No, Revol,' Vassya said.

'No?'

She gave a deep sigh.

'I thought I made my feelings clear on the plane back from . . .' She stopped and looked around. 'Back from Igarka.'

'I only want your professional assistance. Your engineering knowledge of the underground, your great achievement.'

He was not being completely honest.

The lies we tell, his grandmother's voice again, *God hears them . . .*

'I am a detective once more,' he added. 'In a sense, at least. My congratulations on your new role. I mean it.'

She did not reply.

Rossel pointed to the flowers.

'From a friend?'

Vassya shook her head. She began to walk away but stopped and turned.

'No, he's more than that,' she said.

As Vassya disappeared into the night, a single petal fell from her bouquet and blew towards him.

Rossel reached down to pick it up. But then thought better of it.

*

Why spend another night with the Drugovs?

A man could only spend so much time among the dead before he craved the attentions of the living. There would be laughter and dancing at the house of Boris Tarkovsky, Rossel thought.

But when he arrived, there was none.

Tarkovsky tried to push a plate of smoked fish and boiled potatoes into Rossel's hand but Rossel put it on the dining table. 'You are still a skeleton, Comrade Detective,' Tarkovsky said, 'you must eat, you must drink . . .'

Rossel picked up a small portion of potato salad and ate it.

The actor's own apartment was in a wing of the Yusupov Palace that had once, he said, been the servants' quarters. It consisted of three rooms, all in a line: two living rooms – with a kitchen at the end of the first – and a bedroom.

'Time was I had the run of most of the palace. But since the war – since poor Yakov came to such an unhappy end . . .' Tarkovsky said. He kept his voice low while the radio played.

This discreet version of the actor was unnerving.

Some audiences even Boris prefers to disappoint.

'These days my requests to entertain are more and more frequently denied,' continued Tarkovsky. 'The food and drink come out of my own pocket or from favours. My jolly evenings are not what they were. And Party bureaucrats have taken away my key to the ballroom. I was scolded. Never mind,' he whispered, leaning in. 'I have another key.'

Rossel looked around. Compared to the poky rooms and greasy kitchen of his old *kommunalka* it was luxurious, the type of accommodation ordinary citizens such as himself heard about but rarely had the chance to see from the inside. It had carpet and rugs instead of linoleum; comfortable chairs and a sofa; floor lamps; a round dining table . . .

Tarkovsky had heard the bell, descended the stairs, thrown open the door and beckoned Rossel to follow.

Threading his way in and out of the courtyard and through darkened rooms, he had led the way to his private quarters.

Inside, they passed a marble bust of Lenin that was turned to face the wall.

The actor tutted.

'Whatever I do, Vladimir Ilyich always looks so disapproving,' he said.

He turned the bust the right way around. 'But when I have guests, I always invite him, too.'

'You're a wise man, Comrade Tarkovsky,' said Rossel.

As soon as they sat down, Tarkovsky produced a bottle.

'Ah, Schumann,' he said, closing his eyes to a tenor voice on the radio. ' "*Dichterliebe*". "A Poet's Love". Do you know it?'

'I know it.'

> *Das Mädchen nimmt aus Ärger*
> *Den ersten besten Mann*
> *Der ihr in den Weg gelaufen . . .*

Tarkovsky leaned back and crooned along with the singer. At the end of the verse, he walked over to the radio and turned it up ever so slightly. Returning to his seat, he poured them both stiff measures of vodka and stared at Rossel.

'Have you heard of biomechanics, comrade detective?'

Rossel shook his head.

'I studied drama under Meyerhold's system. Please tell me that you have heard of Meyerhold.'

'The director,' said Rossel. Meyerhold had been shot after a show trial in 1940, but it seemed churlish to mention it.

Tarkovsky exhaled, threw his vodka down his gullet, and sniffed. He took a moment to gather himself.

'Biomechanics is an acting method that emphasises the replication of gesture,' he said. 'In essence, when I copy you, I become you.'

Tarkovsky drew his left arm close to the side of his body. His expression changed. Rossel recoiled. The characteristic positioning of the arm, the light, the tilt of the head, the soft smirk . . . whatever it was, there was the face of Stalin. It had not been there before, at least nothing like so clearly. Now it had appeared. That mix of the avuncular and the cruel, the thickness of the lips and the dark eyes set back in their sockets.

When Stalin was twelve he had been injured in an accident and sustained a lifelong disability to his left arm. As a result, he always held it close to his side.

With a broad smile, the ghost vanished.

'You intrigue me, detective,' said Tarkovsky, as if nothing had happened. 'You appear out of nowhere, a skeleton dressed in a suit. A senior army officer – they say he's in military intelligence? – ferries you around as if you were in the Politburo. Yet here you are, drowning your sorrows with me, an almost total stranger who you cannot possibly trust.'

Rossel took his own turn on the vodka. It was fiery on the gums but smelled clean enough. He picked up a morsel of herring with his fingers and dropped it into his mouth.

'You draw the eye of Natalia Ivaskova – and believe me very few men interest Natalia – yet you fail to pursue her.'

The actor finished his analysis. Then sat back in his chair, cradling his drink, expecting an answer.

'I find it puzzling myself, Comrade Callimaco,' said Rossel.

'Should I invite her over? You can be her Orpheus, she your Persephone. I bet she is a wonderful lover. I can tell just by looking.'

Rossel shook his head. 'I just need a good sleep.' He tapped his glass. 'And perhaps a last one of those.'

Tarkovsky regarded him with disappointment, as if Rossel had proven poor company and of dull intellect.

Und wem sie just passieret,
Dem bricht das Herz entzwei.

In flawless German, the actor sang the lines about the poet's broken heart.

Rossel held out his glass.

'Fair enough,' said Tarkovsky. He poured.

Rossel sat back in his seat and closed his eyes.

Two shots to the temple. A body sitting in a chair.

When I copy you, I become you . . .

Who, Rossel wondered, was Koshchei pretending to be?

28

The House of Books was on Nevsky Prospect, directly opposite Pletnev's lair in the Museum of Atheism. Like most of Leningrad's citizens, Rossel had always loved it. They crowded into its rooms and competed for browsing space in an intense, respectful silence. His mother would bring him here when he was young and buy him either children's books or scores from its music department. Something simple for his young fingers by Prokofiev or Rimsky-Korsakov.

Besides the allure of the music and literature, the building itself had a special charm. Before it became a bookshop it had been built for the Singer sewing machine company and the name was still stencilled on its windows: a last capitalist flag left fluttering on a battlefield they had long since fled.

'At the MGB they call this place the House of Bait,' Nikitin said as he and Rossel pulled up outside.

The heavy grey clouds suspended over the city, becoming visible in the morning half-light, hinted at the snowstorm that was coming.

'Why?' said Rossel.

Nikitin switched off the engine and put the keys in his pocket.

'If you're not reading Marx and Lenin, comrade, why are you reading at all? A suspect with the wrong book is already wriggling on your hook.'

*

Inside, the two men made for a door marked *Administratsiya*.

It was opened by a middle-aged woman wearing a green dress and an icy stare. But as soon as Nikitin brought out his GRU card and barked the name of the man they were here to see, she went pale.

'Fourth floor,' she said, pointing to the ornate stairs. 'Comrade Ivashin is checking our stock.'

*

Rossel pushed the stockroom door open and entered, followed by Nikitin.

Books were everywhere: scattered in untidy, teetering piles on tables, chairs and the floor, or crammed into the shelves.

'Can I help you, comrades?' asked a man on the bottom rung of a small stepladder.

Nikitin pushed a tall pile of books off a chair, tipping them all over the floor, and sat down. He removed his gloves, stretching out the fingers of his right hand. The knuckles cracked.

'I suggest you take a seat, too, Comrade Ivashin,' said the major.

Ivashin – a pale, thin man wearing spectacles – did as he was told.

Just out of Ivashin's sight, Rossel leant against a wall. There was dust in the air that irritated his nose and throat, and the beguiling smell of paper. Faint sounds drifted up from Nevsky Prospect. He noticed a patch of damp on the wallpaper.

Not good for books . . .

All around, Marxist historians and social analysts rubbed covers with economic theoreticians, classic nineteenth-century novelists, avant-garde iconoclasts of the Revolution, folk-tale tellers, mathematicians, collectors of Lenin's speeches, of Stalin's speeches, of butterflies and moths . . . Ethnographers, linguisticians, carefully selected foreign poets, chess grandmasters.

And, of course, Pushkin. The poet was the acknowledged master of Russia's soul. *Better the illusions that exalt us than ten thousand truths . . .* Rossel's mother had often recited that line to him when he was a boy. Back then, he had loved the romantic nature of the sentiment. These days, he preferred the truth. Hungered for it.

'We are here about some missing gold, comrade,' said Rossel.

'Gold? I know nothing of anything like that.'

The bookseller's tone was intellectual. And just a little condescending.

'And yet this room feels a little like a vault to me, Comrade Ivashin,' Rossel said.

'A vault?' Ivashin had to turn to look at him.

Rossel nodded.

'To a man of learning like yourself, these books are like gold bars, are they not? To a professional bibliophile, a miser's hoard?'

Ivashin's blue eyes flickered. He made a show of unconcern, scanning the shelves and nodding in return.

'A vault, yes, indeed. Whenever I come to work, step through the door of this building, I feel . . .'

'Rich?' said Nikitin.

Sensing a trap, Ivashin shook his head.

'Rich? No – a venal bourgeois notion. Unless one means that I have been blessed. Spending every day in the company of Tolstoy and Dostoevsky is the greatest of privileges.' Ivashin thought for a moment. 'And among Marxist–Leninist theory and the teachings of Lenin as well, of course.'

Nikitin looked around the room.

'Dostoevsky, you say?'

'Over there.' Ivashin pointed to a pile a couple of metres away. He got up and took two books from the pile, handed them to the major and then resumed his seat.

'*The Gambler* and *The Idiot*,' he said. '*The Idiot* is a particular favourite of mine. The story of Prince Myshkin, whose unworldly goodness is often mistaken for stupidity.'

Nikitin examined the book. Then dropped it onto the small table he and the bookseller were sitting around.

'Unworldly goodness,' he said. 'That's not a concept I'm particularly familiar with, Comrade Ivashin.'

He reached out and took off Ivashin's glasses. The bookseller blinked but did not move. Nikitin balanced the glasses on his own nose.

'These are good, comrade. Very good. With these on . . .'

He closed one eye – his good one. 'Even like this, I can see right inside you.'

The major took off the glasses and began to crumple the frame in his hand.

Ivashin reached out to snatch them back.

'No, I . . .'

The right lens popped and skidded across the floor. The major loosened his grip. Although now buckled, the frames resumed something of their normal shape.

Nikitin leaned forward. 'I have seen your sort a million times in the cells, Comrade Ivashin,' he said through his teeth. 'Read a thousand stories, so they think, "How much trouble can it be to invent a new one to fool this imbecile interrogator."' Nikitin picked up the Dostoevsky novel again. 'This shit-kicking idiot who never went to university, like I did.'

Rossel picked up Ivashin's glasses and placed them back on the bookseller's head. Something about the gesture, its unexpected kindness, touched Ivashin.

He began to sob.

'Coffee, I think, comrade – a warm reviving cup to keep out the winter chills? Then you can tell us everything you know about the gold?' said Rossel.

Nikitin stood up.

'I'll get that frosty bitch downstairs to make us some.'

*

Ivashin was holding on to his coffee cup with both hands as if it was the last lifejacket on a boat in stormy seas.

Rossel took out his notepad.

'We have been investigating the attempted sale of a gold medallion that a welder called Katz tried to sell on the black

211

market. It has the name of a German city, Neubrandenburg, engraved on it. Katz came to our attention by virtue of being murdered and mutilated by the killer every citizen in Leningrad is afraid of. Koshchei the Invisible.'

Ivashin pulled a handkerchief from a trouser pocket and dabbed at his eyes.

'I know nothing of this man, this Katz . . .'

'Your file says you were a committed Communist, member of the Komsomol, that you joined the fight against Hitler in October 1941,' said Rossel. 'You appear to have been in units that followed the front line, which meant that you saw very little fighting until Berlin. Your experience in the capital of the Third Reich must have been a brutal introduction to warfare.'

'It was . . .' Ivashin began. But his memory of that time seemed to defy expression.

'You were in a Guards platoon along with a man called Pavel Grachev. Of course, if I am wrong in any of this, please correct me. And address your remarks to Comrade Major Nikitin, who will be happy to note them down for further investigation. Until we get to the truth, and to Soviet justice, the goal of every investigation.'

Ivashin's imagination regarding the path of Soviet justice would do the rest, Rossel thought.

The bookseller was breathing hard.

'All right, all right. There were six of us – Sergeant Grachev, and five men he trusted.'

'Why did he trust you?' said Rossel.

Ivashin reflected for a moment. 'Different reasons,' he said. 'Akimov was in his own mould: a killer, and none too choosy about who he killed.'

'Akimov?' said Nikitin. The major gave Rossel a look.

'Yes,' said Ivashin. 'He was a cruel man. Said he'd left his family behind in Minsk when the Germans came crashing through. Never bothered to find out what had happened to them, and didn't seem to care.'

He emitted a sound that was more a shudder than a sigh. 'You understand, we were bound together by war. Afterwards there was nothing to keep us together. But . . .'

'But?' said Nikitin.

'Grachev would hold reunions, and for some reason those of us who were still alive would always go. Even though I didn't have much in common with the others, the blood we'd seen together was a bond I could not break. And Grachev liked to talk when he was drunk. Mostly about women he had been with. I suppose he needed an audience.'

'The others, please, Comrade Ivashin,' Rossel pressed him.

The bookseller looked frightened. 'Katz and Samosud?'

'Yes.'

'Volodya Katz was a simple man,' said Ivashin. 'He believed every word in *Krasnaya Zvezda*, he lapped up the agitprop entertainment for the troops. Friendly enough, though. Brave. He trusted Grachev to keep him alive. The sergeant was fond of violence, but he was not entirely reckless with the lives of those under his command.'

'And Samosud?'

'Misha Samosud was another Jew. He'd been one of the first into the death camps. Majdanek, maybe? And had seen plenty of mass graves left by the Einsatzgruppen. It changed him, took something away that had been inside. Grachev replaced it, I think.'

'And you?'

Ivashin hesitated.

'I . . . Well, before you get to me, there was Zvirbulis. Viktor. The only luck poor Viktor ever had was bad luck. It made him wise. He was killed on the very last day of the war.'

'Not wise enough to dodge a Kraut bullet, eh?' said Nikitin.

The bookseller looked down at his hands.

'He was shot by an NKVD officer who mistook him for a deserter,' he said. He was quiet for several seconds. 'Viktor never took a backward step,' he added in a small voice.

Nikitin chuckled.

'I think I understand. You had a soft spot for this Viktor?'

Ivashin lowered his head but did not answer. Sexual relations between men brought a punishment under Article 154a of the Soviet Criminal Code of up to five years' deprivation of liberty. Not expanding on this part of his story would be prudent; silence would serve Ivashin best.

So that was the squad. Sergeant Grachev and his band of Red Army reprobates.

'So how did you get hold of that gold?' Rossel asked.

Ivashin wiped his brow. 'It was in the very last days of the battle for Berlin,' he said. 'Right at the end. It was still savage, mind – young boys and grandads would pop out of nowhere and hit one of us before we could mow them down. Booby traps in every house. But there was time to go looking for souvenirs.'

'Did everyone do that?' asked Nikitin.

'Yes, of course. Some of the military postal depots couldn't keep up. Rugs, clocks, fancy tables and chairs, clothes . . . anything that you couldn't get back home, we'd strip it. It was our due – right, comrades?'

Nikitin nodded and slapped his thigh. 'Yes, comrade. After what those bastards did to us, to our Motherland, the property of the Hitlerites became *our* property.'

Ivashin started to tell his tale with greater enthusiasm.

'So one night we are out on the hunt and we see two or three men next to a blown-up Tiger tank on a bridge crossing a railway line. It was near a station, I remember that. So we opened fire with everything we had. Two minutes later we're going through the uniforms of two dead Nazis. One must've got away. And next to these corpses is a knapsack. Well, we couldn't believe our luck.'

Ivashin rubbed his nose.

'Days of rummaging through the pants of dead Germans for a few cigarettes or photos of darling little Claudia or Heidi and suddenly it's gold medallions all round. One each. And some other stuff. We grabbed it and got the hell out of there.'

'What other stuff?' interrupted Rossel.

Ivashin thought about it.

'*Juno* cigarettes – there was some squabbling over them, I can tell you. A water canteen of some sort, an expensive one. A book. And a picture of a saint, a Russian one; a proper ikon, about the size of a big book, covered in gold leaf – Akimov saw it as a sign. And a dirty postcard from some French tart on the front. That's all.'

Rossel closed his eyes to help him think, then opened them again.

'So who, Comrade Ivashin, got the gold?'

BEN CREED

'Like I said, we all did. One each, and an extra for Grachev. By themselves they were useless. You can't just go out and sell Nazi gold in the Soviet Union. You have to smelt it, mix it with other metals. You have to know someone who can do that without snitching on you or blackmailing you. We agreed to wait a few years until all the fuss over hunting for Nazi gold, art, antiques, weapons, rare books, all that had died down.'

'Looks like Comrade Katz got impatient,' said Nikitin.

'So where is yours?' asked Rossel.

Ivashin didn't answer.

Nikitin cleared his throat and stood.

The bookseller put his hands up. 'All right,' he said.

He went over to the shelves and pulled down a large book. On the front and spine were embossed the words: *Observations on the Use of Mechanised Agriculture on Collective Farms in the Ukrainian SSR, Vol III.*

Ivashin opened it. Inside a circular hole cut out of the pages, which appeared to be largely blank, was a medallion.

Rossel got up to take a closer look. There was the eagle and swastika emblazoned on one side. And the same word round the edge. Neubrandenburg.

'Anything else in that knapsack?' asked Rossel.

'The dirty postcard, like I said,' answered Ivashin. 'And a book.'

'A book?

Ivashin nodded.

'Yes,' he said. 'But I never had the sergeant down as much of a bibliophile. He probably used the pages to wipe his backside with.'

216

Rossel took a step forward. 'You're to come with us, Comrade Ivashin.'

The colour drained from the bookseller's cheeks.

'To prison?'

Rossel shook his head.

'I need you to take us to Grachev's old apartment.'

29

The light was closing in as Rossel, Nikitin and Ivashin stood before what remained of Grachev's former lodgings.

Thanks to the Luftwaffe's nightly bombing raids during the city's 900-day siege, Rossel had seen many buildings like this one. With only the facade still in one piece, it was an enigmatic stone mask concealing a past that had been eviscerated. Its window frames, with peeling paint, containing only shattered glass. Out of one billowed a single white curtain, as if a belated flag of surrender. A table and chairs were visible in a room that now had no walls or ceiling. A huge and twisted steel beam dangled at an unlikely angle: a surreal sword of Damocles hanging over a child's crib.

The street was near the railway lines, which probably explained why it had taken such a pounding from all those Dorniers and Heinkels. It looked as though there had been ten apartment blocks like this one before the war. Now, only three were left standing on one side of the street.

The rest were just holes in the ground, rapidly filling with snow.

'This is it,' said Ivashin. 'We had a reunion here, not long after the war had ended – that time it was just me, the sergeant, Katz and Samosud. We drank a lot and swapped tales of valour, the way old soldiers do. They were rebuilding everything round here. And then one day a couple of years ago – spring of 1950, I think – a labourer working on the site next door to this building took his drill and drilled right into an unexploded bomb. No more labourer, no more building and not much left of the two on either side. That's what Grachev told Katz, anyway. Those two were close. Thick as thieves.'

'Where was his apartment, can you remember?' said Nikitin.

Ivashin shrugged. 'Not the exact position, but it was on the fifth floor, I remember that much.'

'Let's go around the back,' said Rossel. 'There's too much rubble blocking the front door.'

The rear of the block was in better condition. A fire escape had buckled and at its base had peeled away from the brick, but, after a couple of failed attempts, Nikitin managed to hoist himself up, followed by the others. After a storey and a half the floors were in a better condition and they clambered into the apartment block via an empty door frame.

The building was in complete darkness. Using light from Nikitin's torch to pick their way through the debris, they made their way along the fourth floor. From there, an interior stairwell led to the fifth. They turned left and found themselves at the end of a long, wide corridor with doors on either side. The torchlight picked out a mural of workers harvesting sunflowers on the wall, still perfect. At the far end, a glass vase containing dried stalks stood on a small wooden sideboard. Rossel had the strange sense that, at any moment, one of the doors might open and a laughing family, buttoned up to keep out the winter chill, would emerge, heading for a day in one of the city's museums or galleries.

'It's this one, I think,' said Ivashin, stopping in front of the first of two doors on the right.

Nikitin tried the handle.

It was locked.

The major stepped back and kicked at the lock three times. The door buckled in the frame. Rossel pushed it open.

Unlike the corridor, the large communal apartment was badly damaged. There were holes in the floor and the three men had to balance on a steel beam to cross one of them. The layout was similar to Rossel's old *kommunalka* – a big main kitchen, a couple of bathrooms and, off a central corridor, various small rooms. The ones on the right-hand side had all been damaged in the explosion. The ones on the left were in better condition.

Ivashin stopped at the last left-side door and pushed it.

They went in.

Nikitin ran his torch around the walls. Grachev's former bedroom was about three metres by two, reasonably large by *kommunalka* standards. But it had not escaped the explosion – the window had been blown in and glass was scattered across the floor. Next to the window was a gaping hole through which a bitter wind blew. There was a small table and couple of chairs, and a metal-framed single bed with a rotting mattress. At one end was a small stove in the middle of a high bench built into the wall.

Rossel, shivering, looked through the window and clapped his hands together to warm them up. He took a *papirosa* from his pocket and lit it.

'Can I have one?' Ivashin pointed at the cigarette.

'It's my last, but . . .' He handed the cigarette to Ivashin, 'I'm sensing, Comrade Ivashin, that today hasn't been one of your better days.'

Ivashin took the cigarette and sat down in one of the chairs. His hands were trembling. He shut his eyes for a moment, steadying himself with the smoke.

'Here, Rossel, have you seen this? I found Grachev's girlfriend.'

Nikitin shone his torch on the wall just above Grachev's bed, picking out a black-and-white postcard of a naked woman. Rossel reached out and took it. A name was printed on the front. Odette. On the back was something written in French and an address in Germany.

'Odette. That's the name Grachev mentioned to the boy he escaped with,' said Nikitin. 'He swore he was going to find her.'

'Unless he simply meant he was coming back here,' said Rossel. 'Comrade Ivashin,' he called out. 'Does the name Odette mean anything to you?'

Ivashin did not reply.

'Comrade Ivashin, does the name . . .'

As he spoke, Rossel turned to face the veteran.

Ivashin was sitting still in the chair; his head lolling backwards, the *papirosa* sticking to his lip, its tip glowing.

'Hit the floor!' Rossel shouted to Nikitin.

Nikitin did. Then he fumbled for his torch and killed the light.

'Sniper?' he whispered.

'Yes.'

Ivashin's body shook briefly, as though attempting to quell a fit. A second bullet hole appeared in his forehead, only millimetres from the first. He slumped forward and the chair crashed over.

Nikitin rolled his body three times and then, scrambling on all fours, hurled himself out of the room.

Making sure he could not be seen above the bottom of the window frame, Rossel inched towards the door.

An empty vodka bottle next to Grachev's bed exploded.

From the corridor, Nikitin reached in with one hand and, grabbing Rossel by his coat lapels, dragged him out of the door.

Both men got to their feet and started running.

*

Avoiding the last few broken stairs, Rossel leapt from the fire escape, landing almost knee-deep in a drift.

Nikitin jumped after him.

'Fuck your mother!'

'Are you all right?'

Nikitin stood up, grimacing.

'Ankle.' He swore again, putting his hands on his knees.

'I can't run but if I can get to the car, I can use it for cover.'

'Your car is on the sniper's side of the building.'

'Then you'd better kill the bastard, hadn't you, Rossel?'

Rossel pulled out his pistol and started to make his way towards the front of the building.

In the war, the rules to avoid getting shot by a sniper had been simple. Stay in your trench or shell hole, 'keep your fucking head down, comrade,' and, at night, 'don't show your stupid fucking face while having a smoke.'

Pulling out your pistol and charging towards the opposite trench was something only the rawest of recruits might do. Some country bumpkin who had watched *Moscow Strikes Back* far too many times and could hear its soundtrack – Tchaikovsky's Fifth – booming in his ears. A siren voice of heroism.

But what choice did he have?

Rossel patted the seabird on his chest once.

He had survived the bloodiest moments of the war at the Volkhov Front.

Stranded. Pinned down. Refused permission to retreat.

It had been a slaughterhouse.

And yet, he thought, I survived.

He patted the bird again and began to move forward at pace.

After a moment, he reached the edge of the building.

To fire into Grachev's room the sniper had to have been in one of the opposite blocks at about the same height.

Nearly all the windows were dark.

They would have moved. Unless they had an exit planned and could for the time being sit tight, scanning the white street below for slow-moving dark figures.

Luck. In the labour camp, he had made a god of her . . .

Rossel began to run.

He dived behind a van that was missing a wheel, its axle propped up on paint cans.

Hitting the ground, he rolled from the back doors towards the front, hoping the rusting engine would stop a bullet.

On cue, a dull thump.

A hole appearing in the rear wheel arch.

He scanned the ground ahead.

That burnt-out tree – thick enough?

'Hey, you – bastard!'

Nikitin's voice carrying from the other side of Grachev's building. Followed by more curses and taunts.

Enough time?

Rossel got up and ran for the tree, feeling as if time had slowed. He tripped and fell, rolled again, thought he heard something smack into the ground.

Ten paces later he reached the rough walls.

Safe. For now.

He rattled a side door to the building. Only partly on its hinges, it swung open. Pistol in hand, he ran to the stairs, peering ahead into dim light.

Step by step he moved steadily upwards: weapon held high, back pressed into the walls, his breath coming in short, sharp bursts.

Every corridor had half a dozen doors, plus three more on the landing.

At last, he reached the fifth.

He crept along the corridor, pushing at doors to see if any of them gave, but none did.

Then, just as he was about to return to the stairwell, he saw a door to his left, slightly ajar.

He kicked it open. Ran through.

'Fuck your mother . . .'

Nothing. An empty space.

Engine noise. Then a shot.

Rossel thrust his head through an open window.

Nikitin was in the middle of the road, legs apart, blazing away at a retreating motorcycle. The bike teetered as it hit a patch of ice but then, its engine misfiring, turned a corner and disappeared.

*

Ivashin's *papirosa* had gone out but was still hanging from the lips of the dead man. Rossel took it.

'Flying cap, plus a black leather coat. Long. Face covered by a scarf, nice and tight,' said Nikitin.

'That's all you saw of him?'

The major nodded.

'You didn't notice anything else?'

Nikitin shook his head.

'A small man, that's all, like I said.'

Rossel lit the remnants of the cigarette.

'Habits of the camps, eh?' said Nikitin.

'The army,' said Rossel. 'A smoke was never a gift, always a loan.'

Rossel sat down on Grachev's mattress.

'I don't know how I'm going to explain this total *bardak* to the general,' sighed Nikitin. 'He can be an unforgiving man. There are stories.'

'Stories?'

'In Ukraine, in the thirties, when they were closing all the churches: they say he built a bonfire of Bibles and vestments,' said the major, 'and then put the Archimandrite of Poltava on top of it . . .'

Rossel blew out some smoke.

'"Fire goes before Him. And burns up His adversaries round about . . ."' he said.

'I'm not with you.'

'Something my grandmother used to say. And an old Armenian priest I once met. They had things in common.'

Nikitin shrugged.

'Either way, they say the archimandrite sang the Litany like an angel while Pletnev's men roasted him to death.'

The major stood up and rubbed his hands together. He pointed to the little gas stove. 'Fuck, it's cold. I wish we had some tea to boil up on that.'

'Yes, I would . . .'

Rossel's voice trailed away. He stood up and walked towards the stove.

'Give me that torch,' he said.

'Why? What is it?'

Rossel knelt down. Something was propping up one of the legs of the bench that stretched along the wall. A piece of cardboard.

And under that . . . a book.

'Heave this up a notch,' he said.

Nikitin did and Rossel pulled the book free. He held it up and blew the dust from its front cover.

'Something?' said Nikitin.

Rossel showed the major what he had found. It was a slim volume with thick leather covers, with the title embossed in gold.

'*Der Fürst*. Niccolò Machiavelli. *The Prince*, but in German. Grachev hardly read a paper. This must be the book from the knapsack. It has to be.'

'The book Ivashin was talking about is by Machiavelli, too? Koshchei's favourite author? A big coincidence, don't you think?'

Rossel looked at the cover again, his mind racing.

'Or, much more likely, not a coincidence at all.'

He opened *The Prince*. On the first page was an ornate bookplate. At the top were the words EX LIBRIS in white letters on a black scroll. Below that, an eagle with wings unfurled perched on top of a swastika, the latter encased in a laurel wreath.

And underneath, in Gothic type, a name.

Adolf Hitler.

ACT 3
HERO

30

Just before sunrise, with the surrounding pines, firs and birches draped in snow, they waited, slumped on opposite ends of a wooden bench.

'She's late,' muttered Nikitin, sunk deep into his greatcoat.

His words were barely audible but Rossel could see them – puffs of breath marked each syllable.

Captain Morozova, a code and cipher specialist within the GRU, had insisted on somewhere out of the way. Association with Major Nikitin – the Directorate's newest recruit and still tainted by his previous career with the rival MGB – was not much sought-after by his colleagues.

The spot was well chosen. In this far corner of Pavlovsk Park all approach lines were visible. The tracks leading this way were just that – tracks, not paths, nothing a mother pushing a pram would tackle, not in two feet of snow. Most people kept close to the palace and the other imperial monuments nearby.

'She'll come,' said Rossel.

Nikitin grunted, then resumed grumbling. 'I don't trust the GRU and they don't trust me. We shouldn't have told them about the book.'

'We have to show General Pletnev we are making progress,' said Rossel. 'How else could we decipher any messages that might be in it? Like you, I understand barely any German. And even less about codes.'

They sat in silence. Instead of the sun coming up, the dark-grey sky merely grew paler, shade by shade, revealing a light mist hanging at head height.

It was Nikitin who spotted the figure first – an androgynous black stroke against a white canvas.

'There she is,' said Nikitin.

The codebreaker strode towards them. However cautious she had been in their choice of rendezvous, she was making little attempt to make it look like a chance encounter.

Within his coat pocket, Rossel toyed with the safety catch of his pistol.

When the new arrival was twenty paces away, Nikitin stood, shoulders square, glowering.

'Comrade Captain Morozova,' he said.

The woman nodded. She was very short, red-cheeked and hard-eyed.

'Here,' she said.

She took out the leather-bound book and tossed it at Nikitin, who caught it at boot height. She thrust her hands back into her pockets.

'You wasted your time and mine, Comrade Major,' the captain said. 'Nothing in invisible ink, none of the pages can be split into other pages. Too many passages are underlined for anything to stand out, either as marked or unmarked.'

Rossel tugged his coat tight around his shoulders in annoyance.

She hasn't even tried . . .

'What about the numbers at the back?' he said.

The codebreaker looked at him for the first time, apparently not liking what she saw.

'The series of numbers at the back of the book *might* be some sort of code,' she said, 'but unless we have the key – the one-time pad, as it is known – which could be in another book entirely, they are meaningless.'

'What kind of analysis did you run?' he asked.

'The usual – frequency analysis of the most common German letters, patterns of repetition. I gave up after half an hour. It was obvious that further efforts would be pointless.'

Nikitin looked disbelieving. 'Perhaps you missed something? Some little bit of the language, some unusual Fritz phrasing . . .'

'Missed something?' Her voice hardened. 'Comrade Major, I speak extremely good German – but I don't need to,' she said. 'The chances are that this is not even a Hitlerite artefact. A fake of some sort. In the West, there is already a market for memorabilia of this kind, where items are commonly counterfeited. Twenty million Soviet citizens killed by that man and the capitalists just see that as good advertising. The toilet brush Hitler used would set a bourgeois back a month's wages. This is most likely the property of an ordinary officer who plastered in a stolen book plate. Perhaps in the hope of selling it on the black market at a later date. Did you read the inscription on the page opposite the plate?'

Nikitin opened the book at the front and read aloud.

'This bit? *Jetzt . . . bin . . . ich . . .*'

He gave up – 'Rossel, you read . . .'

'*Jetzt bin ich Soldat und Ihr treuer Diener,*' snapped Morozova before Rossel could do so. 'It means "now I am a soldier and your loyal servant". Oberst Halder, 115th SS Panzer Division, 22nd Brigade, March 12 1945. In every detail, nonsense.'

They waited for her to explain.

'Humour us, comrade,' said Rossel.

She turned her back on them.

'The SS didn't even have 115 Panzer divisions,' she said as she began to walk away. 'Thank you for wasting my time, comrades. As I said, your precious artefact is a fake.'

'We need more time,' said Rossel as they watched her walk away.

'We haven't got any,' Nikitin replied. 'The general is a man who wants results, and fast.'

He got up and kicked at the snow.

'She may not have brought us the goods we wanted but that snotty bitch has got me thinking,' he said.

Rossel turned to him.

'Not normally your style.'

'About Koshchei. A small man, you said, from what you saw.'

'Quite small, yes.'

Nikitin reached down into the snow and packed some of it into a ball. Then he half-heartedly tossed it in the direction of the diminutive figure of Captain Morozova.

'Or . . .'

Rossel stood up and, to his own surprise, slapped Nikitin on the back.

'A woman,' he said. 'Of course.'

*

A one-legged man of Rossel's age in a smart blue uniform was bellowing to all passengers that the heavy snowfall of the past two days had caused disruption to the timetable.

The next train to Leningrad took forty minutes to arrive and was three-quarters full. But Nikitin had the kind of face people didn't want to sit next to. So, he had little trouble locating a quiet corner. The major stared out of the window, brooding, as Rossel studied the book.

There were indeed numerous passages underlined. Scribbles in the margin, the work of an agitated hand. Phrases in German that were apparently taken from a different text entirely. Some of those had now been annotated in turn in Russian, presumably by Morozova. From *Mein Kampf*? Or from his last testament?

Occasionally there was nothing but an exclamatory *Ja!* of critical approval and an arrow towards a particular paragraph. As though Hitler – if it was him – was saying, *My thoughts exactly, Herr Machiavelli.*

Flicking through, Rossel saw a dark red line along one section of the text that he had not noticed previously:

Jeder sieht, was du scheinst. Nur wenige fühlen, wie du bist.

The codebreaker had taken the trouble to translate it:

Everyone sees what you appear to be. Few experience what you really are.

As the train moved through a thickening blizzard back towards Leningrad, he began to doubt Captain Morozova's dismissal of *The Prince*. He turned it over and over with his broken hands. Rationally, it was just another war trophy. A Nazi bookplate made it neither more or less than a collection of paper. But its link to Grachev, to the murdered men . . . the inscription, the numbers in the back.

It had an aura, like a sacred object. Or a satanic one. In his hands, it felt like a mythical chest that he could not open. But he was certain that within it lay the answer to his quest.

Rossel stared down at the underlined quotation. His thoughts travelled to the besieged bunker near the Reich Chancellery in April 1945, and the mind of the man who most likely had drawn the line. Hitler, too, must at some point have gazed down at this exact page. Perhaps when all around him Berlin was in flames and Marshal Zhukov's soldiers were only days away from dragging him out into the light and . . .

Everyone sees what you appear to be. Few experience what you really are.

Rossel glanced around at his fellow train passengers. Sombre, mute and inscrutable. At the very end, he wondered, did the little Austrian corporal who had set the world on fire understand the impossibility of ever truly knowing another human being? And see it as the ultimate means of escape?

The train halted at a signal. Rossel stretched out his limbs as far as he was able in the confined space.

Something else was bothering him. The sniper. *How did I not realise she was a woman?*

'In the Great Patriotic War, the People's Commissariat of Defence set up special Sniper Training Schools,' he said. 'I remember *Pravda* crowing about it. "Brave Soviet women cradle their rifles as they would their children." That kind of thing. Heard of them?'

Nikitin nodded. 'That girl, what was she called? Comrade Shanina. I think she was one.'

Roza Shanina had more than fifty kills to her name and had received the Medal for Courage before she was killed in action. For a while, all the snipers, men and women, were lauded and lionised throughout the Soviet Union.

'The main school was in Moscow but they trained a few of them up here during the blockade,' said Rossel. 'They closed everything down for the women even before the end of the war.'

Still feeling pleased with his own detective powers, Nikitin smiled.

'Of course they did,' he said. 'But a sniper would never forget her training.'

31

Back in his apartment, Rossel stared out at Koshchei's mist-covered realm, where more than half a million souls lay in Piskaryovskoye Cemetery. He remembered his grandmother and her friends sharing the tale of 'the Deathless, the Immortal'. How their eyes would gleam when they talked of the diabolical spell that protected him, relishing the terror they inspired in a small child.

How Koshchei would hide his soul in nested objects to preserve his immortality. In one version, in a needle that was hidden inside an egg, which is carried by a bird who flew away so no one could catch it.

The snipers he had been thinking of were all men. Vasily Zaitsev, Ivan Sidorenko, Semyon Nomokonov. Heroes of the Soviet Union, their tales often repeated in newsreels and the papers.

But what would Koshchei do differently if she was a woman?

His own prejudice had blinded him. The locket should have opened his eyes. What stung his pride most of all was that Nikitin had seen it before he had.

The sniper must have been tracking Ivashin and had followed them to Grachev's old apartment. Did she know about the book?

A murderer who puts the words of Machiavelli into the mouths of her victims, following them to a place where they discover a unique copy of *The Prince*. The two cases seemed to fit together.

Perhaps, Rossel thought as he took a step back from the window, one is nested inside the other? Hidden away like Koshchei's soul.

*

Rossel walked back to the piano, lowered its music stand and shut the lid. The watching Drugov family had haunted him long enough. Now he needed their help. He had been plonking out one of Medtner's piano sonatas to help him think.

It hadn't worked.

He slapped his damaged left hand down on the lid. He needed a composer who could make a virtue of simplicity – Prokofiev, perhaps. Maybe he could prevail upon the composer to create a piece specially tailored to his own unique needs – 'Concerto for a Man with Missing Fingers' – and to make it a stumbling, jazz-like reverie filled with lost hopes and bleak, discordant frustration. Although, in composing such a piece, Prokofiev would need to take care to avoid the Soviet crime of 'formalism'; not produce the 'muddled, nerve-racking' sounds for which that brutal arbiter of taste Andrei Zhdanov had condemned him and so many other composers.

Since Zhdanov's decree, the soul of a Soviet artist could only soar upward in a pre-agreed direction. The rubber stamps of Party bureaucrats had smudged black ink on their hearts.

Photographs of each member of the missing Drugov family stared at Rossel from the top of the piano. Like a detective in an English country house murder mystery, he had assembled his audience.

Captain Morozova's observation was still troubling him – *'The SS didn't even have 115 Panzer divisions . . .'*

Nikitin had confirmed this as they had parted company near the Admiralty. 'Just under forty, depending on how you count them,' he'd said. 'Most of the later ones were cannon fodder, made up of Hitler Youth or pensioners or desperate foreign collaborators who preferred to be slaughtered in battle than face Soviet justice. I was one of those who had to root them out, get them to confess, bang heads together, and sometimes . . . Well, you get the picture. So that's how I know. At the end, entire German armies existed only inside Hitler's head. I should have realised, but she's right. There was no 115th SS Panzer Division.'

Rossel walked over to a little stove he had set up. He warmed his hands on a teapot and his insides with the tea. The apartment was still very cold. Bureaucrats decided when the district's heating was turned on and off and had finally relented a few days ago, but it took time for the entire block to warm through, even with, as now, every radiator throbbing.

He lit a *papirosa* and started pacing up and down.

'Let us assume that it is not a fake,' he addressed the Drugov family members in turn, showing them each the book. 'Who props up something with Hitler's copy of Machiavelli's *The Prince*? Most people would use a piece of cardboard, or half a brick, or a piece of wood. But Sergeant Grachev *would* prop up a table with a Nazi copy of *The Prince*, because he took it from a dead German in Berlin and brought it back to Leningrad without having the first idea of its value.'

He took a sip from his cup.

'In sum, is it plausible that this book came back from Berlin with Sergeant Pavel Grachev, but that he was indifferent to it because it wasn't a gold medallion with a swastika on it? Yes, it is plausible. The sergeant's kitchen stove was unsteady and he used what was to hand to solve the problem.'

The museum director stared back at Rossel, hostile and disdainful. Had he, Drugov, been afforded this level of reasoned inquiry at his own trial – if he'd even had a trial? Of course not.

Rossel appealed next to Madame Drugova, stout and matronly with a kind face.

'At the end of the war, members of the SS took off their uniforms and tried to pretend they were regular army or civilians,' he told her. 'But Oberst Halder, Commander, purportedly of the 115th SS Panzer Division, 22nd Brigade, which did not exist, was happy to inscribe his name in a gift to the Führer himself a matter of days before the Third Reich ended.'

Now Rossel looked into the bright, hopeful eyes of the young teenage violinist, Anna, his favourite of the family. A handwritten note near the bottom of the picture frame read: 'Alas, our little Anna loves only Borodin, Schubert and Arensky!' The note was adorned with three kisses.

'The key point, dear Anna, is this. If the book is significant and if Oberst Halder is real, then consider the fact that when inscribing a gift to the Führer, a German officer does not get his own Panzer division wrong.'

Rossel sat down and stubbed out his cigarette.

'Unless, of course, he did it on purpose.'

32

'I need a German speaker.'

'At this time?'

Tarkovsky was still half asleep and bewildered to be roused at five a.m. He was also, Rossel could tell, a little relieved to see that it was him, and not the people who usually came knocking shortly before dawn.

It had taken hours of staring at words he didn't understand before inspiration struck. Hours of examining *The Prince* in German, from cover to cover, looking for something that the GRU codebreaker had missed in her impatience.

The clue, when he saw it, was so simple that he'd spent several minutes berating himself before throwing on his coat and setting out for the actor's apartment in the Yusupov.

'It's to do with your old friend Machiavelli, if that piques your interest, Comrade Callimaco,' said Rossel. 'A quick translation and then I will be gone.'

Tarkovsky thought for a moment.

'I'll need my glasses,' he said, opening the door a little wider. 'Whatever it is, it's got to be better than the horse-shit they have been writing for me at Lenfilm recently And I'm not back on set until eleven.'

*

'I want you to read from this page for me.' Rossel tapped a finger on the book, which lay open on a small coffee table between them. They were sitting in Tarkovsky's living room, next to his piano.

Tarkovsky picked up the book.

'Page 115?'

Rossel nodded.

Captain Morozova had found the cipher, or part of it. She just hadn't realised it.

A German officer does not get his own Panzer division wrong.

Back at the apartment, the insight had finally led him from 115th Panzer to page 115. 22nd Brigade? That had stumped him for a while. Then he had counted down 22 lines from the top, to find nothing of significance.

But 22 lines up from the bottom . . .

'See that heading,' he pointed it out for Tarkovsky.

Von der Grausamkeit und Milde, und ob es besser ist, geliebt oder gefürchtet zu werden.

'Can you translate it and the text beneath it for me?'

Under it was a lone unmarked passage. An island of virgin text in a sea of scrawlings, underlinings and margin notes:

Denn man kann von den Menschen insgemein sagen, daß sie, undankbar, wankelmütig, falsch, feig in Gefahren und gewinnsüchtig sind; solange du ihnen wohltust, sind sie dir ergeben und bieten dir, wie oben gesagt, Gut und Blut, ihr Leben und das ihrer Kinder an, solange die Gefahr fern ist; kommt sie aber näher, so empören sie sich.

'Let's have some music?' said Tarkovsky, pushing his glasses further up the bridge of his nose.

He turned the radio on.

'*Swan Lake*. Of course. The epitome of banality, perfect for pacifying the masses. When is it not *Swan Lake*?'

Yet it would do nicely to mask their voices from any eavesdroppers.

The actor beckoned Rossel closer and cleared his throat.

'*Von der Grausamkeit und Milde.* "On Cruelty and Kindness. Or whether it is better to be loved than feared."'

Tarkovsky paused, straightened his back, and assumed what he presumably imagined to be the bearing of a fifteenth-century Italian diplomat. He picked up the book with his left hand and turned the palm of his right out, as if delivering a lecture. Then, translating as he read, he began to declaim in the manner of a sorcerer intoning a spell.

'"Because one can say this in general of men,"' he continued. '"That they are ungrateful" . . . not sure about that next one, something about stumbling – faltering? "False, cowardly in the face of dangers, and mercenary. As long as you benefit them," so, er, as long as you are good towards them, "they are to you beholden," or maybe devoted, "and will offer you," as I said above, "goods and blood, their lives and that of their children, as long as the peril is far away. But should it come closer, so do they turn on you."'

Tarkovsky removed his glasses with a flourish. 'That's it,' he said.

Rossel looked around for a pencil and some paper.

'Can I write on this?' he asked, holding up a copy of *Literaturnaya Gazeta*.

Tarkovsky shrugged. 'It is dangerous, even illegal, for an ordinary Soviet citizen to possess *The Prince*, is it not? So I might as well allow you to deface the principal cultural organ of the Soviet establishment as well. Anyway, over the years they've never been particularly kind to me.'

'Say it all again, please.'

As Tarkovsky translated the paragraph for the second time, this time with more precision, Rossel scrawled on the newspaper.

He read it back to himself. It was something, he was certain of it.

A step forward.

But he didn't feel that much closer to Pletnev's mysterious hoard of gold.

'Turn off the lights when you leave,' said Tarkovsky.

The actor stood up, put the book down, switched off the radio and walked towards his bedroom. 'I don't understand the attraction of *Swan Lake,* do you?' he said. 'The message of it, I mean. A swan that wants to be human? A life spent climbing the greasy pole as opposed to one floating regally across a lake. I mean . . . why would you?'

Rossel pointed at the book.

'Men are ungrateful, false and mercenary. I think Comrade Machiavelli agrees with you.'

*

Just over an hour later, the streets were starting to fill with the early shift workers, their headgear rammed tight down against the cold. A few were hopping up into Rossel's tram, adding more bodies to the press. Chunks of snow fell off their boots, turning the metal floor wet and muddy. One half of the carriage emptied at Nevsky while the other half filled up with new passengers. The tram rattled on under the blazing streetlights, up to the Field of Mars, where he got off. Over the Fontanka at the intersection of canals, down Mokhovaya, which was deserted, and to the corner of Liteiny and Nekrasova.

Back to his former life in the militia and Station 17.

He knew she would be early. She was the most conscientious officer in the station. That was why they always had got on.

Lidia Gerashvili was small and half-Georgian, with dark hair and darker eyes. She used to dye her shoulder-length hair blonde but had let it return to its natural colour. Her pupils were more guarded and introspective than when he'd first known her; the side-effect of a previous temporary incarceration and subsequent release by the agents of state security.

'Lidia. Comrade Senior Sergeant now, I see,' he said, glancing at her insignia.

For the briefest moment, Gerashvili paled. She stared at Rossel as though she had been walking through a cemetery and encountered an old friend climbing out of one of the pits. But she had the presence of mind not to yell or take flight when he placed a hand on her elbow.

Recovering, she led him straight inside, where she demanded the night officer bring them tea from the samovar.

As they walked down the corridor, doors closed. He saw a couple of familiar faces but they immediately turned away. He might as well have been marked by the plague and ringing a bell.

Fair enough, he thought. What could Comrade Albatross – a former senior member of Station 17, who had crossed swords with Beria and ended up in a labour camp – bring them but trouble? If he was in their place, he'd be thinking the same thing.

Treachery can be catching.

*

They proceeded to the archive room. Gerashvili's domain. They sat without speaking until the tea arrived, after which they sipped and blew and sipped again.

Rossel glanced around the boxes of files that lined the shelves, and at the metal cabinets that were also full of them. When he had been senior lieutenant here, he had made nightly pilgrimages to spend time with the files of the missing: those kindred spirits of his lost twin sister who he felt – in some way he was unable to explain – kept Galya company.

She had left him, he knew, because of what she believed he had done to their mother and father. Informed on them. Whether he had meant to or not was immaterial. In the Soviet Union, it was the most unoriginal of sins. Babayan's words about Vustin came back to him: 'That's why the boy liked you, Rossel. He was jealous of your soul's burden.'

The image of Galya's face on the night he had last seen her came to him again. He had watched her from a window: curious, uncomprehending. His sister had stepped out from beneath a light and disappeared. Been enveloped by the dancing flurries.

At that moment, he thought, she became a shade to me.

An ever-accusing finger. One of the old priest's shadows in the snow.

'Are you all right, Revol?' Gerashvili asked. 'You've gone missing.'

'Yes, sorry. I'm fine.'

He wasn't. But he gave the briefest of smiles anyway.

The last time he had seen Gerashvili, almost exactly a year ago, she had been a rank lower. She had also been mentally broken as the result of a prolonged spell of interrogation at the hands of Nikitin's MGB colleagues – former colleagues, he corrected himself. Not many who were that far gone managed to find their way back again.

That was something else they had in common.

'Would you be able to check all the files available on the two sniper schools for women in Moscow and Leningrad that operated during the war? Particularly the Leningrad school.'

He watched her reaction as she turned over the request in her mind, looking for danger. 'It is not official work,' he added. 'You should feel free to refuse.'

'What would I be looking for?' she asked.

'Anyone who had a particular way of killing. A kind of signature.'

Gerashvili nodded. 'We are allowed to request access to Red Army files in certain circumstances. I will do so. But it might take a little time.'

'Thank you,' he said.

'Is that it?'

Rossel shook his head.

'No, sorry. Lidia, I need something else, too. You have a reasonable grasp of German,' he said.

She inclined her head.

'I was right to suspect you hadn't come to ask me to go dancing at the Hotel Astoria,' she said.

'Next time, I promise. And during the blockade, you carried out radio and signals duty for a while?'

She nodded again. 'Well, they gave me the radio to look after. I was only a teenager when I was sent to the front for the first time. I learned and listened out for words such as *Angriffsziel, Unternehmen Nordlicht* and *feindliche Truppen*. A notch or two above the standard words like *Hände hoch* and *Scheisse*.'

'How about for codes and ciphers?'

She hesitated. 'I did my best. At least, I tried to spot words that might signify that a code was being used. Or any apparently innocent message that might have another meaning.'

'I see,' said Rossel. 'And a signals unit had to send coded messages as well as intercept them. Correct?'

'Yes.'

Rossel took out the copy of *The Prince* and outlined his reasoning so far.

Gerashvili listened. Then picked up the mugs from the table.

'For this,' she said, 'I'm going to need more tea.'

33

The book lay between the two mugs. It was open at page 115.

'As I told you, the numbers 115 and twenty-two led me to this section of the book,' Rossel said, showing her the relevant passage. 'So, the numbers are significant. Next comes the date – 12 March 1945. I feel that must be important, too, but that's where I am stuck. I can't see why.'

Gerashvili frowned.

'Everything they have used so far is about numbers. So maybe this is, too?' she said.

'Not March, not the month itself?'

She shook her head. Distracted, she straightened some files on her desk. Tapped a finger on the side of her cup. Once, twice, three times . . .

She grabbed a pencil, scribbled something down on a notepad and pushed it across the desk towards him.

'1, 2, 3, and 45. March is the third month. So perhaps the correct way to read this is the very simplest one – numerically.'

'A sequence,' said Rossel. 'You're a genius, Lidia.'

Suddenly he felt weary. He stretched out his arms and yawned. But helping to fight his fatigue was the thought that another obstacle was crumbling.

'Now I see it. The man who wrote this wants us to look at a sequence of some sort. Every word in turn.' He looked up at her. 'But how?'

Gerashvili shrugged.

'I don't know. What else do you have to show me?'

Rossel turned to the back of the book and the jumble of numbers on the inside back cover.

Someone had already taken a look and dismissed this part, he explained. 'I was told by the GRU that these numbers were so random they could not be deciphered. That you would need a particular text, a separate text, that would give you the key. But that you could only use such a text once without compromising its security. And there is no chance of us ever getting that text.'

'Then we are at a dead end,' Gerashvili said. 'And not even a third cup of sweet tea will help us.'

Rossel leaned back and looked at the stacks of files all over the room. He had spent hours here, leafing through missing person's records, of which there were still so many. Immersed in stories, tragedies and mysteries.

'Unless.'

She tapped the side of her head.

'It would be perverse on the part of whoever wrote all this in the book to set out a clue on the opening pages, indicate the significance of a passage in the middle, and leave a row of random numbers at the end,' Gerashvili said.

'Lidia, I am no longer your superior officer,' he said. 'Please speak freely.'

'It looks to me like the cipher and its key are meant to be all in one place.'

'Please explain it to me.'

'You have reminded me of my wartime radio duties,' she said. 'The most basic military cipher was to assign numbers to letters. The simplest would be to take the first letter of a sentence and replace it with the number one, the second letter and replace it with the number two, and so on.'

'The Germans used that?'

She shook her head.

'No, they had sophisticated machines. Our job was to pick up phrases indicating that they were sending messages using those machines. You know – *Hans, there's an important message coming, wake up*. That fact alone might suggest an attack was coming. We used this method all the time, though. When we needed to get a simple message from one place to another – something to act on quickly, a secret that would be useless an hour later – we would sing the first lines of a revolutionary song or a nursery rhyme over the radio. Something every Russian would know but the Germans would not. And we'd say the number three, which was an instruction to note down the third letter of every word and write them out in a row. Then the recipient would substitute those letters for numbers and wait for us to send a numerical message by runner.'

Rossel tried to imagine this. But failed.

'Then why send a runner? Why not just read out the numbers on the radio?'

'The Germans took prisoners,' she said. 'Prisoners can be persuaded to sing revolutionary songs or nursery rhymes when their fingernails are being torn out.'

'Runners get shot by snipers or tread on mines,' Rossel said.

'There was always another runner.'

Rossel stared at the book. An act of desperation. Perhaps the sender was in a hurry. Perhaps the gold medallions were a calling card – a sign of the sender's seniority? And the book contained instructions on how to find something more important. Use keys the other side won't know, like the numbers of SS Panzer divisions. And then indicate that it's a simple sequence. Put in a dirty postcard and some *Juno* cigarettes to distract attention from the main prize.

But what if you had only one book and one courier, and the message never got through?

'Let's try it,' he said.

Gerashvili pulled open a drawer, took out a notebook and got to work.

Denn man kann von den Menschen insgemein sagen, daß sie, undankbar, wankelmütig, falsch, feig . . .

'If it's just a sequence and the sender is keeping things very simple, then the letter d will be 1, e2, n3, n4, m5, a6, n7 . . .'

Rossel pulled a lamp closer to her.

She frowned. 'Wait.'

'What is it?'

She pointed to the jumble of numbers at the back of *The Prince*. 'The highest number here is twenty-six. And it occurs repeatedly. That is a big clue that this is an alpha-betical cipher in German. But in such a case, one would be more likely to use only the first occurrence of each letter in order. So we give the letter n only one number.'

Gerashvili kept up her rapid scribble before stopping. She stabbed the pad and cursed.

'Nonsense,' she said. 'Let's try the numbers in reverse order.'

Rossel closed his eyes, listening to the scratch of pencil on paper.

'So,' she said, just as he was dropping off. 'Are you ready? This might not work – we may have missed a clue. Or it might be an instruction to take the first letter, then skip two, then three, four five, and then back to one.'

'We should know within a few numbers,' he said. 'Though my German is not good, I warn you, so we may need a few sentences for me to be able to distinguish actual words from gibberish.'

'Then take this. I'll turn the numbers into letters and read them out. You write them down – do rows of ten at first.'

She began.

'D. E. N. N. D. E. R. G. O . . .'

There were seventy numbers in all and it took only a few minutes for Gerashvili and Rossel to work their way through them.

They scanned the results:

```
D E N N D E R G O T
T E R E N D E D A M
M E R T N U N A U F
S O W E R F I C H D
E N B R A N D I N W
A L H A L L S P R A
N G E N D E B U R G
```

'Does it mean anything to you, Revol?'

Rossel looked at the letters. At first, they just swam in a sea of gibberish.

But then . . .

WALHALL . . . GOTTER, or rather GÖTTER . . .

'Yes,' he said. 'It's from an opera. By Wagner.'

She suppressed a laugh.

'Opera? Was this opera about war? Are there tanks on stage?'

Rossel stared at them again. He was no expert on Wagner but students of orchestral instruments at the Leningrad Conservatoire were given a gruelling education in the symphonic and operatic repertoire, and he had done long stints rehearsing a couple of Wagner's major works, including *Götterdämmerung*. It had not been a hardship: the music was divine, shattering, intoxicating. He'd even taken the score out from the library, spending a couple of evenings revelling in its brilliance.

But *here*?

'This bit doesn't fit,' said Gerashvili.

She pointed at a line of letters and numbers at the bottom of the page. They might have been written in the same hand as all the other numbers, but it was hard to be sure.

15OSRD18B

'Not with number substitution anyway,' she said. 'You get ZPOSRZLGB. Or possibly IOSRDSB, if 1 and 5 are 15, and 1 and 8 are 18. Either way, it isn't German, or any other language.'

Gerashvili tore out the pages of her notebook on which she had done her workings and handed them to Rossel. Then she replaced everything in her desk drawer.

They both stood.

'Thank you, Lidia,' Rossel said.

'It might take me a week to get the records for the sniper school. Can you wait that long, Revol?'

'No,' Rossel said. 'But I suppose I will have to.'

As they walked back down the corridor, Rossel tried not to look through the door to his old office, but it was slightly ajar and he could not resist. The only thing he glimpsed was the dark fireplace with the engraved metal decoration, including the outline of the seabird that he used to touch for luck.

So far, he thought, it hasn't really brought me much.

*

Major Nikitin was waiting in the Drugovs' apartment, seated at the dining table like a suspicious spouse.

'General Pletnev is getting very impatient, Rossel. I hope you have made progress.'

Rossel needed to sleep. He yawned to see if Nikitin would take the hint but the major just stared back at him. With a sigh, Rossel pulled up a chair and took out the scrap of paper on which he had written the letters. He smoothed the paper on the table so Nikitin could see it:

> *Denn der Götter Ende dämmert nun auf.*
> *So werf' ich den Brand*
> *in Walhalls prangende Burg*

'Which means?' said Niktin.

Rossel wrote out the translation in Russian:

> For the end of the Gods draws near,
> So I throw this torch
> onto the shining walls of Valhalla.

'Wagner,' Rossel said. 'It's from Wagner.'

Nikitin grimaced.

'That's . . . that's *everything*?'

'So far. That, and a small but impenetrable jumble of words and numbers, which I still have no idea about.'

The major gnawed at his upper lip.

'Tell me about bastard Wagner, then,' he said.

'The text is from his opera *Götterdämmerung*,' said Rossel. '*The Twilight of the Gods*. The final scene. The very last bars of *The Ring*, his epic operatic masterpiece in four parts.'

'More,' said Nikitin.

'Brünnhilde, a Valkyrie who became a mortal, sets fire to the funeral pyre of her lover Siegfried. She rides her horse into the flames. At the same time Valhalla, the home of the Norse gods, disappears for ever. A new era begins. A celebrated scene, one of the most famous pieces of music ever written. The Nazis adored it.'

Before the Great Patriotic War, the authorities had tolerated performances of Wagner in the Soviet Union. After it, even whistling the 'Ride of the Valkyries' on the tram was risky.

'But is it enough?' muttered Nikitin.

'Enough?'

The major scowled. 'For Pletnev.'

'I don't know. It's all I have got.'

Nikitin jabbed a gloved finger into Rossel's chest.

'Get some sleep, comrade. An hour only. Then we report to the general.'

34

A dull headache tapped like a Morse code signal at his temples.

Rossel rubbed a porthole into the misted passenger window of Nikitin's Pobeda and stared out at morose afternoon pedestrians with heads lowered into the whipping breeze. Daylight was one of many winter scarcities in Leningrad. The weather was often fickle, with blizzards and bright sunshine alternating without warning.

As they arrived at his office in the museum, General Pletnev was in conclave with two officers. He looked up from their deliberations, his face pale.

'News?' he said.

Several paces from the desk, Nikitin saluted and stopped, placing a hand on Rossel's arm. Shaking it off, Rossel walked straight up to the officers, took out *The Prince* from one coat pocket and the gold medallion from the other, and threw both on the desk.

'Yes,' he said.

The general looked down at the book and back up at Rossel.

'Comrades,' he said to his officers. 'A moment, if you will.'

The officers left the room.

'You should know your place, comrade,' said Pletnev.

Behind him, Nikitin stifled a cough.

But the general opened *The Prince* and inspected the bookplate.

'Who was Oberst Halder, Comrade General?' asked Rossel. 'And why is someone ready to kill, and keep on killing, for this book?'

Pletnev's eyes moved between the two objects but he did not answer.

'Like all the other dead men, the war veteran Ivashin had kept his gold medallion,' said Rossel. 'He had no clue that it was in any way significant. I wager that none of the victims did. Under torture, the first one screams out the name of the second one, who does the same for the third one, and so on. But none of them gives the killer the information they seek. Because they do not understand what they have.'

With the crooked forefinger of his left hand, Rossel tapped the desk.

'But I think you do.'

Pletnev leant over, resting on his elbows, collecting his thoughts. Then he straightened up. He marched over to a table in the corner to retrieve his coat and cap, which he put on with care.

'And have you reached any other conclusions, Comrade Detective?' he said.

'I have,' said Rossel. 'Using a code he wrote into the book, Oberst Franz Halder, whoever he was or is, was issuing an instruction,' answered Rossel. 'A command to set fire to Valhalla. A coded message to bring about the end of the world. The next question is: a message to whom?'

Pletnev finished doing up his buttons.

'Comrades,' he said, 'follow me.'

*

Just ahead of them, in the dying light, a platoon of down-trodden conscripts was shambling its way towards the vast Palace Square, oblivious to the presence of one of the Soviet Union's most senior commanders. Underneath the triumphal arch that led into the square, the general slowed and watched them.

'Just look at them,' he said, pointing to the young soldiers. 'Already we are weak. The Motherland is losing her resolve and discipline. I foresaw as much when we reopened some of the churches. The Americans and British at our borders, always probing, preparing for invasion . . .'

He resumed his walk. The conscripts, orders yelled at them by a fat captain in the middle of the group, veered right.

Pletnev strode forward several more paces, glanced around the square and stopped. He looked up for a moment at the Alexander Column, the monument to Russia's victory over Napoleon. On the far side of the square was the Winter Palace. Away to the left, the gilded spire of the Admiralty, once headquarters of the Imperial Russian Navy. This place had once been the centre of tsarist power. Now it all belonged to the Soviets. In theory, to the workers.

'Franz Halder is a man we have sought since the final weeks of the war,' the general said. 'A German aristocrat. A fighter ace. The commanding officer of the elite Jagdgeschwader 26: a group of more than one hundred fighter pilots flying Me-109s. He was an officer who inspired complete trust and loyalty.'

He turned back to watch the conscripts performing a slovenly drill and cursed under his breath.

'But then Halder was reassigned to work on the Luftwaffe weapons research facility at Peenemünde, on an island in the Baltic Sea,' resumed the general. 'Rockets and missiles. Some of which were devastating, most of which were expensive failures. When military intelligence agents conducted their interrogations of leading Nazis after the fall of Berlin, they established that Halder was in effect number two to Albert Speer, the Third Reich's armaments minister. An uneasy relationship, by all accounts, but they put up with each other.'

Pletnev took off his hat and ran his right hand over his scalp.

'Indeed, Halder's position was such, and he was so highly thought of, that he became an adjutant to Hitler himself. We believe he was in the Führer's bunker until the very last hours of the war.'

Nikitin whistled. 'Hitler's adjutant,' he said.

'And a way for Speer to keep an eye on what the Führer was up to,' said Pletnev. 'Speer spent the last weeks of the war countermanding Hitler's orders to raze Germany to the ground. Blow up bridges, destroy factories, set fire to crops. Speer stopped that. Well, most of it. He wanted to be the leader of a new Reich, not of a wasteland.'

The conscripts trundled off Palace Square behind the Winter Palace, their captain administering kicks to the backsides of the stragglers.

'You were once a musician were you not, Comrade Rossel?' said Pletnev.

'A student, yes,' said Rossel. 'Of violin, at the Leningrad Conservatoire.'

'One with a future? A career in music?'

'People said so.'

After one of Rossel's examination recitals, the head of the strings faculty had stopped him in the corridor and told him he had never heard a finer performance of Beethoven's Kreutzer Sonata.

'But I never got to finish my studies,' he added, to forestall the next question. 'The defence of Leningrad came first.'

'As a musician, even a former one, this detail will interest you then,' Pletnev said. 'The last time we saw anything of Halder was in April 1945, at the final wartime concert of the Berlin Philharmonic. The Reichstag had not yet fallen but we already had spies all over Berlin. One of mine was looking after the coats of important fat Krauts who were about to become a lot less fat and significantly less important.'

He gave the ground a kick. 'We were already in a race with the Americans to find Hitler's scientists, rocket designers, chemical and biological weapons manufacturers . . . But many threw themselves into the arms of the capitalist West.'

Pletnev pulled out his watch, checked it and replaced it in his jacket.

'At the concert,' he said, 'our agent observed Halder deep in conversation with Speer, though he could not overhear what they said. Speer, of course, was captured, but Halder disappeared. For years we assumed he had been killed, or had committed suicide, or fled to Argentina or Brazil. We sent out agents but they heard not so much as a rumour.'

The general began walking again. Rossel and Nikitin kept pace.

'Speer was a defendant at the Nuremberg trials, was he not, Comrade General?' said Rossel.

'Yes, but the man is a charmer. Someone who could not only talk the birds down from the trees, as they say, but then persuade the trees to lie down next to them. A gifted story-teller who managed to convince the judges he was not a Nazi but a saint. Through his penitence, he escaped the noose. Which, to be fair to him, was indeed some kind of miracle.'

After the war, the papers and radio broadcasts had been full of the Nuremberg trials – the denunciations by Soviet prosecutors, who had demanded justice for the heinous crimes of the German leaders and their people. They condemned the Western judges as Fascist collaborators for jailing some of the leading Germans rather than hanging them. *Nazis who garrotted Soviet heroes and hung them from hooks in their torture chambers for the spectacle of it. Yet the capitalists show mercy to these animals.*

'What happened to him then?' said Nikitin.

'Albert Speer is one of seven senior Hitlerites residing in Spandau prison in Berlin. They are guarded by us, the British, the French and the Americans, on rotation. But Soviet wardens are always present. The other three powers cannot be trusted with the prisoners. They will bargain with them, offer them freedom for any last scraps of intelligence.'

Pletnev tugged his coat tight and checked his epaulettes. 'If Herr Speer has one last secret to impart, then I would wager that he knows the fate of Oberst Franz Halder.'

As they arrived at the entrance to the General Staff building, two huge guards standing outside came to attention and saluted as Pletnev approached.

'I want you to go to Spandau, comrades,' said Pletnev. 'Find out from Speer whatever he knows about Halder, whatever he knows about the message in that book.'

The general took it out from his greatcoat and pressed it back into Rossel's hands.

Rossel was struggling to take this in. For most people, a trip to the West was unheard of. Only the most trusted citizens were permitted foreign travel.

'Why would he talk to us, Comrade General?' he asked.

'Because you will be conveying a personal offer from me,' replied Pletnev. 'In exchange for intelligence that leads us to Halder, I will make representations at the highest levels of the Kremlin that will help reduce his sentence.'

Rossel looked straight back at the general. This was an unexpected commitment. Even more surprising was that the general was entrusting the message to him and Nikitin.

'Forgive me, Comrade General,' he said. 'I am still thinking this through. Halder's message in *The Prince* includes an instruction to set fire to Valhalla.'

'Yes.'

'One interpretation of that instruction is to order an attack of some sort?'

A guard opened the door to the General Staff building, revealing more soldiers lining the corridor. On sight of the general they saluted in unison.

'That would not be an entirely foolish interpretation,' said the general. 'As well as being Hitler's adjutant, in the last months of the war Oberst Halder was also a senior official in the Fascists' programme to develop an atomic weapon.'

From somewhere within the building Rossel heard raised voices and an unexpected burst of laughter. Pletnev checked a button and adjusted his cap.

'That, comrades, is the real gold I seek,' he said.

The general swivelled on his heel and marched inside.

35

In the dusk, under the yellow streetlights, snow whipped over the roads and round the corners of buildings.

At last, a tram came. Rossel and Nikitin got on board and found seats away from the handful of other passengers.

Nikitin slumped down in his.

'This could put you back in the camps, Rossel, and me alongside you. Or worse,' he said. 'Failure will condemn us.'

Rossel kept silent.

It makes no sense.

Within the confines of the Soviet Union, the GRU, as a military entity, was nothing like as powerful as the MGB. On foreign territory, however, it had carte blanche. It would be quicker and easier for General Pletnev to order GRU agents already located in Berlin to convey his offer to Speer, especially when it was the turn of Soviet forces to take responsibility for guarding Spandau.

On the other hand . . .

The only possible explanation was deniability. A former MGB officer of uncertain loyalty, acting with a former militia officer and camp inmate of complete political unreliability. With a record of challenging Soviet authority. If they failed, they could be quickly removed. If they were caught, they could be disowned with ease.

The tram clanked to a halt.

Rossel stood up but Nikitin pulled at his arm.

He could see something in the major's eyes. Something he'd never seen before. Fear.

'It's my wife and son, and my daughter, Svetlana,' Nikitin said. 'They'll come for them, too. Little Sveta has already been through enough. She couldn't cope with the camps as well . . .'

Rossel looked down at Nikitin, disgust welling up in his stomach. He thought of the terrified pleas of the hundreds of people the major had dispatched to the care of the GULAG. Or beaten senseless in the cells of the Bolshoi Dom.

He shook off the major's hand.

'My stop,' he said.

Then he exited the tram in a hurry.

*

Dr Maxim Bondar emerged from the morgue at The Crosses prison to greet Rossel in his office.

He opened a desk drawer and pulled out the locket.

'I am a pathologist, not a jeweller, but I can tell you that this was mass produced,' said Dr Bondar. 'No fingerprints. A little residue from some oil, probably gun oil.'

He dropped the locket. The chain uncoiled from his palm and cascaded onto the desk.

'The hair inside was a little more interesting,' Dr Bondar said.

'A family memento, perhaps?'

The pathologist shook his head.

267

'I highly doubt it. When a person dies, the pallor of the skin, the temperature of the body, the stiffness of the muscles, the breakdown of the cells, all these things happen rapidly and tell their own story. But the hair, apart from the root in the follicle, is already dead. You cut your hair and it doesn't hurt, yes? It can last for years, centuries, longer, provided it is relatively dry and free from fungal attack. Mummies have been unearthed with their hair intact . . .'

'Hair lasts a long time. I get it,' said Rossel.

Dr Bondar smiled.

'But,' he said, 'hair can still tell a story. The follicle is linked to the blood supply, so any toxins in the blood can show up in the hair. It is an excretory tissue, as we say.'

'Have you found poisons?'

'No. Something else.'

The pathologist paused for effect.

'Max, please.'

Dr Bondar grinned.

'Gunpowder, traces of zinc and copper, and one or two other substances that point to the owner of this hair having been shot in the head at close range.'

The kill shot. A sniper's work? But a sniper operated from range. More likely an executioner's shot, thought Rossel. As for the hair – a trophy taken from a victim? Or a keepsake from a friend or lover. Or a talisman. A reminder that vengeance was demanded.

'On the subject of the hair itself, I can tell you that it was human hair, from the head, probably European. This lock was hacked off rather crudely – jagged edges, no follicles – so it wasn't ripped out. It was also slightly redder than yours or mine, though that's because the red pigment pheomelanin hangs around after death more than the darker pigment. Our victim was no redhead, more a coppery brown. Very fine hair – only thirty-five or forty micrometres. I'd say it belonged to a relatively young person.'

'Can you tell when that person was killed?' asked Rossel.

Dr Bondar shook his head. 'No. Not recently, but it's not ancient either. I would be guessing if I tried to be more precise.'

Rossel thanked him.

'Not at all,' said the pathologist. 'You're looking a little fuller than the last time I saw you, though just as pale.'

'An occupational hazard,' Rossel said, 'for men like us who spend too much time in the shadows.'

*

Nikitin gave him no respite. As soon as Rossel was back at his apartment, the phone rang and the major declared he was on his way to pick him up.

'Where are we going?'

'Tarkovsky,' said Nikitin. 'I'll explain as we go.' The line went dead.

They did not exchange a word for the first few minutes of the journey. Not far from the river, a lorry swerved into their path. They both aimed a barrage of invective at its driver – a moment of release that thawed the ice.

As the two of them entered Tarkovsky's apartment, they found the actor cradling a bottle of cognac, recumbent on a chaise longue. He opened an eye, gave a soft moan at the sight of Nikitin and, closing it again, began to mumble.

'I can't sing,' he said. 'I have to sing at the Anichkov Palace and I can't hit a single note.'

'I don't know about the Stalin prize for acting,' said Rossel, 'but they should definitely give Boris's liver the Order of Lenin. From what I've seen since I moved in here, its daily labours are more heroic than anything Pletnev ever undertook.'

'So, the words you decoded are definitely from Wagner?' said Nikitin.

'Yes, and definitely from *Götterdämmerung*.'

'A flying bomb?' said Nikitin. 'Like the ones at the end of the war?'

Rossel shrugged. 'How else do you set fire to Valhalla?'

'Wagner, at his best, I always found sublime,' Tarkovsky said in a loud voice. He had sat up on the chaise longue and looked at the two of them with pleasure – as if his guests would take his mind off his troubles. 'Before the war there was talk of a Soviet film of the Ring Cycle with Lev Kuleshov directing. I was offered the part of Siegfried. Was going to take it, too. But then I saw a lecture Kuleshov gave all about how the only important element of filmmaking was editing and knew that little shit would cut all my best scenes out. It was filled with endless close-ups of plant pots.'

He snorted. 'After the war started, of course, Wagner was *kaput*. I'm glad I didn't take that part now. Otherwise, the MGB might have come to visit me one night and done a little editing of their own.'

'The major and I are going on a little trip to Berlin, Boris,' said Rossel.

'Berlin?'

Rossel nodded.

'Yes, and we need a guide.'

'A guide?'

'A translator. I don't speak German and neither does the major.'

Rossel took out a *papirosa*, lit it, took a hard drag and looked over at the still-befuddled figure on the sofa – a terrible singer who nevertheless had a talent for singing Schubert and Schumann in German.

'But I know someone who does.'

Nikitin followed his gaze.

It took a moment for Tarkovsky to understand.

'What? No. No, no, no. Berlin, me? No thank you, comrades. I turned down Kuleshov so I have no difficulty in turning you down. Kuleshov was a real big shot back then, I can tell you. It took a bit of nerve . . .'

Nikitin took off his jacket and hung it on the back of a chair.

Rossel walked across the room and sat down next to the actor.

'You should have taken that role, Boris. You would have made a wonderful Siegfried. So brave, so handsome. Slayer of dragons, seducer of Valkyries . . .'

Nikitin began to roll up his right sleeve.

'Though I suspect,' Rossel added, 'that the noble knight may have fared less well if he had ever sallied forth to meet Major Nikitin . . .'

36

By the time their flight landed in the late afternoon, Berlin's Schönefeld Airport was shrouded in drizzle and darkness. As they were towed to the aircraft's berth, the long lines of runway and perimeter lights were gradually extinguished. Only the main terminal building remained illuminated as they disembarked, soon separating themselves from the other twenty or so passengers – mostly military or diplomatic staff returning from home visits, along with a party of grim-faced low-ranking politicians from First Secretary Ulbricht's East German government who had boarded from a connecting Moscow flight.

East German guards, a couple of them holding back Alsatians on leashes, patrolled the arrivals area.

'Documents, please,' said the German officer seated at a large desk in front of the only door out of the hall for arrivals.

'Smirnov, Senior Lieutenant,' said Tarkovsky in a firm voice as he came to a halt in front of the desk. 'Camera operator, Special Information Films Unit, Soviet Army.'

'I've never heard of it,' said the German officer, meeting Tarkovsky's glare without flinching. His Russian was excellent.

'Of course not,' replied the actor. 'We are here on what is known as active measures. If you had heard of us, something would have gone wrong.'

The officer leafed through every page of Tarkovsky's passport, travel permit and military identification. Then he started again. Rossel stared straight ahead; Nikitin looked bored and impatient. Other passengers had caught up and joined them but besides the panting of the dogs the hall remained silent.

Finally, Tarkovsky and Nikitin were waved through.

The German officer leant back in his chair and looked Rossel up and down.

'Where are you based?'

'In the Leningrad Region,' answered Rossel. '19th Guards Rifle Division.'

'I thought that was a fighting division,' said the officer, fixing him straight in the eye.

'Your knowledge of the Soviet military is impressive, comrade. It *is* a fighting division.'

'Your documents say Special Films Unit? That does not sound very warlike to me.'

'The Special Films Unit was formed by the Defence Ministry in 1948 and consists of politically reliable and technically accomplished officers with excellent war records,' said Rossel. 'There is more than one way of waging war, comrade. Control of information is vital.'

Even to himself, his voice sounded too rehearsed.

The officer thought for a moment. Then he turned to a statuesque uniformed woman who was sitting behind him sorting through a pile of documents.

'Hey, Irina.'

She looked up from her paperwork.

'I always said you should be in the movies. There is a Special Films Unit here. Now's your chance to audition.'

Irina gave him a frosty stare in return. She slammed a rubber stamp down onto a travel permit, but said nothing.

The officer turned to Rossel and shrugged.

'The film business, eh?' he said.

With a little more force than was necessary, he took hold of his own stamp, applied it to Rossel's passport and handed it over.

'You lucky bastards must get plenty.'

*

The driver was fat, middle-aged, and smelled like he'd been fried on a griddle with some bratwurst. But the smell of onions was not his least appealing feature. He would not stop talking in a coarse pidgin Russian.

'Over there, comrades,' he said, pointing to a pile of bricks, 'that was a cinema. Der silberne Stern. I went out with an usherette from there before the war. Tits like zeppelins. And in bed . . . *Es war unglaublich . . .*'

'It was crazy what she did,' said Boris, translating.

The driver pointed at another heap of rubble, tidied into a pyramid. 'St Hedwig's Church, bombed in forty-three.' And again. 'The Lessing Theatre. Bombed in forty-five . . .'

Rossel looked out at a city that was half-missing: wide open spaces of flattened gravel and concrete punctuated by damaged buildings, of which only one or two sides might remain, or neat piles of bricks placed here and there by optimistic construction workers. Their driver had appointed himself tour guide to a Berlin that no longer existed.

What the Germans did to Leningrad, he thought, came back to haunt them.

Actual buildings had become more numerous as they drove further into the city, but so had the evidence of the war – once-grand blocks that were occupied in one half yet charred, twisted ruins in another; others that were little more than husks. Almost anything that was still standing had been left alone, for the time being at least, while the rubble around it was cleared away. Here and there – scaffolding, cranes, wire fences – signs of some reconstruction were in evidence.

After a few more minutes, Nikitin tried to shut the driver up.

'Who needs a travel guide, eh, comrade, when all that's left of Berlin is fresh fucking air?'

The man started laughing. 'Not much of that either, Ivan, when you live next to a sewer plant in Hellersdorf like me.'

He began to whistle a jaunty tune.

'Where are we staying?' asked Tarkovsky to no one in particular. He sounded as weary as Rossel felt. 'The Kaiserhof? The Kaiserhof used to be quite the thing . . .'

The driver chuckled. 'Only if you want birdshit on your head while you sleep,' he said. 'Also hit by bombs. Lots.'

'What about the Adlon? That was the best of the best, wasn't it? Sergei Eisenstein told me he stayed there before the war.'

'Survived,' replied the driver. 'Then some Red Army boys got pissed in the wine cellar and torched it. Nothing left now.'

Tarkovsky turned to Rossel. 'Then where?'

Rossel didn't answer. He looked back out of the window and stared at every face that went past, whether on a bicycle or peering out from a crowded tram. Berliners looked much like Leningraders, he thought. Gaunt. Tough. Tired.

'Welcome to Hotel Beatrice,' said the driver as the cab pulled up.

Nikitin wiped away the moisture on the window. The three men stared out at its grubby façade.

'Perhaps it's nice inside,' said Tarkovsky.

*

Like the Kaiserhof and the Adlon, the Beatrice had once been frequented by Berlin high society. Unlike them, it had the virtue of still having walls and a roof. It was now a dark and creaking edifice, a long way from its luxurious past but with pretensions of grandeur nonetheless, including a portly major-domo. He was short, with an oil slick of black hair brushed from the back of his neck over his balding pate. There was also a suspicion that he was topping up his bonhomie with the odd shot of schnapps. He introduced himself as Herr Bernard.

He had once, he said, worked at the Kaiserhof. 'I met all the big stars back then,' he told them via Tarkovsky, who was the only one showing any interest in his tales. 'Chaplin and Clark Gable at the Kaiserhof. Marlene Dietrich stayed when she was filming *The Blue Angel*.'

The three of them had convened in the Beatrice's gloomy restaurant, which was deserted save for themselves and a table of Red Army colonels making their way through several bottles of Beaujolais.

Bernard leaned towards Tarkovsky and lowered his voice. 'A local Schöneberg girl and occasional sister of Sappho. I brought some flowers to her room in the morning and . . . well, let's just say even the roses started blushing.'

He bowed and left. Rossel watched him go, being bullied all the way to the kitchen by the Russian officers still determined to put any Germans in their place – 'Hey, Fritz, fetch us another bottle of the Moulin-à-Vent – and be quick about it.'

The major-domo was, he thought, a bit like the Beatrice's tangled crystal chandeliers or dented oak panelling: a relic of the heady days of the Weimar Republic, a piece of bourgeois driftwood washed up on the most unexpected of shores.

Bernard was not long in bringing their food. Chicken was the only meat on the menu, accompanied by ersatz puréed potato and some lacklustre beans.

'Berlin seems quiet,' said Rossel, elbowing Tarkovsky for the translation.

'Yes and no. Tensions are rising,' said Bernard, doling out the beans. 'Since the blockade and the airlift – when was it, two, three years ago? – people are crossing over to the West all the time. The roads are being blocked. Guards are demanding papers and passes. But there is still the railway, and the S-Bahn.'

'We know all about blockades, Comrade Bernard, we're from Leningrad,' said Nikitin. 'A million dead, remember? Did you even know? If you ask me, it's good to see you Fritzes getting a taste of your own medicine.'

Tarkovsky kept silent and Nikitin did not insist on a translation.

'But you are still here, Herr Bernard,' said Rossel, risking a few words of German.

Bernard smiled, pleased at the effort.

'This is my place,' he said. Then he bowed to them, each in turn. 'But perhaps your friend the major is right and we Fritzes must . . .'

He delivered a stage wink.

'. . . learn to enjoy our punishment. As, I'm told, they used to in a special upstairs room at the Eldorado nightclub in the twenties. Great days. Back then, it was known as a workers' city – the reddest city after Moscow. Now the eastern half is red once more. *Plus ça change*, as the French say.'

Bernard began to sing. '*Politicians are magicians who make swindles disappear, the bribes they are taking, the deals they are making* . . . That tune is by a Russian composer, *kameraden*,' he said. 'Mischa Spoliansky. "It's All a Swindle". Spoliansky was in Berlin before the Nazis. He was a friend of Dietrich's. I think of that song often these days.'

He glanced at the table of colonels just as one of them threw an empty bottle against the fireplace.

'In Berlin, regimes come and go. But the music remains the same.'

37

Two turrets stood on either side of the gatehouse to Spandau prison, a small block that was dwarfed by the keep looming over it. To the right of the gates stood a gaggle of Soviet officers in caps and coats – relaxed and cracking jokes until, at an unseen signal, they all turned to look up at one of the watchtowers.

A Soviet soldier ascended the stairs, walked past the French sentry without a word and took up position, AK-47 strapped tight to his body. The Frenchman disappeared from sight – the cue, it seemed, for a Soviet column of about twenty men in three lines to tramp its way towards them along the wire perimeter fence that ran parallel to the heavy red stone walls of the prison.

This was where the opposing sides of the Cold War came to dance.

All eyes watched the column come to a halt outside the gates. It waited.

Almost immediately, the French detachment emerged, though with less frantic energy. They marched through the gate and took up station directly opposite the Soviet force. Their commander, an avuncular man in his sixties, handed over a file, shook hands with the Soviet commanding officer and saluted. Then the French were on the move once more, wheeling smoothly right along the perimeter and towards two buses that would ferry them to their own zone of the city.

For the next month, the Soviet Union would be in control of the seven most notorious prisoners in the world.

Among the less formal group of officers, Major Nikitin leaned towards Rossel so that their heads were almost touching. He leant out again, chuckling, and patted Rossel on the shoulder. Trying his best to look at ease.

By contrast, Tarkovsky looked stern, hefting his bag of camera equipment and ignoring the furtive glances of men who had been through the war and who had a good recollection of what Stalin's disgraced son Yakov Dzhugashvili had looked like. Here's 'spoilt Yakov' again, some of them must have been thinking; a little fatter, a little less hair, a few more wrinkles, but large as life. Even though they all knew the Nazis had imprisoned him in a concentration camp and then shot him.

Or perhaps, they were wondering, that's just what we have been told?

*

'Comrades, I do not believe I have been notified of your arrival,' said the warden.

Nikitin saluted.

'I am Major Nikitin, this is Captain Ivanov and Senior Lieutenant Smirnov, all normally of the 147th Guards Rifles, ultimately of the 8th Army, now on secondment to the Special Information Films Unit. We are here to interview

Albert Speer for a propaganda film on senior surviving Nazis, on the order of the Defence Ministry . . .'

The warden looked shocked. 'I have received no advance warning of this.'

'It was all requested at short notice,' said Nikitin. 'We will be in and out before you know it.'

'Absolutely out of the question,' said the warden. 'Access to the prisoners is limited and only granted by permission of the governorate, which means obtaining the agreement of all four powers that run the—'

'Call Defence Minister General Pletnev,' said Nikitin, pulling out a piece of paper from the file tucked under his arm. 'This propaganda mission is of the utmost importance. Part of a broader plan to discredit the Western occupying powers, expose the German denazification process for the charade that it is, and reveal American and British complicity in permitting Adolf Hitler's most loyal henchman to escape . . .'

He paused for breath. 'Of course, if you think this is a bad idea you are most welcome to address the general himself,' Nikitin added.

The warden swallowed.

Rossel took a piece of paper from his own pocket. 'Or Lieutenant Colonel Timofeyev, the head of active measures in the Foreign Ministry in Moscow. Or his deputy, Colonel Kirillov. I have their numbers here,' he said.

Nikitin took it from him and waved the paper in the warden's face. The man tried to swat it away but Nikitin pressed it upon him.

'It would be extremely irregular,' the warden said. 'Under the regulations, only the governorate can determine who can visit a prisoner and—'

281

'For private visits, yes,' said Nikitin, slipping into a smoother gear. 'We are here as representatives of the Soviet Union at a time when the Soviet Union has control of Spandau. I would, of course, be more than happy to consult with the Soviet governor of the entire sector here, Major Viktor Alabyev, who is aware of our mission . . .'

The warden's eyes darted about. To say 'no' was to risk incurring the wrath of General Pletnev. To say 'yes' would be to go against procedure. The punishment for an incorrect choice would be severe.

But Nikitin had given him an escape route.

'Major Alabyev knows?' he said. He pulled at his lower lip, considered his options and nodded. 'In that case, comrades, you are most welcome. Major Alabyev is very angry at the Americans over recent anti-Soviet lies in the Western press about Spandau.'

And Major Alabyev could therefore take the blame. The warden turned and led the way into the prison.

38

Boots clanged on the metal stairs as the warden and two Soviet guards led the way up to the third level of the prison.

'Prisoner Four is in there,' the warden said, gesturing to a cell door as they passed by.

'Which one is he?' asked Rossel.

'He is Prisoner Four. That is all they are now. A number.'

'And before, who was he?'

'Grand Admiral Erich Raeder. He speaks excellent Russian, incidentally.'

'Which number is Speer?'

'You mean Prisoner Five. You are not permitted to address him by name,' said the warden.

'He doesn't even deserve a number,' said Tarkovsky. 'These Fascist scum were fortunate not to be executed.'

The actor was warming to his role and the guards looked like they approved of this sentiment.

'This is a big place for seven people,' said Rossel. 'How many cells are there?'

'There are 132 cells,' said the warden. 'At all times, there are seven wardens by day, five by night. Guarding the prison are forty-four sentries, plus sergeants and officers.'

Soviet newspapers had printed tens of thousands of words about the Nuremberg trials. *Now, when as a result of the heroic struggle of the Red Army and of the Allied forces, Hitlerite Germany is broken and overwhelmed, we have no right to forget the victims who have suffered. We have no right to leave unpunished those who organised and were guilty of monstrous crimes* . . . The Soviet prosecutor had demanded a Soviet response, his every word transcribed for the grim approval of Russian readers.

And in summing up: *I appeal to the tribunal to sentence the defendants without exception to the supreme penalty. Death.*

There were other trials – of captured Nazi party officials, German military leaders, members of the SS, German and non-German. And thousands of collaborators, Russian, Ukrainian, Belarussian, Polish, Latvian, Estonian, Lithuanian, Romanian, Bulgarian . . . In courts throughout the Soviet Union, they had been tried, sentenced and executed with neither mercy nor delay. Some had followed Göring's example, cheating their captors and accusers by killing themselves before retribution could be taken.

And then there were the seven who had been spared the noose. The seven prisoners in Spandau.

The party marched down a corridor and came to a halt outside another metal door studded with locks.

'It is now 08.35,' said the warden. 'The prisoners normally have work until 11.45 before they have their midday meal but in the winter this rule is relaxed, depending on the weather and the health of the prisoner. All except Prisoner Seven, of course, who refuses to do any work.'

'Prisoner Seven?' said Rossel.

'Rudolf Hess.'

Tarkovsky flexed his right fist, a gesture he had copied from Nikitin. 'Give me a minute with him,' the actor growled.

Careful, Boris. Don't overact . . .

'Physical punishment is forbidden unless a warden or guard needs to protect themselves, which is unlikely. These are old men with bladder problems. Once they ruled the world. Now they don't even get to choose the times in the night they get up to take a piss.'

'Does Number Five speak any Russian?' said Rossel.

'A few words only. In any case, according to the regulations you are only permitted to speak to the prisoners in German.'

The warden moved aside to allow one of the guards to open the door. Behind it lay Hitler's favourite architect and the Reich Minister of Armaments and War Production. A man who had once seen himself as successor to the Führer.

Speer had escaped one bunker only to end up in another.

39

Prisoner Five had a receding hairline and prominent ears, accentuating a broad forehead. Below his thick eyebrows, the face still had traces of youth – strong, even features and the ghost of a conspiratorial smile. He took another puff of the pipe that rested on his lower lip and crossed his legs, appraising the unexpected visitors at leisure. But as he analysed the possible implications of a Soviet delegation led by a figure who looked like Nikitin, his shoulders hunched a little.

The warden snarled at him in German.

'He is telling him to stand up and put his pipe out,' Tarkovsky translated. 'Prisoners must be respectful at all times.'

Albert Speer got to his feet and tapped out his pipe on a metal ashtray.

'My National Socialist German Workers' Party number was 474481,' he said with a curt bow. 'Now I am Prisoner Number Five. If only from a purely numerical perspective, gentlemen, I have of late risen in the world.'

This elicited another volley from the warden. Speer responded by holding up the book he had been reading.

'Dostoevsky,' said the Third Reich's former Minister of Armaments with a wry smile. '*Schuld und Sühne. Crime and Punishment*. Ich hoffe, das findet Ihre Zustimmung.'

'He says he hopes we approve,' said Tarkovsky.

'The *svoloch* is all yours,' said the warden, as he left. The bolts clanked shut behind him.

Speer smiled at them, but his eyes flickered from one visitor to the other. Then he held out his hands as if to express uninhibited cooperation.

'Tell him that we are making a documentary about the final days of the war,' Rossel said to Tarkovsky. 'Specifically, we are interested in the movements of the leading Nazis in the very last days. Not just Hitler, but his closest aides also.'

Tarkovsky relayed the question in a voice that echoed around the cell. He looked Speer in the eye as he was talking, playing a dual role – part ardent Bolshevik and, with his excellent German, part interrogator for the Gestapo. Or perhaps the Stasi, the recently formed East German secret police, thought Rossel. The methods of both organisations were likely to be very similar.

Boris was convincing.

Most people would have been intimidated. Especially with Nikitin sitting next to him and glowering across the table.

Speer did not seem cowed. Perhaps he was unsure of the situation – if a trap was being set, if a punishment was being prepared. Or if they were telling the truth. His expression was . . . not blank, exactly. Expectant. A confidence perhaps born of having tiptoed through the minefield of the Nuremberg trials and having avoided detonations.

'A documentary crew, eh?' said Speer, through Tarkovsky. He looked at each of them in turn. 'Which one of you is Sergei Eisenstein? I would have hoped that the great Soviet cinematic maestro was the least I deserve.'

Tarkovsky, unable to resist, leaned forward and assumed an air of eager friendship.

'What was he really like?'

'He?'

'Hitler. Who else?'

Speer thought for a moment.

'On reflection – and as you can imagine, I have had much time for that – only a man, like you or me. Who for some reason known only to itself, History had decided to listen to.'

Speer picked up his empty pipe and tapped it on the table.

'By the end, however, he was a different man to the one I had once known. If the Führer – if Hitler had had his way, Germany would have burned. Everything gone – industry, infrastructure, transport networks, the German people themselves, everything. Had I not disobeyed him, thwarted his desires, it would have been . . .'

'A *Götterdämmerung*?' said Rossel.

Speer gave him a sharp look.

'That is one description.'

He waited for Tarkovsky to catch up before adding: 'A musical reference. Does that mean you are a musician?'

'A violinist,' said Rossel.

'Do you still play?'

Rossel held up his left hand and removed the glove, showing the missing fingers.

'Regrettably not,' he said.

'A war injury?'

'Something like that.'

Rossel replaced the glove. 'You are still an architect at heart, I see,' he added, pointing to the large piece of paper that took up practically all of the only table in the cell. It was a detailed scheme of what appeared to be an enormous building, embellished with Gothic lettering.

'A fanciful castle,' said Speer. 'Rather in the style of Ludwig II of Bavaria. Given your reference to Wagner's music, one should remember that Ludwig was Wagner's greatest and richest admirer. My own work here is a homage, if you like, to the mad king. When you have fourteen years left to serve behind bars, a man needs to kill time. So I design buildings that will never be built, worlds that cannot be, empires that exist only in the mind.'

Rossel stared down at the plans. The dutiful servant of a mad king. That was how Speer had portrayed himself at his trial.

'Prisoner Five, a story that I have heard concerns the music of Wagner,' he said. 'A concert that took place on April 12 1945. Less than a month before the Third Reich's capitulation. Can you remember what was on the programme that night, Comrade Speer?'

Speer's expression did not change as Tarkovsky relayed the question, but a tiny note of recognition crept into his eyes.

'What makes you think I was even there?'

'You were there,' said Nikitin.

Speer cut short the translation with an irritated wave.

'The Beethoven violin concerto,' he said. 'Performed by the orchestra's leader, a young and gifted man. He was the only member of the orchestra who accepted my offer of help to leave Berlin. Half an hour after his performance he was in a car on his way to Bavaria. The others stayed. Too proud to leave their city.'

'Was that it?' asked Rossel.

Speer tilted his head – *do not treat me as an idiot.*

'A short section from *Götterdämmerung*. Brünnhilde's Immolation Scene, from there to the end. But it is evident that you already knew that. And Bruckner's Symphony Number Four. That piece was my signal to a select few. If they heard the Bruckner on the radio, it was time to leave the city. Via certain checkpoints manned by guards who also knew to listen out for the musical code.'

Speer stood and leant backwards, pressing a hand into the small of his back.

'Bruckner was a wonderful writer for strings,' he continued. 'The Führer adored him – even more, I believe, than he admired Wagner. And no one knew better than Hitler that admiration and adoration are two very different things. One gets a man a little respect, the other allows him to conquer worlds.'

Rossel gave what he hoped was an encouraging smile.

'Messages within music,' he said. 'Always fascinating. But I was thinking more about the Wagner. The symbolism. Valhalla in flames.'

Speer did not reply.

'Was the ending of *Götterdämmerung* a message of some sort, too?'

'From whom?' asked Speer, toying with his pipe. 'To whom?'

'A message from Oberst Franz Halder, Hitler's Luftwaffe adjutant, to the Nazi resistance,' Rossel said.

Speer picked up his tobacco and began to fill the bowl.

'A documentary crew, eh?' he said, tamping down the tobacco. 'I don't recall Leni Riefenstahl asking so many pointed questions before she made *Triumph of the Will*.'

Picking up a heavy steel lighter, he put the pipe to his mouth and tested the draw. For half a minute, he did nothing but regard his visitors, lips pursed. His calculations made, he spoke.

'The Russian cooks here are worse than my mother, and bless her, she couldn't bake a Zwiebelkuchen tart without cremating the onions.'

Speer smiled at Rossel.

'A Sachertorte,' he said. 'Do you know what that is?'

Rossel waited for Tarkosvky to translate. Then shook his head.

'A Viennese chocolate cake. That's my price for talking to you a little more, comrade.'

Speer looked up at the cell's little window.

'As memory serves, just one morsel will feel almost as good as climbing over Spandau's walls.'

*

'No,' said the warden as he leapt up from his office chair. 'Absolutely out of the question. The seven Spandau prisoners get the same calories as ordinary German citizens, as stipulated on their ration cards. But you want to give Speer a Viennese chocolate cake. Fuck your mother.'

Rossel held up a hand to silence him.

'It is a test,' he said. 'We need to demonstrate to Speer that we have some influence here.'

The warden didn't look convinced. Rossel went in for the kill.

291

BEN CREED

'We will, of course, be sure to mention your cooperation and invaluable assistance in our report to the defence minister,' he said.

The warden sat back down again.

'All right,' he said. 'Spoil him if you need to. But next thing you know, that stuck-up bastard will be asking for some cream.'

*

'Your cake is on its way,' said Rossel. 'Though the warden insists that you eat it out here. It took a little persuasion for him to allow your request.'

Raised beds full of black soil and neat lines of plants ran in rows of thirty or forty metres, some pruned almost back to the root, others allowed more leeway to lie dormant and sagging. Trellises ran up the bricks of the prison walls. In one distant corner a greenhouse stood at a slight angle, misted up. Large areas were dug over and covered with matting, old carpet or mulch. Transported to a collective of Russian dachas, Rossel thought, the ensemble might have earned a coveted *ideal'nyi uchastok*, or 'model plot' award, a plaque that inveterate dacha dwellers displayed with pride on the side of their huts or houses.

But this little garden was tended by men who had dreamed of ruling the world.

Speer nodded.

'Thank you.'

For a winter's day it was bright and sunny, but Speer still slapped his hands together to ward off the cold before wandering over to a garden bench. Then he sat and surveyed

292

the movements of the other middle-aged or elderly men scowling amid the shrubbery.

'That's Dönitz,' he said, flicking a finger in the direction of the white-haired former admiral, who sported a sneer above his jowls. 'The man he is pretending to ignore is Admiral Raeder. They are inseparable, really, though they pretend on occasions not to get along. The one sitting on his own is von Neurath, the former Protector of Bohemia and Moravia. Very ill. Heart, he says. Unlikely, since I've always suspected he doesn't have one. Another aristocrat who cannot abide a hint of dirt beneath his fingernails.'

He pointed again. 'There you have Prisoner One. Von Schirach. Head of the Hitler Youth and Gauleiter of Vienna. Who else? That's Funk. Odious man. But very musical. Sometimes he plays the organ at our Sunday services. Yes, we have those, comrades. The battle to save our souls never ends. Perhaps, when I die, the Good Lord will make me his Minister for Munitions. I have little doubt I would be able to rapidly increase production of both hymn books and holy water.'

Speer sat back.

'Hess?' said Rossel. 'Where is he?'

'He refuses to do any work and is wary of setting foot outdoors in case you Russians force him to do any. No one likes him, anyway.'

Speer nodded at von Schirach.

'Unrepentant Nazis like von Schirach say that Hess betrayed the Party by fleeing to Scotland. The rest of the world simply sees him as a horrible unrepentant Nazi. Rudolf doesn't get many invitations to parties these days.'

'But you are repentant? Battling to save your soul. Is that what *you* are doing here at Spandau, Comrade Speer,' said Rossel, taking out some cigarettes and offering one. 'A penance?'

Tarkovsky translated. Speer gazed into the middle distance for a moment.

'When I married Margarete, my mother felt I'd married beneath me and would not allow us to visit her for seven years. That was a penance, I think. Its sting never fades. This is merely a purgatory, of sorts. I can survive it. Besides, *tout comprendre, c'est tout pardoner, n'est-ce pas?* A sin explained is a sin forgiven. I intend to write a book. My side of events. Every man's story can, after all, only ever really be that.'

Rossel was already on alert. The familiar prickle on his neck, under his jaw where his fading fiddler's mark lingered; the skin, once dark red from constant playing, now a tinge of pink. A mark that mocked him every time he looked in the mirror. And he could hear the change in Speer's voice – the same subtle difference he had heard as a prelude to so many confessions. His skill was in listening, in letting others fill the silence.

'Atonement, then,' he said. 'Have you something to offer the world by way of that? That might be of interest to people who watch our film?'

Speer seemed about to reply. But then something caught his eye.

A Soviet corporal was walking towards them holding a porcelain plate on which rested a silver fork and a large piece of cake.

'Look at them.' Speer gestured to the other prisoners in the garden. Each man had straightened his back, turned his head towards this astonishing gastronomic spectacle. 'The last time they eyed up something as hungrily as that was, I'll warrant, an empty seat next to Hitler at the Führer's dining table.'

*

Speer dropped the fork onto the plate with a clatter. He wet the tip of his little finger and then used it to pick up a last crumb of Sachertorte.

'*Wunderbar*,' he said. 'Not only was it delicious, but it has also allowed me a few much-needed moments of reflection.'

He looked up at the other prisoners going about their gardening and noticed von Neurath frowning at him. Speer smiled.

'In our little realm of Spandau, gentlemen, the most a man can hope for is to be king for a day. For when he wakes each morning, he once again discovers he no longer possesses even his own name.'

He leaned back and turned down a finger.

'Now, to business. Here you are, a mysterious Russian delegation who haven't so much as touched their cameras or microphones or lighting gear, but have heard something about Oberst Franz Halder, *nicht wahr*?'

For a moment Rossel held his tongue. Then he nodded.

'They cut out many references from the papers they let us prisoners read,' Speer said. 'But they miss some things. Mentions of the leading lights of the Kremlin, for instance. Beria, Malenkov, Khrushchev, Kaganovich, Pletnev. Molotov less so, thus I assume he has fallen from grace.'

Speer picked up the fork and inspected it for traces of icing as Tarkovsky translated.

'I know better than most that leaders do not last for ever,' he continued. 'Stalin is an old man. His inner circle will be making calculations and dreaming of taking his place. I assume that you represent one of them. Whoever sent you, I want a deal. I have another fourteen years in this prison and Stalin won't last that long. When he's gone, I simply ask whoever you represent to remember that I helped him.'

A sparrow flew close by. Speer watched it skimming low through the air before soaring round the building and out of sight. He dropped the fork back onto the plate.

'I will request that your assistance is recognised, Herr Speer,' said Rossel.

Speer sat back and nodded.

'In my current circumstances, that's the best I can hope for,' he said. 'The wisest beggar is the one who understands he still has a tin cup to shake. You know about the concert, and the Bruckner and the Wagner, and that both myself and Halder were present. I take it that Franz Halder has never been found?'

'No, he has not,' said Rossel.

'Yet he has apparently not made use of the information he was charged with concealing and delivering to the underground resistance.' He looked up at the Russians. 'I also take it our glorious German resistance never actually resisted?'

Rossel and Tarkovsky shook their heads. Nikitin curled his lip.

'It was a ridiculous idea, anyway,' said Speer. He examined his nails. 'But, even at the very end, the Führer was convinced.'

'What was the information in Halder's possession?' said Rossel.

Speer waved across the garden at Funk, who ignored him. The others were also turning their backs.

'While we were all awaiting trial,' he said, 'the Americans dropped their bombs on Japan. The world changed in that moment.' He sat up straight, pressing the small of his back, wincing. 'But the American bombs were as nothing compared to what our scientists had designed,' he said. 'It was a design only, of course. Had it been tested and built, Moscow and London and New York would have been eradicated. Yet the Yankee bombs proved, too late, what our scientists had been saying. The big bang was possible, and if it was possible then a bigger one was also possible. Calamity would breed ever greater calamity.'

Two of the guard towers had sight of the gardens. At least one of the Soviet guards had his eyes on the prisoners at all times. The other might turn away to scan the world outside but only for a few moments.

Over by the heavy doors that led from the main prison block to the garden, the Soviet warden emerged. He kept his distance but Rossel could sense they were running out of time.

Opening one of the cases containing camera equipment he had no idea how to use, he pulled out *The Prince*.

'Herr Speer,' he said. 'Halder encrypted a message to the German resistance. This was the key text.' He read the lines from *Götterdämmerung*. 'Was that his meaning? To create this new weapon?'

Speer took a moment.

'The guards here talk. I'm told that in Moscow General Pletnev is highly thought of,' he said. 'The coming man.'

Rossel nodded.

'He is. And I'm sure if we bring him good news back from Spandau, the general will also think highly of you, Herr Speer.'

Speer sniffed the air. Considered. Then smiled.

'Yes,' he said. 'To destroy the old order and build a new one. That was the instruction. To create a bomb of unimaginable power.'

Rossel opened the book at the back and showed Speer the last numbers.

1 5 O S R D 1 8 B

Speer took the book and squinted at it.

'Aha. I was wondering when we would get to this,' he said.

Rossel waited for Speer to elucidate but he did not.

'I think this is the code for a location,' Rossel said. 'A place with nine letters, perhaps. Scrambled through one of the Nazi code machines . . .'

'*Nein, nein,*' answered Speer. 'A location, yes. You are right about that. But the answer is simpler than you think.'

He looked into Rossel's eyes, his expression almost tender.

'It is a map reference,' he said. 'The Luftwaffe system. Oberst Halder was in the Luftwaffe.'

'How does it work?'

'It is a grid. A series of grids, in fact, each one fitting inside the other. Rather like your Russian dolls. Look at this.'

He pointed to the first few characters.

'You start with 15 OS, or Ost Sud. East South. A pilot would know instantly, but my guess is that it is a large piece of Europe.'

Rossel waited for Tarkovsky to translate.

'And the rest?'

'Then the grids get ever smaller. So 15 Ost Sud is divided into a twenty-by-twenty grid, and the letters RD identify a particular square. The north-west corner is AA, then AB, AC and so on as you move across to the east on the map. You get to letter number twenty and then start again for row two – BA, BB, BC and so on.'

'So RD would be . . .' Rossel had to think for a moment. 'Bottom left – south-west?'

'Yes, I suppose so. It has been a long time since I stared at maps with the Führer, or anybody else,' said Speer.

'And then what?'

'Then the square RD is itself divided into nine – three by three. Then nine again, and then the smallest square.' He looked at the paper once more. 'So, the one means the top left square within the grid RD. The eight means the middle bottom square within *that*, and the last reference is B. I suppose B would be top middle, after A.'

'How accurate was it?'

'If I remember, the smallest unit of the grid system was about one square kilometre.'

Nikitin threw up his arms. 'That's not exactly pinpoint- ing our destination, is it? Not exactly X marking the spot, comrade . . .'

Rossel reached out a hand and placed it on Nikitin's left arm.

'Where is this location, Herr Speer?' he said.

Speer bared his teeth. Picked at a small morsel of food stuck between the front two. Then he shrugged.

'Without a map I can't help you,' he said. 'I have told you all I know. But I can offer your general one more name that might be of interest to him. That of a scientist, a physicist. *Ein Kernphysiker*. Baron von Möllendorf. Hitler sometimes called him "the man who knows too much".'

Then all his humour left him, as if it were dust he had brushed from his sleeve. Albert Speer got to his feet.

'Two places in Vienna claim to have invented the Sachertorte,' he said. 'The Hotel Sacher and the Café Demel. In the thirties they went to court. As far as I know, they still haven't settled it. In my humble opinion, gentlemen, the Führer understood human nature all too well. We human beings were not placed on this earth to peacefully coexist.'

Speer's finger located a last crumb on the plate.

'Why, just think of the Sachertorte,' he said. 'Two men in Vienna bake a cake and then, a short time later, go to war over it.'

He turned and walked away.

40

Back at the Hotel Beatrice, Rossel wandered about in search of the major-domo, Herr Bernard. Tarkovsky took a nap. Nikitin fumed, muttering curses at Speer.

The hotel was silent, save for some rhythmic and angry grunting behind one door on the second floor and the strumming of a guitar behind another on the third. The crimson carpet might once have been a fixture to be proud of. Now it was threadbare and stained.

He ran Bernard to ground on the fourth floor, polishing the brass buttons of the lift.

'Comrade Bernard,' Rossel began. 'I recall you saying you could get your hands on anything a guest needed.'

The major-domo gave his instinctive bow.

'Anything, comrade.' He gave Rossel a wink. 'Or anyone?'

'Perhaps another time,' Rossel said. 'For now, however, I am hoping that you know where to find some old Luftwaffe *Kameraden*. For once, the Soviet Union has need of them.'

Bernard looked pensive.

'I imagine they might be reluctant to talk to you,' he said.

'There is no need for them to meet us,' replied Rossel. He explained what he needed.

Herr Bernard beamed.

'By tonight, comrade.'

*

After a small plate of chicken, which Rossel devoured but the others barely touched, the three men drank some schnapps.

Nikitin had gone from angry to morose. Tarkovsky was subdued. Rossel waited until the restaurant was empty of the same group of noisy Soviet officers, knowing that Bernard would not deliver his package before then.

On cue, the major-domo materialised with what looked like a rough, oil-stained tablecloth. Rossel thanked him.

Nikitin's cheeks were flushed. 'More schnapps, Bernard,' he shouted after the retreating German.

Rossel pushed their glasses aside and unfolded the map. Across the top, on either side of an eagle gripping a swastika in its claws, were the words *Luft-Navigationskarte in Merkatorprojektion*.

Rossel dropped his notepad next to it.

'We are looking for 15 Ost Sud, RD, and then 1, 8 and B,' he said.

Sure enough, *15 Ost S* encompassed a chunk of territory on the right of the map – a section of the Baltic Sea and, below that, northern and central Germany. The place names were faint under the grid lettering, but in the south-east corner of this section Rossel could make out Kattowitz, which he assumed was Katowice, and below that Oswiecim, which he didn't know.

On the south-west side were Fürth and Nuremberg.

The map section yet further east, *25 Ost S*, ran from Warsaw almost to Kiev. The westernmost edge of the map, at that latitude, was Kursk. At one time, all of this – every number, letter and place name – had been within range of the Luftwaffe's Dorniers and Heinkels and every other plane at Hitler's disposal. And everything within the confines of *15 Ost S* had been fought over.

For a moment, Rossel lost himself in the towns and cities of the immense battlefield that had been the main theatre of the Great Patriotic War.

'So where is RD, then?' said Nikitin, his voice slurred.

They searched, Rossel running his finger down from AA to RA. Names of towns swam before his eyes.

'Gerolzhofen. Ebrach.'

'Never heard of them,' said the major.

RB. 'Bamberg.'

RC. 'Strullendorf. There's RD. What's next?' said Nikitin.

Even Tarkovsky was showing an interest.

'The top left,' said Rossel. 'Imagine a grid of nine and choose the first square – number one. And if the next number is eight, it should be at the bottom of *that* square in the middle.'

Nikitin sighed. 'You're making as much sense to me as one of the *mudaki* who work in the GRU archives.'

Rossel tapped a finger at a place on the map. He stared down at it. The lettering was on a crease and had faded, but he could make out the first letter and the last half of the word.

'Oberst Halder, I have you,' he murmured.

'You do?' said Tarkosvky.

Rossel looked up.

'This Halder is a warrior, a Wagnerian, and a man unable to resist the power of symbols.'

He tapped the map.

'Tomorrow, we go to the West. We go to Bayreuth.'

41

'Gutenfürst! Gutenfürst! Have your papers ready!'

The conductor's warning to passengers was drowned out by the steam engine's shriek but he lost no opportunity in repeating it as he progressed along the passenger wagons. He was Rossel's idea of a German conductor: burly but jovial, with a moustache that must demand considerable attention every morning.

A few kilometres back they had slowed for the *Sperrzone* – the restricted zone that gave advance warning of the inner German border. Before that, East Germans without passes to the West had got off the train in droves. Locked out of half of their own country.

Since then the locomotive had trundled along, steam and smoke whipping past the windows. Reaching the edge of the Soviet Zone, the barriers became increasingly formidable – a fence, then a trench. A control strip for vehicles. A watchtower.

Tarkovsky shrank into his greatcoat.

'More trouble?' he said.

'No trouble,' said Nikitin. 'Until six months ago this crossing was under our control. Officially, we have handed it over. But Fritz knows who is really in charge.'

Two dozen branch lines between East and West Germany had been closed in the past year, the woman in the Berlin station ticket booth had informed them, cursing all Communists as the enemies of freedom. That meant that crossings like this one, even sleepy Gutenfürst, were well stocked with East German soldiers and plainclothes spies. But none was brave enough to challenge a GRU major. The young officer from the *Grenztruppen* who had inspected Nikitin's ID had even saluted.

A few hundred metres beyond the border, the Americans didn't even come out of their guardhouse, merely waving at the Class 52 locomotive as it crawled past. Through the guardhouse's little window, Rossel could see them playing cards.

A minute later they picked up speed.

The rhythm of the train and the enveloping trail of steam was comforting. But nothing was more comforting than the thought that no one in the Soviet Union had any idea where he was. Nikitin seemed on edge, never taking his eyes off him and Tarkovsky. Eventually, Rossel understood why. The major feared that one or both of them might make a run for it, might follow the millions of East Germans who had tasted Communism and didn't like it.

The German countryside meandered by. Yes, Rossel admitted to himself, the thought had crept up on him. He looked through the window and wondered if he would be happy here. No Siberian camps, no MGB, no Stalin. None of the cruelty of Bolshevism.

But they had gone mad here too, hadn't they? One world war had ended and the promises of eternal peace had been made, only for insanity and slaughter to resume two decades later, but worse.

More than that – he was Russian.

If he defected, he would be setting himself against his own country. He was a Leningrader, and his fight to save Leningrad would be meaningless if he could never see her again.

Would any of that matter?

If he jumped from the train, Nikitin would be finished, of course. But so would the major's family. Tarkovsky wouldn't stand a chance, either.

And Galya? His missing sister would be gone for good.

If he quit the city, the country, the Union of Soviet Socialist Republics, his chances of ever tracking her down would be over.

At Hof they switched trains, swapping the Deutsche Reichsbahn of the East for the Bundesbahn of the West.

'For Bayreuth you'll need to change at Neuenmarkt-Wirsberg,' another ticket seller had told Tarkovsky, amused by his over-the-top gallantry and formality. 'No need for the airs and graces, your highness, you're in Bavaria now . . .'

Another hour went by. Tarkovsky was asleep in his seat opposite Rossel and Nikitin. As the train came to an unexpected halt it juddered and woke him. He stretched and sat up.

'Explain it to me again, Rossel,' he said.

'What exactly?'

'The bit about the grid reference.'

'All right.'

Rossel shifted in his seat to stop one leg from going to sleep. 'The Luftwaffe grid is accurate enough for an aerial attack, a bombardment, perhaps a landing zone. But not for a particular building, let alone what we are looking for. A square kilometre is a lot of ground to search.'

He thought back to Gerashvili's reminiscences as a radio operator. If you were a Red Army soldier humming Russian revolutionary ditties, a Wehrmacht radio operator would be left clueless. Conversely, if you were a Nazi Wagner fanatic quoting a few lines from *Götterdämmerung*, what were the chances any Slavic savage would be any the wiser?

'But let's say you were in the know. Let's say you knew something about Wagner. Then you would understand that he persuaded a mad German king to build him a huge opera theatre in the town of Bayreuth, which became the place of pilgrimage for his acolytes and the venue for an annual festival of his works.'

'That takes us to Bayreuth,' said Nikitin, raising his chin. 'But what are we looking for when we're there?'

'I'm not certain,' said Rossel, 'but Speer gave us another name, remember? Von Möllendorf. A baron. A man who knew too much. My guess is that there is something in Bayreuth connected to this von Möllendorf. It's a place to start.'

42

The three Russians tramped southwards towards the Hofgarten, just as Halder had instructed. A thick directory at the train station had given them their destination. There were only two von Möllendorfs, and only one of them was listed with a title.

Bayreuth was quiet. Also beautiful, Rossel thought. A town built like a stage set, waiting for an audience to arrive, a conductor to pick up a baton, singers to respond to their cues.

They entered a long boulevard, gazing at the tall, stocky Franconian buildings, their sloping roofs flecked with snow. At ground level, a cluster of stalls wrapped in multi-coloured lights offered steaming drinks and what looked like outsized twisted biscuits.

'It's like stepping back in time,' said Tarkovsky. 'You know, I have always wanted to play Peter the Great. Riding boots, gold epaulettes and, perhaps, a powdered wig. This place would make a perfect location for that movie. I can see the poster now – "He conquered an empire but not himself!"'

'Yes,' said Nikitin wearily. 'You're an actor. I get it.'

Once or twice as they looked down a side street, they glimpsed a still-ruined church or a historical building propped up with beams and boards. But for the most part, under the yellow gas lights and a blanket of snow, the Bavarian fairy-tale town had come back to life. Bayreuth may not have been made whole again since the bombing raids but American money had already wrought some miracles.

'Quiet,' said Rossel. He pointed. 'Over there.'

In the midst of the stalls, a quartet of Amercan GIs were drinking from large steins of beer. One, a large black man, broke into song. His words had an irresistible sway and swagger to them, even though they could not understand their meaning.

They took the nearest exit into a warren of side streets. As they walked on, the man's voice – something about *boogie woogie boogle* – began to fade.

The dark was drawing in. Soon they were lost.

Tarkovsky spotted an elderly man about to enter a narrow pink building. He stopped and asked him for directions to the address they had found in the directory.

'Down that street, which is Friedrichstrasse,' he said, reporting back. 'Go left when we see Ludwigstrasse, then we'll see the park.'

They set off in the direction the actor was pointing.

'The boogie woogie bugle boy,' said Tarkovsky, laughing. 'I think I might like America . . .'

*

'Ludwigstrasse.' The actor read out the sign.

They took the turn and almost immediately followed a path towards the park.

Nikitin pointed through the trees and across a small lake. 'On the north side, the man said – we need to go that way.'

They followed the line of a long, palatial building that in style was like one the Romanovs might have built. Then they went right again.

'There,' said Rossel.

It was an L-shaped mansion with a circular summer house in the courtyard. The smaller of the two wings had suffered extensive bomb damage. At the main entrance to the grander structure, a coat of arms was carved above the door. A knight's shield containing an eagle. The bird held a sword in one claw and a book in the other.

Beneath it, the family name. Von Möllendorf.

Rossel looked up at it.

'Let's hope he knows as much as Hitler thought he did,' he said.

*

'Locked,' said Nikitin.

He banged on the door but there was no response. If any lights were on, they were not visible. Shutters shielded the interior from prying eyes.

'Let's split up. There must be a hole in the wall somewhere near the bombed section,' said Rossel.

Most of the courtyard was gravel, which had been raked even. The grass and hedging that bordered the mansion was neat and well cared for. Someone was looking after the place.

Nikitin and Rossel went in opposite directions, each surveying the length of the mansion in the hope that an entrance would present itself. As he reached the end Rossel looked back but he had lost sight of both the others. He was about to walk down the side of the building and along the back when Tarkovsky's voice reached him.

'Here!'

Rossel could see a dark figure waving an arm. He walked back at a brisk pace to see the double doors at the front were open.

'Welcome to the palace of Peter the Great,' Tarkovsky said, bowing low. 'The back door is hanging off its hinges.'

Nikitin marched straight past him.

Rossel shook his head.

'You just can't resist making an entrance, Boris,' he said.

*

Inside the mansion of von Möllendorf, whoever he was, an entrance hall led straight to a wide marble staircase, one banister of which was missing. They struck out to the left, finding themselves in a grand ballroom that was almost empty. In one corner, a huge crystal chandelier lay like a collapsed constellation of stars on the parquet floor.

'This place is huge,' said Tarkovsky. 'But it already looks like it's been stripped of anything of value.'

'I can't see a thing,' Nikitin complained.

Guided by a thin moonlight that had been let into the room when one of them had pulled back the curtains, Rossel reached the far end and stood before a beautifully carved door.

'We will have to do this the old-fashioned way,' he said. 'By splitting up and . . .'

He pulled the door open and then sprang back, fists raised at the spectre staring back from the other side of the threshold.

The figure had its fists raised in return but they were shaking – with frailty, Rossel realised, rather than fear.

Behind him, Rossel heard a sigh from Tarkovsky and an oath from Nikitin, who strode towards him.

'Who the fuck are you, Grandad?' said the major.

Hands still raised, the figure took a small step forward. In a soft, low voice, it spoke German.

'He says only the stupidest thieves break into an empty home,' said Tarkovsky.

The man shuffled forward, moving into the moonlight.

Tarkovsky took a step back.

Nikitin swore. '*Kakoi-to prizrak*,' he hissed.

But it was not a ghost.

*

Rossel fetched a chair from the corner of the room and offered it to the man who, after a moment's pause, sat.

He was cadaverous, his shirt and trousers hanging off him. He was deathly pale save for a livid pink that covered half of his face – all of the brow, most of the left cheek, sweeping under the chin and across the neck. Malnourished. Neglected. Much of his hair was gone but some was left in clumps.

Rossel stared at him. To his own surprise, he reached out with two fingers to touch the affected skin on the man's face and neck, which was everywhere peeling. The man did not flinch. He did not move at all.

'Scar tissue,' said Rossel. 'He's been burned.'

'Are you the baron?' Nikitin said to him. "Are you von Möllendorf?'

Before he could answer, Rossel shook his head and pointed to the walls. They were covered in black scrawl from an obsessive hand. Pen, charcoal, paint. One word, repeated over and over.

Neubrandenburg.

He called for Tarkovsky to translate.

'I would like to say I do not believe that the past can return to haunt us, but events have proven to me that they can,' said Rossel. 'And you, Oberst Franz Halder, of the town of Neubrandenburg, have just discovered the same thing.'

At the sound of the name, the man closed his eyes. In the silence, Rossel could hear Nikitin's breathing.

Then the German straightened his back and drew his heels together.

'Yes. I am Oberst Halder,' he said. 'Are you here to kill me?'

Halder peered at them through pink, watery eyes. He spoke as though each syllable shocked him, as though every word was a feat he no longer expected to be able to perform.

A click of the fingers. 'No, I am being foolish,' he added. 'Goethe said that one is inspired only in solitude. And yet it seems that I am still found lacking, even after so much time alone.'

Halder scratched at a patch of dry skin on his cheek.

'You have discovered who I was and want to know what I know.' He sighed. 'The British imprisoned me for two years without knowing who I was. They kept me in solitary, hoping to break me. Question after question. In some ways, they succeeded. But I never told them anything. Why would I tell you?'

This much speech appeared to tire Halder. He went quiet again.

'At last, I've found a part I would not wish to play,' whispered Tarkovsky to Rossel as he stared at the German.

Life flickered once again in Halder and he bowed to the actor with military precision. 'In that British prison I at least learned something. Each man rules his own realm, however small,' he said. 'No man who realises that is in need of pity.'

Rossel took a step forward.

'In Leningrad, we found a copy of *The Prince*. Hitler's copy,' he said. 'It was in the possession of an ordinary Red Army soldier, a man who would only have taken it as a trophy. It has your name in it. You were using it to send a message to someone. We would like to know what is here in Bayreuth, and how we may find it.'

Halder shook his head.

'You deciphered it?' he said. 'Well, I was merely a Luftwaffe pilot, not a spy. I was with the Führer in his bunker. The telephone lines were down, the radio was not safe. I had to improvise a cipher . . . something a German would know.'

He began humming. Rossel tried to listen, but the sound was without tune or tonality.

'Then with Bormann and his friends – Axmann and some others – we all tried to get out of Berlin,' Halder continued. 'We ran into some Russians. Marauders, trophy hunters. Bormann was killed. I escaped. But I lost my knapsack. I assumed the Russians took it. A day or two later I was captured further west, by the Americans.'

'We haven't got all night, Rossel,' said Nikitin. 'Let me talk some sense into this Hitlerite bastard . . .'

Rossel shook his head.

'It was taken, Oberst Halder. They found the book, your postcard from Odette. Your gold medallions. But I need to know about the book. The lines from *Götterdämmerung*, and the grid reference, leading here. What is in Bayreuth?'

Halder prodded at his face again, dislodging some flakes of skin that fluttered to the ground.

'Odette,' he said.

His face crinkled.

'A very beautiful woman.'

'Rossel . . .' said Nikitin.

'Your friend is impatient,' said Halder. 'So why don't I show you?'

'Show us what?'

Halder stood up.

'This way,' he said.

*

Halder led the way through the mansion. Almost at the end of one wing, he ascended a narrow flight of stairs with surprising ease and disappeared at the top. Rossel, Nikitin and Tarkovsky chased after him. At first, they thought he had made a run for it.

But then a door opened at the opposite end of the room, which turned out to be only a few metres across. Halder had returned with a lantern.

'My home,' he said, holding up the light.

Rossel looked around.

More scrawl on the walls. The same word on every surface.

Neubrandenburg.

Halder traced a finger over one of them.

'It was my battle cry,' he said. 'But, these days,' he touched his face, 'my nerves aren't what they were. Neubrandenburg is known as the City of the Four Gates,'. 'When I was young my dead father would sometimes appear to me in my dreams and say, "The gates are open, Little Franz, walk through the gates with me."' He traced a finger over one of the words on the wall. 'At the end of the war, I was offered a cyanide pill by a girl from the Band of German Maidens. Almost every night since then I have wished that I had swallowed it. So that I could be with him.'

'Oberst Halder . . .' Rossel began.

'What you seek is a secret hidden within a secret. At one and the same time gigantic, of a size beyond comprehension, and yet it derives from something so small that you could look for eternity and never find it,' he said. 'Atoms within atoms, worlds within worlds. A cosmos of dots. The three of us – Speer, myself and the physicist, von Möllendorf – managed to hide a universe within a single room.'

As Tarkovsky translated, Halder smiled.

'Or, to put it more prosaically, hide it inside a score hidden inside a piano,' he added.

'A piano?' said Rossel.

They all looked around the room. There was no piano.

Halder began to chuckle.

'It has not been here for years,' he said. 'In the summer after the end of the war, the Red Army trucks arrived.

317

Bayreuth was in the American Zone but they had been allowed in to take some German art and artefacts. Cultural looting. The locals are still angry about it. They still talk. That is how I know.'

'So they took it? Russians?' said Rossel.

Halder nodded.

'They were emissaries of a high-ranking Soviet. They went to the Hermitage Castle and the Opera House. Then they came here. Instruments, music, even the velvet curtains from the opera house. And before the war the von Möllendorf family had taken ownership of one of Wagner's pianos. The maestro's own instrument. It was their pride and joy. A piece of musical history. The Red Army carried it away and every score in this mansion.'

'But who?' said Nikitin. 'Who was this Russian?'

'Oberst Halder,' said Rossel, stepping in front of the major. 'Please. The name.'

Halder glanced up at the words written on the wall.

'"The gates are open, Little Franz,"' he whispered. 'Perhaps, if I tell you, I can, at last, make myself walk through them and be with my father.'

Seized by a coughing fit, he fought to regain control of his breathing.

'The man we duped,' he said, wiping his mouth. 'The man to whom we Germans promised friendship. And then invaded his country. A man who, I suppose, sought a petty recompense. Your former foreign minister, Comrade Molotov.'

43

Leningrad's temperature had risen, turning everything to slush and ooze, and then abruptly fallen again. Dirty, shrunken snow that had been piled at random along pavement edges had turned into rock, while icicles the length of a Cossack *shashka* dangled from the eaves of buildings, forming lines of frozen sabres posed to impale the unwary or unlucky. The city's roads were cracking up under the pressures of expansion and contraction.

At the late hour of their aircraft's arrival, most taxis had given up for the day. Though several other smartly uniformed individuals were picked up by limousines as they arrived at the airport, no such greeting awaited the three of them.

Rossel, Nikitin and Tarkovsky had to walk more than a mile to the nearest bus stop and endure a long journey into the city centre, where they had parted company under a broken streetlight. Tarkovsky had grumbled all the way. He looked shattered, and announced his intention to go to bed. Nikitin stomped off without a word. Rossel was reluctant to return to the Drugov residence, but he'd spent enough time with the actor.

Without the score, they had nothing.

All they had was an ageing Nazi's word that Molotov had it.

And if Molotov had it, Pletnev did not.

As soon as Rossel got back, fighting his tiredness, he picked up the phone and called his old militia station, asking for Gerashvili.

'Anything, Lidia?'

'Something, I think,' she said. 'I only got the files yesterday. I can't . . .'

She stopped herself.

'Can you meet me tomorrow?' Rossel said.

'Of course. About eleven. Where?'

Rossel looked out of the window.

'I know the perfect place.'

*

Even in the grip of winter, survivors of the Siege of Leningrad came to lay bouquets on the mounds of frozen earth that marked the mass graves of Piskaryovskoye Cemetery. They brought pictures of the victims of the Siege, too, on white ceramic disks. They pinned them to trees or tied them to small wooden staves and, where possible, stuck these into the icy ground – as if Piskaryovskoye had in places become a field of mournful flowers, seeded from the half-million or more corpses in its ground.

Elsewhere, blocks of granite and bags of sand lay strewn around, proof of plans to turn the cemetery into a memorial worthy of the great sacrifice of the Hero City.

Gerashvili, wearing her militia uniform under a trenchcoat, was waiting for him near the cemetery's main entrance.

'I see what you mean about the perfect place,' she said as he approached. 'For you, anyway, Revol. A man who used to spend nights at the station browsing the files of the missing. It makes sense you would come here to make friends with the dead.'

He shrugged, but was pleased to see that the old spirit she had once had in abundance was returning.

He reached out with both hands and tapped her twice on both shoulders.

'For a little while, you went missing yourself, Lidia,' he said.

Her cheeks coloured. Then she took out her notepad, tore a sheet from it and gave it to him.

There were three names written on it:

Irina Bok

Mila Kitsenko

Lada Vinogradova.

'That's all I've got,' she said. 'Army files are a mess. When the women's sniper academy closed, individual records got lost or were sent to a hundred different places. Most of what I have managed to acquire are records of exceptional valour. Also some misdemeanours – not reporting back on time, minor insubordination, that kind of thing. At first, I thought they would be of no use to you. But I stayed up the last few nights to go through them anyway.'

Rossel folded the paper and put it in his pocket.

'And the three names?' he said.

'I found a report of a reprimand. All three were mentioned in it.'

'What had they done?'

'The three of them must have been close. They trained together and went to the front together. Apparently, they even referred to themselves as the *troika*. A sisterhood of three. Perhaps it's not surprising they got into trouble together.'

'How and when?' he asked, trying to contain his impatience.

'Towards the end of the Battle of Stalingrad,' Gerashvili said. 'They were reported for a breach of discipline.'

She pulled her coat tighter.

'After the Soviet counteroffensive in November 1942, pockets of German soldiers became isolated. For the snipers, it was the easiest kills they ever made. On December 3 1942, the *troika* set up three positions from which they could cover as wide an area as possible, according to their training. They shot an entire platoon dead. But then they climbed down from their hiding places and shot them all again in the head.'

Pulling one hand out of his pocket, Rossel gestured at the burial grounds around them.

'Considering the scale of suffering in the Great Patriotic War, not the worst of crimes.'

Gerashvili nodded.

'I agree. But it was ill-disciplined. They gave their positions away. They wasted ammunition. And their commanding officer reprimanded them formally.'

Like bullets, rifles and battleplans, discipline was something that had sometimes existed only on paper in the defence of Stalingrad. Yet it had also existed in reality, and in large enough doses to bring victory.

'And your killer has a habit of a double shot to the head. And like a sniper, Koshchei is invisible. And, so you tell me, possibly a woman. So I thought—'

'It is excellent work, Lidia,' he interrupted.

Her face lit up. He thanked her and prepared to leave, eager to pass on the news to Nikitin.

'Aren't you going to ask me who their commanding officer was?' she called after him.

He stopped.

'You have found that out as well?'

'Major Anastasia Firsova,' she said. 'She trained them and then joined them in Stalingrad.'

Gerashvili handed him another piece of paper.

*

Major Firsova lived in a communal apartment near the Vitebsky railway station. A note on the wall outside gave the doorbell codes for each of the five households that lived there. He rang three times for Firsova.

She was in her fifties. Despite her civilian clothes, everything about her was military – her formality, her posture, her short-cropped red hair.

'Ah, the school,' she said. 'The happiest time of my life. I have found it hard to adjust to life since the war. But I am not alone in that.'

'Where was it?' he asked her.

'Partly in a large hut in the grounds of the Peter and Paul Fortress,' she said. 'That was for theory, learning to strip and reassemble the rifles, movement, how to work in teams. Timing your shots to mask them. Making a hide.

Many of our principles were formulated by the great Vasily Zaitsev. We sometimes had the honour of his personal instruction. We learned from him how to understand the minds of our opponents. That the hunter must become the prey.'

She smiled at the recollection. 'But we would go out into the countryside for practical experience. Until the Germans imposed the siege. And then we were learning on the job, if you like.'

Rossel took out the list of names Gerashvili had handed him.

'Do you remember these women?' he asked.

The major took some wire-framed spectacles from her pocket and held them up to him.

'I scored 307 kills before I became an instructor. If you gave me a rifle now, I couldn't hit the tram that brought you here.'

She put the glasses on and read the names on the paper. Then she looked up.

'Yes. I taught all of them.'

'What were they like?' Rossel asked.

'Young and foolish, naturally. Especially Irina and Lada. Barely adults. But dedicated. And excellent shots – after they had done their training, excellent. They notched up sixty-seven and thirty-two kills respectively before . . .'

Major Firsova sighed.

'Before?'

'They were both killed in Germany, in hand-to-hand fighting near the end of the war. Not far from Berlin. I believe it was the 5th SS Panzer Division, the *Wiking*. The girls were forced into one of our trenches, which was overrun. The SS cut their throats. A good sniper always knows the way out, knows where the exit is.'

The major sighed. 'They forgot what I taught them.'

'When was this?'

She thought for a moment. 'Right at the end. March 1945, I'd say.'

As Rossel pointed to the third name on the paper, he felt his mouth go dry.

Both killed, he thought. *It has to be . . .*

'What about Kitsenko? Is she still alive?'

'Mila? I don't know. We lost touch after the war. I never heard of her being killed. I heard of her killing a lot of other people, though. She came from the Urals and was as a patient and as still as the mountains themselves. I've met corpses that blinked more. And what a shot. Her father had been a hunter and took her out with him when she still a child. In terms of shooting, there was not too much we needed to teach her – I mean, 277 kills and she made it through to the end. Only Lyudmila Pavlichenko and one or two others managed more, and that includes the men.'

'But there was a disciplinary matter,' Rossel said. 'A formal reprimand?'

Firsova picked up her cup and pressed it to her lips, looking at him over the rim, taking a little longer than she needed to. She wasn't sure. The encounter might now have taken on a different character. Matters of discipline, or perhaps of insufficient discipline, could come back to old soldiers and create problems.

'There was,' she conceded, setting the cup down again. It rattled a little in its saucer.

'Which organisation did you say you . . .'

'I am from the Defence Ministry,' Rossel said.

'I understand, but which . . .'

'Can you explain the circumstances, please, Major Firsova?'

She picked up her teacup again.

'Elite snipers aim for one shot, one kill,' she said, sitting upright. 'The closer you are, the easier it is, but it is also more necessary. When you are close, your shot will be heard, your position will be easier to pinpoint. They broke this rule. It seems there was a . . . competition.'

'An extra bullet to the head,' said Rossel.

'You have heard about it? Yes.'

'And you were the officer who reprimanded them?'

She hitched her shoulders back. 'I had to,' she said. 'For a sniper to lose discipline like that can be fatal. The irony was that Mila was the one to survive.'

'Irony?'

'Yes. She was the one to instigate the game. If one can call it that. And yet it was the others who were killed.'

Rossel leant forward.

'How can you be certain, Major?'

'Oh, I knew my girls very well,' said Firsova. 'She was the ringleader. And something inside her was never the same as the others, comrade. She became obsessed with death. Infatuated with it.'

In the sudden silence came a distant boom – the traditional midday artillery shot from the Naryshkin Bastion of the Peter and Paul Fortress.

'Perhaps she thinks death is something that only happens to other people,' said Rossel. 'If you are Koshchei the Immortal, after all, you might well come to believe that.'

44

Fighting to keep his balance on the iron pavement, Rossel slipped and skated along the banks of the Moika towards the Yusupov Palace. He was already anticipating what Tarkovsky called his 'Ottoman gold', the rich Turkish coffee he served in a copper pot. As well as telling Nikitin the news about Mila Kitsenko.

A subdued party of schoolchildren was filing into the main entrance of a school. Further down the road, a militia officer was plodding along towards them, head bowed against the cold. Probably one of the *uchastkovyi,* the local militia officers whose job it was to know their neighbourhood as well as anyone could know it.

As his gaze turned to the little side door that led to Tarkovsky's apartment, he stopped in his tracks. A figure in a fur coat with a violin case by her side was standing at the door, hesitant, not pressing the bell.

Rossel crossed the road.

'Vassya,' he said.

She turned and recognised him with a small smile. She lifted up the violin case.

'I kept her safe for you, Revol.'

Seeing his old instrument was like seeing a long-lost family member.

'Thank you,' he said. 'How did you know I was staying here?'

'I asked Ilya to enquire . . .' She coloured a little. 'He has some influence in the Party.'

'Ilya?'

'The man who buys me flowers.'

'Ah, yes.' For a moment he was at a loss. He fumbled for the key Tarkovsky had given him. She looked like she was feeling the cold, so he added: 'Do you want to come in?'

She shook her head and held out the case.

'No, I just wanted to give you . . . sorry.' The apology was not to him but to the militia officer, who had doubled back on his beat and was now trying to pass by on their side of the pavement.

The officer stepped behind them and stopped. He turned and pointed something in Rossel's direction. The gleaming muzzle of a Makarov pistol.

'That's what I always hated the most about you, Rossel,' said Pavel Grachev, sergeant in the Red Army; sergeant in the militia; survivor of war, purges, labour camps and the long, long walk to freedom across Siberia. 'Always chasing pussy like the rest of us pricks . . .' He shoved them inside. 'While all the time pretending to be some kind of fucking saint.'

*

'Who is she?' said Grachev, waving the Makarov at Vassya.

He had shoved them down the corridor into Tarkovsky's private quarters.

'She is just a violinist from the conservatoire,' said Rossel. 'I'm giving her lessons. You and me, she has nothing to do with that. Let her go.'

Grachev's pistol hovered between them. He moved his bony hips in and out a couple of times and leered.

'Lessons, yes. I bet.'

Grachev's features were twitching and contorted. He was already anticipating the blood to come – could hardly wait for it. In the war, Rossel had seen men get like that. Licking their lips. Flaring their nostrils as if Death wore an alluring scent.

But before the kill, he needed to preen, needed to rub Rossel's nose in it.

'Not many make it back from Vorkuta,' Grachev said. 'Brain two guards with an axe, shoot a third, take their weapons and go. That was the easy part. You'll know that. As a former zek.'

Of Tarkovsky there was no sign. Rossel hoped that the actor had gone to Lenfilm and was well out of the way. Unless Major Nikitin turned up soon – and they had not set any specific time to meet – Grachev would kill both of them. He knew how to control two people, and how to finish them off. He would kill one. Make the other one watch. Then finish it.

'You went north instead of south,' Rossel said. 'That was what I would have done. You persuaded that boy to go with you. If you made it far without anyone picking up your trail, he could be the *myaso*. Provide you with a meal or two in the middle of the taiga. But they were after you faster than you'd bargained for. So you sent the boy into the forest as a decoy while you hid out for a while. In one of the mines, was it? You could burn a fire there without being seen.'

The sneer on Grachev's face curdled into a look of cold contempt. Rossel knew he had got it roughly right.

'Then you doubled back. Made it back to Vorkuta and bluffed your way onto an aircraft.'

'Always the great detective, you smug bastard,' said Grachev. 'But you didn't see me coming today, eh?'

'Pavel, it wasn't me who—'

'It's amazing what you can do if you wander around in a militia uniform,' said Grachev. 'All this shit about Koshchei. I hear chatter about a corpse at Lenfilm, of all places. So, I stand guard there – literally stand guard, like a statue. A few days later you walk straight past. I follow, and you are staying at the Yusupov Palace. Living in a fucking palace. You always did think you were a cut above . . .'

The journey back from Siberia, Rossel noticed, had taken its toll on the sergeant. The dry skin on his face was rough and reddened, the lobe of his left ear was gone. It was a reasonable assumption he'd lost a toe or three. He looked tired, too. Exhausted.

Maybe I can jump him.

Grachev's lips sank backwards to reveal dark brown teeth. He tried to imitate Rossel's voice.

'*Pavel, it wasn't me who* . . . You think you can lick my arse like you did with Captain Lipukhin or one of those idiot superior officers in Station 17?'

'No,' said Rossel. 'And I had nothing to do with—'

'You informed on me!' Grachev yelled, leaping forward, a heartbeat away from putting a round in Rossel's face. 'I know it was you. That's why they sent me to the fucking *camps*.'

Vassya was sitting and had not moved a muscle. Her hands rested on the table. She looked straight at Grachev.

'It's impressive what you did, escaping like that,' she said. 'Not many men could do it.'

'No,' Grachev said, settling a little. 'Not many men could. But if you think you'll save your neck just by making me think you want to suck my *khui* . . . Every whore we booked in the cells in the station used to try that trick.'

He tapped the Makarov.

'Four bullets for you and one for the bitch,' he said to Rossel. 'But before I kill her, I'm going to fuck her.'

Grachev's right forearm was in range.

Now make a—

An object came hurtling out of the shadows. Rossel threw up an arm to parry it. As it smashed into his shoulder and deflected into the middle of Grachev's face, Rossel still had time to recognise it – the bust of Lenin that Tarkovsky hated, the one he would turn to the wall.

There was a deafening retort – Grachev's pistol firing as it dropped from his hand. Tarkovsky stood pale and motionless in the corner of the rooms, unable to believe what he had done.

The Makarov slid across the floor.

Rossel dived for it.

Vassya hurled herself at Grachev.

The sergeant threw her off him and kicked her twice in the face. Rossel's hand was under a sideboard, groping for the weapon. Grachev leapt on top of Rossel, dirty fingernails clawing at his face.

Rossel's own fingers closed on the Makarov. He pressed the pistol against Grachev's temple.

Fired.

At the last moment, Grachev pulled his head back and rolled. The bullet missed and removed a chunk of brick and plaster from the wall. Then Grachev scrambled to his feet and started running.

A moment later, the apartment door slammed shut.

*

Up ahead, Rossel heard the main door to the street smack against the wall. He raced down the corridor and out into the light, which was blinding against the ice and snow.

The detective scanned the street.

Left. Right. Nothing.

There.

Grachev, a way off to the right, heading along the Moika towards Isaac's Square. A group of children and adults spilled out onto the street from the school. A little girl screamed when she spotted Rossel with his pistol levelled.

He lowered the weapon and set off in pursuit, pushing through the frightened crowd. Grachev was limping. He must have hurt his leg in the fight.

Rossel was closing but the embankment curved at this point and his target was always just out of sight.

Twenty metres.

Ten.

Five.

Where is he?

Grachev exploded from a doorway, going for Rossel's throat rather than the pistol. His body pinned Rossel's right arm to his side and knocked the weapon from his fingers.

They twisted and turned together. In a slow, ungainly *pas de deux*, they toppled over the embankment rail.

Picking up speed, they plunged through the ice.

*

Blackness.

He blinked twice.

Still black.

Above him nothing but a roof of white. Below and around him, only freezing murk.

Follow the bubbles. Upwards, towards the light.

Rossel clawed at the ice, his palms and knuckles sliding without effect on the white crust that had become his coffin lid.

But the Moika was narrow. If he got lucky, he'd find the granite bank.

If I get unlucky?

On hitting the freezing water he'd gasped – the reflex that killed so many ice fishermen who trod in the wrong spot and went through, sucking in water.

He already had no air in his lungs but plenty of foul liquid in his mouth and stomach.

A distant, muffled pounding.

A few last apologetic notes. A disappointing final aria . . .

Black spots multiplied on his vision like ink spreading on paper.

He had become a score. Or some strange being that hid inside it.

The pounding grew louder, like the crashing of the percussion. A last dazzling whiteness before the fade to black.

Hands pulling at his clothes.

Angels will take us, Revol. His grandmother's voice. *Angels will carry us up to heaven . . .*

Rossel lay on his back on the bank and vomited black, grainy liquid all over his own face.

His ears drained themselves of water, only to fill up again with the sound of someone screaming. His arms were being pulled out of their sockets as he was rolled over onto his front. A knee to the ribcage made him vomit even more.

Vassya was kneeling next to him. Beside her was a twisted chunk of broken metal rail that she'd used to smash a hole in the ice.

Angels will take us, Revol. Angels will carry us up to heaven.

45

Vassya tugged hard at his coat, tearing it free. A shove in his shoulder blades to propel him further along the corridor and into Tarkovsky's ornate bathroom, with its plush carpet on the floor.

Helpless, teeth chattering, he let Vassya remove his jacket and shirt. She sent the actor to fetch more towels and steered Rossel into the bathroom. Turning on the shower, she started to pull at the buttons of his trousers but he fended her off and clambered into the bath, straight into the scalding stream.

After a couple of minutes, the bathroom door opened again and more towels were thrown in. Ignoring them, Rossel sat on the bath floor, arms across his knees, and let the hot water cascade over him.

Still shivering, he closed his eyes.

Black spots again. Ink on paper.

Another image came to him.

A cosmos of dots. Worlds within worlds. The gigantic hidden within the shell of the infinitesimal.

A sound, too.

Sung by a madman to the dark Siberian skies.

A single leitmotif.

*

Rossel and Ilya Koshkin were about the same height, though Koshkin's waist was a little larger. As befitted a Party man.

'Thank you, comrade,' said Rossel.

Koshkin grunted. He was handsome, with piercing blue eyes and straight black hair that was turning grey. He wore a permanent half-smile that seemed to flit between friendship, aggression and deference. He was, Vassya had said before his arrival at Tarkovsky's apartment, a senior manager in the Ministry of Machine Tool Building.

It must be the engineer in her, Rossel thought. When they're in bed, they get to exchange pithy anecdotes about quotas and five-year plans.

Koshkin eyed the clothes Rossel was wearing.

'I bought that suit last summer.'

'It fits well,' said Rossel. He was hoping it was Koshkin's best.

'I bought boots, too, and a coat, just as Vassya asked.'

'Thank you again.'

Vassya reappeared with a teapot in one hand and the coat in the other, which she tossed at Rossel. Koshkin did not protest. A well-connected Party man could always get another coat.

'I must go. Work,' said Koshkin. 'They're building a new tractor-part factory out near Chudtsy. I have to attend the opening ceremony.'

Vassya nodded at him.

She turned to Rossel. 'Are you still in trouble?'

He blew on his tea. Then nodded. 'Unless I can find a way to see Comrade Molotov.'

'Don't ask him questions, Vassya,' said Koshkin. 'Not ones we don't need to know the answer to. When you have opened one tractor-part factory I can assure you, Comrade Rossel, you have opened them all. But, as I believe you already know, there are worse ways of spending a day in our glorious Soviet state. Your past is well known to me. For many, Igarka is a one-way ticket . . .'

'You have no need to worry,' said Rossel. 'Our investigation appears to have reached a dead end. Access to Comrade Molotov is unlikely to be granted to me.'

Koshkin drew himself to his full height and pulled on his gloves.

'Molotov, you say? Pah. Yesterday's man,' he said. 'I hear he has fallen so far out of favour that his wife has been arrested and sent into exile. Molotov himself is merely counting the days until his own fate is sealed.'

With an effort, Rossel sat upright.

'How do you know?'

Koshkin turned to face him.

'If you want rise in the Ministry of Machine Tool Building, comrade, you need to develop a keen ear for more than just the sound of the carburettors on the new MTZ2s they are producing in Minsk. And a keen eye, too. An eye for the tallest stalks of corn. Especially the ones that have been marked out for the harvest.'

Koshkin put on his *ushanka* and centred it.

'I gather Comrade Molotov has fallen so far they have even taken his Party dacha away. They say he has been forced to retreat to his own country residence, where he now awaits Soviet justice.'

'But where is it?' asked Vassya. 'His own dacha, I mean.'

Koshkin walked across to her and kissed her.

337

'An ugly little smear on the map called Valdai. He's there now, apparently. Brooding. He has no power in Moscow and no friends in Leningrad, so it is appropriate for him to languish halfway between the two, welcome in neither. Nothing to do there but fish. And wait.'

46

'You know what, in my opinion, is better than having friends in high places?' the minister said.

Nikitin shrugged. 'No.'

'Loyal comrades in low ones.'

The minister seemed pleased with his joke.

It was the same room in the Astoria hotel as last time. He wore a big coat, just like his underling. Unlike him, he filled it.

'And we are still friends you and I? I'm right about that, am I not, Major?'

'Of course, Comrade Minister.'

But he hasn't come all the way to Leningrad just to see me, thought Nikitin.

Something else must be about to happen.

'Excellent. I gather that you, like me, are from peasant stock. I myself am from a village so poor the peasants there couldn't even afford a sign. Herded cows and sheep as a boy.'

He lifted the sleeve of his coat and gave it an exaggerated sniff.

'Sometimes I think I can still smell the cowshit.'

Nikitin leaned forward.

339

'My wife, Comrade Minister. My son. My daughter. You will still intervene on their behalf? As your representative has promised me?'

The minister sat back.

'Later on, I worked down a mine, and then in a chemical factory. I can see from the scars on your face, your accent, the way you lump about the place, that you are hoping the next *apparatchik* who walks past will spit in your face just so you can give them a good kicking.'

He sniffed his sleeve again. 'And I can tell that you can smell the cowshit too. You're a man like me, who's not ashamed of having done peasant work, of having dirty hands. Or a dirty conscience. Am I right?'

'My wife, Comrade Minister. My son, Dima.'

The minister did not reply.

Sometimes, a man breaks easier when he is still allowed a little hope.

The minister understood that, too.

Finally, he nodded.

'Yes, I'll keep them safe. Providing . . .'

'Providing?'

'You continue to keep me informed.'

His eyes creased at the corners.

'So, tell me a little more about this man Halder . . .'

47

Grey-white sky above, dirt-white road below.

Small, three-hut villages raced past the car's misted windows and became dots in Rossel's rear-view mirror.

Valdai. *An ugly little smear on the map.* But also a place of recreation for second-tier members of the Party, according to Koshkin. Lakes, spas, a smattering of summer dachas for middle managers and bureaucrats. Very few people there at this time of year. Easy to find, and nowhere to run. A perfect place to hunt down Molotov, cocooned in bourgeois luxury, waiting for Stalin's axe to fall.

Nikitin had barely raised his voice to question Rossel's request to take the car. He seemed distracted, on edge – on the verge of another meeting with General Pletnev.

After four hours, Rossel was skirting Lake Ilmen and the town of Novgorod, once a rival power centre to Moscow. Until Ivan the Terrible had sacked it and slaughtered or deported its inhabitants with Stalinist thoroughness.

The light was fading. He pulled in for petrol, receiving assurances that he was on the right road but that it would take him another three hours.

For a while he sang to keep himself awake – an old peasant song about fortune tellers. A little hymn offered up to Fate.

Without a map and by now in the dark, Rossel had to guess the turning and guessed wrong, necessitating several stops for assistance from tiny settlements amid the thickening forest. A tractor driver returning to his *kolkhoz*, respectful but sullen, set him straight for a while. Soon lost again, he saw in his headlights a peasant woman gathering wood.

'Valdai? Comrade Molotov?' he asked her through the window. She was bent almost double by years of physical toil. She pointed down the road and then, with a jerk of her whole arm, towards the left. He followed the road until, sure enough, there was a left turn.

The road grew rougher and the wheels of the car began to spin against the deepening snow.

There it is.

A fine, two-storey wooden dacha, a mere couple of hundred metres from the lake, with a bright moon flashing on the water.

Between the house and the lake, silhouetted by light from a long wooden veranda, a man sat lost in contemplation on a small wooden bench. He turned to face the car. If he was alarmed he did not show it.

Rossel stopped the car and got out.

Head to one side, the First Deputy Chairman of the Council of Ministers waited for him to approach. Wearing a dark fur coat, Molotov was flat-faced, with a moustache that had starred in a thousand newsreels and newspaper photographs.

'I have been waiting for you,' Molotov called out, his tenor voice quavering. 'But you don't look like Mercader.'

Rossel kept walking towards the bench, hands out of his pockets and by his sides.

'Mercader?'

'Ramón Mercader. The man who put an ice axe in Trotsky's head.'

Rossel stopped.

'I'm not here for that. And I'm not here from them – the MGB. Besides . . .'

Rossel glanced around. Pine and birch encircled the lake, which was ice until the last few centimetres before the water lapped against a beach.

'As far as I can see, this isn't Mexico.'

Molotov stared out at the lights that dotted the distant shore.

'No,' he said. 'It's a lot closer to Moscow than that.'

The two men faced out to the water, taking a moment to revel in the silence and stillness, both grateful for a moment of peace.

'In Stalin's court, every prince sleeps with his head on the block. If not Beria, who sent you?' said Molotov.

'General Pletnev. I came for some information, comrade. Information vital to the security of the Soviet Union.'

Molotov stood.

'Pletnev. I see. You have had a long journey, comrade, I can tell,' he said. 'Let's eat.'

48

Inside the dacha, three walls of the main room were covered with paintings in the Russian folk style. For the most part they were winter scenes. One was particularly impressive: a downed stag impaled by arrows. Alongside happy peasants in the fields, there were more scenes from fairy tales and landscapes of forests and lakes. The curtains and furniture coverings were a riot of red berries and gold leaves. A subdued fire crackled in a simple brick fireplace.

The fourth wall was covered in books from floor to ceiling – hundreds of them. At least three and a half rows were taken up by musical anthologies and biographies of great composers.

Molotov walked over to an ancient gramophone and began to wind it up.

'No staff?' Rossel asked.

Molotov snorted.

'In the Kremlin, every day you learn to take the temperature,' he said. 'How blows the wind today from Gori, we ask ourselves.'

Gori was Stalin's birthplace.

'For some time now an unexpectedly cold breeze from the Georgian mountains has required me to take particular care when buttoning up my coat.'

The needle dropped onto the record.

'I sent my staff away last week,' Molotov continued. 'Just because I have caught a cold, doesn't mean they have to.'

The music began to play.

'Glazunov,' said Rossel. He caught Molotov's eye. 'I studied violin at the Leningrad Conservatoire.'

'The conservatoire? So we have the appreciation of music in common.'

For the first time, Molotov smiled.

'Have you ever seen the portrait of Glazunov by Ilya Repin? He looks so severe. A priest confessor who has ceased to believe in the concept of mercy.'

Rossel shook his head.

'No,' he said. 'But from your description, I think I'd quite like it.'

They listened to a few more bars.

'I myself dabble. I have attempted this concerto,' said Molotov, 'but it demands more attention and talent than I can give it.'

To play the Glazunov concerto required an advanced technique. Molotov was a man possessing some unexpected gifts.

Through a door off to the right, Rossel could see a long dining table, large enough for a dozen people. But set for only two.

'You were already awaiting a guest?'

Melancholy passed over Molotov's face.

'My wife, Polina,' he said. 'She was exiled to Siberia over the matter of Jewish settlement of the Crimea. I was forced to denounce her. Yet I set the table each night so we might one day dine as we used to.' He took off his glasses and then replaced them. 'There's a little hope in ritual, I find.'

'Exile is not death, at least,' said Rossel.

Molotov laughed. 'Mostly, it is death,' he said. 'But let us eat while we can.'

*

For several minutes the two men had chewed away in determined silence, grunting or jabbing a fork into the air to indicate their approval.

After a second helping of the *pelmeni* Molotov had brought from the kitchen and another enormous dollop of sour cream, the old Bolshevik poured out two glasses of vodka.

'To the artists, musicians, directors and writers of the Soviet Union,' Molotov said, raising his glass.

He took a sip, and then a longer, greedier gulp, setting the glass back down on the table and rubbing his cheeks.

Rossel drank his vodka down. The warmth of the alcohol cheered him.

Molotov pointed at Rossel's left hand. 'There's a story in your hands, I think. A violinist with missing fingers. Someday I'd like to hear it. But not tonight. Let's get down to business.'

In the next room, the Glazunov was halfway through the finale: a joyous, rumbustious dance. And a challenge, Rossel remembered. Left-hand pizzicato, harmonics at considerable speed, and you needed a free, supple bowing arm.

'You are in possession of a piano,' he said. 'Brought back to the USSR from Bayreuth. One that used to belong to Richard Wagner. And with it, a musical score that must have accompanied the instrument. The latter is of interest to Defence Minister General Pletnev.'

Molotov swept a hand several times across the table. The old Bolshevik thought for a moment. In the centre of the table was a white plate on which were the last of the dumplings. Three of them were round and perfectly formed. The fourth was small and stunted, a runt the chef had made from the last scraps of dough.

Molotov picked it up.

'So why doesn't the general simply place a call to me? Or send a platoon. Why send you?'

Rossel shrugged.

'I am a person of no importance. The general does not confide in me. I am simply here to do his bidding.'

Molotov frowned.

'"I am a person of no importance." I might print that phrase on a card and hand it out to the next people who come calling at my dacha. That way, I might live a little longer.'

He tossed the dumpling in the air and caught it again.

'Permit me to pass on some news that may not have been in the newspapers,' he said. 'A few weeks ago, the Americans carried out the first successful test of a hydrogen bomb, somewhere in the South Pacific. Do you know what a hydrogen bomb is?'

'No.'

Molotov held the palm of his right hand flat so that Rossel could see the dumpling.

'The bomb they dropped on Hiroshima was 16 kilotons. That is equivalent to 16,000 tons of TNT,' said Molotov. 'In that explosion, about 140,000 people died.'

347

He picked up one of the bigger dumplings with his left hand and held it out.

'Our people estimate this recently detonated hydrogen bomb was 10 megatons. That is equivalent to 10 million tons of TNT.'

Molotov raised up the larger dumpling in his left hand.

'That's Moscow, gone. Leningrad, gone. Sverdlovsk, Chelyabinsk, Omsk, Gorky, Stalingrad, Kuibyshev, Vladivostok, Kazan. Not a brick left, not one child's cry, not a single mournful bird singing in a tree.'

His eyes were round and set well back in his face. He spoke with long pauses to complete the calculations taking place in his mind. Rossel began to see why he had survived for so long when so many of Lenin's comrades had slid beneath the quicksand of the revolution.

The record crackled to a stop and Molotov rose again to replace it.

He took a while with his choice. Then the mournful opening bars of Mozart's 'Requiem' drifted into the room. Still a Russian favourite, even in the atheist's paradise.

'Immediately after this new American bomb, Stalin held a meeting of the Politburo,' Molotov said, resuming his seat. 'Myself, Kaganovich, Khrushchev, Beria, Mikoyan, Pletnev, Malenkov, a few others. The Great Leader screamed at us. Called us useless fools. He worked himself up into such a rage I thought his heart would give out. When he was finished, he sat back and was silent. He looked very old in the way people do when they have seen too much and become a little tired of living.'

Requiem, the basses rumbled.

The tenors agreed. *Requiem aeternam*.

'Without our own hydrogen bomb there will soon be no Union of Soviet Socialist Republics, was the main point he was making. As we sat at the table and looked across at Stalin's grey skin and glassy eyes, every man there suddenly understood – Stalin won't be around forever. And the man who builds that bomb will most likely take his place.'

Et lux perpetua luceat eis . . .

Molotov got to his feet and gestured towards the door of the next room.

'And now here you are, comrade. Sent by General Pletnev. In pursuit of a piano that was shipped to me, along with many other items of musical interest, from the Bayreuth house of the German nuclear physicist, Herr von Möllendorf.'

*

Molotov led the way into a large, homely living space with more books on all sides. And a Bechstein piano resting on a green-topped table in one corner.

'There,' he said.

Rossel stared at it. It was a rich walnut brown, sleek and polished, its only fault being that it looked like someone had cut the legs off.

'I had expected something more imposing.'

'The composer had more than one piano, of course,' said Molotov. 'After all, he was Richard Wagner. But this was the instrument on which he composed *Götterdämmerung*. So they tell me, at least. A table piano. Simple to move from place to place. Practical. And yet an artefact.'

From the gramophone, the choir sang of judgment and resurrection.

'And talking of the Twilight of the Gods . . .'

Molotov gripped Rossel's elbow and led him to a central section of the bookshelves.

It was an extensive collection of musical scores. Rossel could see long rows of symphonies and concertos; music for solo piano; a vast collection of violin works . . . and about two metres of operatic scores, mostly Russian. There was Rimsky-Korsakov, Glinka, Tchaikovsky – even the out-of-favour Prokofiev. And the banned Rachmaninov.

There it is – the Ring Cycle.

The four music dramas, *Das Rheingold. Die Walküre. Siegfried. Götterdämmerung.*

Molotov reached out and picked it up.

'Sometimes the wind from Gori will chill a man's bones no matter how many buttons he has done up. Do you understand, comrade? Tonight, you were not who I thought you might be. But tomorrow . . .'

'There maybe somebody else,' said Rossel.

'Precisely.'

Molotov handed the score to Rossel, who opened it.

It was monumental.

'Tell General Pletnev that this comes not from me but my wife, Polina. Do you understand? That with this gift he is in her debt.'

Rossel nodded.

'I will impress that fact upon him, Comrade Molotov. That whatever happens, he must set her a place at his table.'

*

A gentle snowfall had resumed. 'Be careful on the road,' said Molotov, leaning into the window of Rossel's car, his face half in light, half in darkness. 'This snow will only get heavier.'

The minister stepped back and looked out towards the bench on which Rossel had found him sitting. 'Your name, comrade? It sounds foolish but I was born in Kukarka, where peasant superstitions once reigned before Soviet modernity swept them away. I did not want to ask you when you arrived, in case you were indeed a shade and the sound of the words alone might have stopped my breath.'

'Rossel, Comrade Minister Molotov. Revol Rossel.'

'Revol. A good name. *Revolyutsionnaya Volya*. The Will of the Revolution. Your family must have been greatly committed to the cause.'

Rossel nodded.

'When they gave me the name, yes. Later, circumstances may have convinced them something else may have suited me better. They were both sent to the camps.'

Molotov sighed.

'As Marx said, "There is only one way in which the murderous death agonies of the old society and the bloody birth throes of the new society can be shortened, simplified and concentrated, and that way is revolutionary terror." It is regrettable but we Russians have had to make many sacrifices for the great peace to come. I must soon make mine.'

Rossel started up the motor. It took a couple of tries to get it going.

'One last thing, since you work for General Pletnev,' said Molotov, leaning into the window again. 'A word of caution. In April 1945, at the Seelow Heights, the First Belorussian Front was taking a beating.'

'I know,' said Rossel. 'Everyone knows that General Pletnev saved the day.'

'But listen,' said Molotov, pressing a finger to his lips. 'Zhukov was throwing more men into the fray but the Germans had burst a dam to flood the ground. A brilliant defensive move. Everything was sinking into the mud. It's true what people say. Pletnev reorganised the assault, the artillery tactics, the tank formations. Broke through, raced forward to the outskirts of Berlin. And halted.'

'To let Zhukov through,' said Rossel. 'To let him have the honour of capturing the Reich's capital city.'

Molotov drew a rough circle in the snow with his foot, and then dragged his heel to make a line next to it.

'No, Comrade Rossel. General Pletnev halted there because that was the approximate range of the *katyusha* rockets he had available. Nine kilometres. He lined up every mortar regiment in the First Belorussian Army – every *katyusha*, every howitzer – and opened up. His intention was to obliterate everything between him and the Reichstag.'

Molotov stepped onto the circle.

'He maintained fire for approximately twenty minutes before Zhukov could get through on the telephone and ask him what the hell he thought he was doing. Apparently, the answer was, "What Hitler wished to do to Leningrad I will now do to them."'

A breeze was getting up, skating off the lake and shaking the smaller branches of the trees. Molotov's jacket whipped open but he was content to let it flap as he took a step back out of the car's way.

'Beria is the poison that runs through Stalin's veins,' the Old Bolshevik said. 'But Pletnev is the knife at his throat.'

He shoved his spectacles up the bridge of his nose and peered through them at Rossel.

'Polina, comrade. Be sure to tell the general about her.'

*

After half a kilometre, Rossel pulled over and grabbed the score.

> *Denn der Götter Ende dämmert nun auf.*
> *So werf' ich den Brand*
> *in Walhalls prangende Burg.*

Brünnhilde's great soprano aria came right at the end of *Götterdämmerung.*

In the thin light provided by the overhead bulb, Rossel could barely see the music or the words. He clambered out of the car and used the headlights instead, half-blinding himself until he got the angle right.

A fusion of instruments and voice, music and drama, gods and men – dozens of leitmotifs converging for the climax.

And amid the notes, a line of Brünnhilde's aria. *Denn der Götter Ende dämmert nun auf. He* followed it to the climax. A massive fanfare on the word *Burg* in the wood-wind and brass, dominated by the trumpets.

Protons. Electrons. Neutrons . . . Even smaller particles, and smaller still.

A cluster of notes that looked darker than the rest.

Perhaps a dozen.

Black spots again. Ink on paper.

He removed the glove from his withered left hand and traced them with his forefinger. The nerve endings were long dulled but the sensation was evident and undeniable. Lost in the cosmos of ink, a short fanfare of notes, which, like Braille, were raised from the paper. Almost imperceptible bumps that gave off tiny shards of reflected light.

The gigantic hidden within the shell of the infinitesimal. Worlds hiding within worlds.

And within each of them, the power to destroy this one.

ACT 4
GODS

49

Nikitin drove his reclaimed GAZ through a dilapidated arch into a courtyard somewhere in the middle of Vasilievsky Ostrov – the island district of the city, out west, where every building looked like every other building.

That was the point. When on Soviet territory, GRU agents had every army base in the Leningrad Oblast to hide in, so that was where they were expected to be. But on occasions, a hideout in the city that Beria's Ministry for State Security did not know about was safer.

As they got out and headed for the elegant, pre-revolutionary apartment block, both men had to step from side to side to avoid the puddles of slush that pockmarked the courtyard. For all that, they moved with purpose and pace.

Outside, up four flights of the stone staircase, a man in blue overalls stood to attention.

'My balls have shrunk to one kopek pieces,' muttered Nikitin as he rapped on the door. 'Hurry up, *ublyudki*, it's fucking freezing out here.'

From inside came the sound of a complicated lock being turned.

Now that he was back in Leningrad, Rossel could not shake off the fear, real or imagined, that a sniper's sights were trained on the back of his head. He remembered a moment of quiet while jammed into a crater with another soldier during the Sinyavino Offensive, right in the depths of the war – a moment when both sides were reloading and the sun came out. They had shared half a damp cigarette and memories of childhood before a sniper had picked the man off. It was not for several minutes – as Rossel lay face up, pressing his shoulder blades as far as he could back into the mud and slime – that he discovered a small grey piece of the man's brain stuck to his right lapel. As if it was a badge.

Snipers, he thought, usually preferred the distance kill. But Koshchei was different . . .

'Something on your mind?' said Nikitin.

Rossel tried to stop feeling as if he was being hunted.

'Something Molotov told me,' he said.

'Which was?'

Beria is the poison that runs through Stalin's veins. But Pletnev is the knife at his throat.

Rossel shrugged and took a step forward. The door swung open.

'Nothing important,' he said.

50

The room was large but still filled with the fug of smoke from imported Bulgarian cigarettes – better quality tobacco, for those who could get access to it.

In a corner was a pink-tasselled standing lamp. On one wall was a black-and-white photograph of a man standing next to an ageing elephant: a once-beloved beast named Betty that was killed by German bombs at the very beginning of the city's wartime bombardment. This room, Nikitin had told him, used to be the elephant keeper's apartment. The GRU had long ago appropriated the building, though for some reason had maintained the animal theme for the décor. On another wall was a tapestry of deer grazing in a forest, similar to the one Rossel had seen at Molotov's dacha but not as well executed.

At a large, polished table in the centre of the room sat a small, thin woman with neat black hair and horn-rimmed spectacles. Rossel recognised her – Captain Morozova, the GRU codebreaker who had been so dismissive of the markings and clues within *The Prince*. She had the score of *Götterdämmerung* open before her – at its final pages. Next to her was a microscope with some cumbersome attachments.

'A pleasure to meet you again, Captain Morozova,' said Rossel.

She acknowledged him without enthusiasm.

'Likewise, comrade,' she said.

At the far end of the table sat two more people, a man and a woman, going over outsize sheets of photographic paper on which were printed images of documents. Three men, dressed in suits and ties, were peering over their shoulders. All five were whispering to each other. They looked excited. Rossel did not have the spy's facility for reading upside down but the images looked like pages of typed paper, in Roman script, interspersed with handwritten equations and rough diagrams.

Sitting behind them on a stool against the wall was a bald man in his late thirties with a small red goatee and doleful eyes. No one introduced him.

'Captain Morozova,' said Nikitin to the codebreaker. He was as agitated as ever. 'How long before everything is ready?'

A door that Rossel hadn't noticed opened. Beyond it was a dark red gleam. He caught the whiff of chemicals – a strangely pleasant scent.

'Microdots, when all is said and done, are photographs,' said Morozova, who looked displeased at having her name said aloud. 'You take a standard photographic image of your chosen document on a high-contrast film. Then you take that negative, which is already smaller by approximately ten times, and you reduce it again – shining a bright light on it from where the eye would be, through a lens to shrink it another thirty times or so, and focus the positive image onto a glass plate coated with a special emulsion . . .'

Nikitin sighed. 'It doesn't sound very simple.'

Morozova picked up her cigarette from a metal ashtray and took a thoughtful drag – a gesture that seemed to suggest that simplicity was a relative concept, dependant on the intellect of the beholder – before continuing:

'Then you cut out the emulsion from the backing – a slightly enlarged hypodermic needle is favourite for doing that, to stamp it out. *Pozhaluista* – you have a *mikrat*.'

'A *mikrat*?' said Rossel.

'A microdot. The Hitlerites were masters at it.'

Nikitin was losing patience.

'I don't need a detailed lesson in how microdots work, comrade. All we need to know is, have you found anything significant yet?'

Morozova coloured a little. 'To preserve their clarity, we have a two-step enlargement and development process.' She jabbed a thumb in the direction of the room with the aroma of chemicals, and Rossel realised it was where her colleagues were developing and printing the film. 'There are more than 250 pages here. We are up to page . . . page twenty-three. Please allow us to do our work, Comrade Major Nikitin. Once developed they must be fixed into slides – we'd blow them up bigger but there isn't that amount of quality photographic paper in the city. Only a sample are being turned into larger images.'

She looked at Rossel.

'You can hide a microdot anywhere,' she said. 'On the hem of a doll's dress. In the full stop at the end of a love letter. In a packet of tobacco. Under a stamp is a favourite.'

She leafed through the many pages of *Götterdämmerung*.

'In an opera the size of this one there are hundreds, thousands, maybe tens of thousands of places you could put one. How did you know to look on this particular page?'

Rossel lent forward and tapped a finger on the score.

'I started studying the violin at the age of four,' he said. 'Over two decades of training I learned a few things about what composers wrote, and what they meant. And I had some further direction from the ghost of a man we found in a haunted house. How long until everything is ready, Comrade Morozova?'

'Four hours should do it.'

Nikitin checked his watch.

'It is 11.30. You have until 15.00. I must report to General Pletnev by 16.00 and not a moment later,' he said.

Morozova reattached her eye to the microscope.

'I will go as fast as I can, comrade. But no faster . . .'

*

'Where are we going?' asked Rossel, yawning.

'Tarkovsky's place,' answered Nikitin. 'You need rest. And you won't get any in that room. In a couple of hours, it is going to have half a dozen GRU officers in it, all the general's men, plus all those scientists we saw and a few more besides.'

Red and gold banners streamed from buildings and lampposts, bearing rousing slogans and images of Stalin.

Rossel and Nikitin passed a *Produkty* with a long queue outside, citizens pulling up their collars and clutching their string bags in anticipation of some *kolbasa,* or tinned fish, or some other delicacy for the evening meal. Many of them would be queuing because there was a queue to join, happy to find out what was on offer once they were inside. A car coming the other way lost its hold on the road and slid diagonally towards them. Rossel could see the eyes of the driver as he whirled the steering wheel in his effort to regain control. They missed each other by inches.

'You saw the man with the red beard?' said Nikitin. 'That's Dmitri Fironov. Two years ago he was expelled from the main nuclear research team that reported directly to Beria.'

'Not so smart,' said Rossel.

'Wrong. He is now the lead scientist on this project. He got the boot because he fell out with the project's leader, Igor Tamm, and its star physicist, Andrei Sakharov. They set up the entire thing from scratch, on the site of an old munition factory. Place called Sarov, officially known as KB-11. Fironov told them their design was flawed and that they were on the wrong track. He got reported for defeatism.'

'Then he was lucky not to be shot,' said Rossel.

'In forty-two, he was in the air force when he noticed that American academics had suddenly stopped publishing anything public in the field of nuclear physics. Now why would they do that, he asked himself. More importantly, he asked the question in a letter to Stalin. It turned out to be a very good one. He had correctly deduced the capitalists were building a bomb. When you do something right in Stalin's eyes, even Beria sometimes has to wait before he puts a noose around your throat.'

'And Pletnev took him in?'

'Yes,' said Nikitin. 'He did. He likes to take in the occasional stray mongrel. In case we prove useful.'

*

Nikitin turned right, onto the embankment, heading for Lieutenant Schmidt Bridge.

'The snowploughs have been out at last,' the major said.

Rossel stared at some of the saltwater-stained hulks moored on the river, but began to close his eyes. He was exhausted, and the cough that had plagued him in Igarka had returned.

After a few minutes, he felt the car begin to slow down. Then roll to a stop. His eyes blinked open.

'Visitors,' said Nikitin in a low voice.

Rossel sat up.

About fifty metres away, he could see two black vans parked outside the entrance to Tarkovsky's apartment. Six men in the blue-banded caps of the MGB were bringing the actor out of the front door. They bundled him into the back of the van that was furthest from Rossel and Nikitin.

Rossel pointed at the van that was closer to them. Sitting in the passenger seat was a thin, grey-haired man.

'Fadeyev,' he said.

The Head of the Writers' Union looked rather pleased with himself. Like someone who had been putting off tidying a messy bookcase for some time and had finally got around to doing it.

'Poor Boris,' said Rossel. 'Tonight was going to be his big night at the Anichkov – Tarkovsky sings for Stalin!'

Nikitin shrugged. 'Be honest,' he said. 'He was never going to get close to any of those high notes.'

The major revved the car and they set off again.

'We'd better make for the Drugovs' place instead,' he said. 'Let's hope it's safer than here.'

51

Four hours later, after a restless sleep that had made Rossel feel worse, he and Nikitin returned to the GRU safe house. This time, it was crammed full of gleaming belt buckles and cap badges.

Good news, Rossel thought. In the GRU, like the militia, senior officers always make an appearance when it turns up.

A large piece of plywood, recently painted white, had been nailed to a wall. Morozova was feeding slides into a holder, marking the edge of each with red pencil and cataloguing them in an exercise book.

Professor Fironov was rubbing his hands together in excitement, telling a tall, middle-aged man with red cheeks and a weathered face whom he addressed as Colonel Zotov that even he had no idea what to expect from the images that had just been developed. A young man smelling of chemicals was fiddling with the slide projector. A German brand, labelled *Liesegang*. Sleek, minimal, efficient.

Rossel barely noticed the short opening speeches of congratulations, though at one point Nikitin dug an elbow into his ribs and he realised that everyone was looking at him. The lights snapped off and soon Fironov was waving his hands through clouds of smoke, the light from the projector dancing through them like flashes of sunlight on an overcast day.

To Rossel, all the slides looked the same. Technical drawings, impossibly long equations, pages and pages of theoretical physics. His tired brain could barely follow Fironov's simplified explanations to the GRU senior officers, let alone the technical details.

A GRU officer soon lost patience and demanded assurances that this was important information. His epaulettes denoted a colonel.

The room seemed to be full of them. 'What I want to know is, how is this different from Sakharov's work for Beria? Sakharov claims he is close to the hydrogen bomb.'

Fironov removed his tiny spectacles and dabbed at his brow.

'For years, it has been our thinking that it would be the neutrons from the first atomic explosion that would compress the fuel sufficiently for the secondary thermonuclear explosion. But this Hitlerite document tells us it is the radiation. The radiation all along . . . This, and the more complex design, will send the necessary shock wave towards the centre.'

'How can you be certain, Comrade Fironov?' asked yet another officer. A thin man with dark eyes.

'Certain? That is not a word I would use. You have different types of physics in play, all interrelated; multiple reactions and effects happening in impossibly short timescales. Flow of fluids, heat transfer, pressure inwards, pressure outwards.'

Fironov thought for a moment. 'Every reaction has to happen in precisely the right order for the next one to occur. Put crudely, the pressure that will force the particles together for the second reaction must take place at sufficient scale before the whole contraption is vaporised by the first explosion. Sakhorov's "layer cake" design has never solved that. But I believe this one will do so.'

The projector clicked through more slides – more equations. Fironov was encouraging the projectionist to get to one slide in particular.

'Here it is,' the scientist said.

The slide was entirely taken up by a drawing of a large cylinder on its side. At the top were three concentric circles. Below them was an open-topped container with sloping sides, inside of which was another cylinder.

Fironov rubbed his hands together.

'This is the missing part. *This* is what Minister Pletnev will want to see and understand. The principle is similar to that pursued by Sakharov's team. Fission to create fusion, to create fission again. But Sakharov's layer cake doesn't work – not because the physics is wrong but because of the order in which the reactions take place.' He tugged at his goatee. 'Get those reactions in the right order and . . .'

'How big?' demanded Colonel Zotov. 'The explosion, I mean.'

Fironov looked around the room. 'The bombs the Americans dropped on Hiroshima and Nagasaki were small compared to the hydrogen bomb the American imperialists tested on November 1. It reached more than 10 megatons . . .'

Rossel sat up. What did he mean, the hydrogen bomb the Americans had tested?

'Some of us have seen the film,' said the GRU colonel who had not been identified. 'I did not believe it at first. Is this the same design?'

'Hard to be sure,' said Fironov, 'but I believe so. And as to Colonel Zotov's questions, the explosive power of a hydrogen bomb is theoretically limited only by the availability of the fuel. We could make a king of bombs, with the right materials and design. One to strike fear into the hearts of the capitalists.'

'What film is he talking about?' Rossel said to Nikitin in an undertone. His question was masked by the chatter around the room.

'I have not seen it,' said the major. 'But a Soviet spy ship took some film of the American test. I am told it looks like the fury of the gods.'

'Silence!'

Colonel Zotov had lost patience. 'Comrade Fironov, you are confident that Sakharov's design, this layer cake, cannot achieve such explosive yield?'

'It cannot,' said Fironov. He took off his jacket. His shirt was soaked through. 'It might destroy Manhattan. This' – he gestured at the screen – 'could annihilate the whole of New York city and flatten most of New York state in the process.'

The room fell silent. Only the whirring of the projector could be heard.

'A two-stage weapon,' said Fironov. 'With a core of fissionable material inside the fusion fuel to provide a third reaction: an added dimension to a blast of already extraordinary power. We still need several things, though. The material for the core. The composition of the inner casing and the calculations for the reaction between that substance and the radiation. And how they have countered the instability. Next slide, please.'

'Comrade Fironov,' said Morozova. She was examining her notebook and looking at the projectionist, who nodded back at her. 'There is only one more slide.'

'What?'

The projectionist pressed the button and the cartridge of the Liesegang clunked, throwing the last image upon the wall.

A small photograph of a man. In his army uniform, with hair swept back from his forehead, he looked every inch the Teutonic Knight. He had hooded eyes and a sad expression.

And a short, white scar above one eye, such as might have been made by a sword in a duel. Printed beneath the photograph was a small coat of arms. An eagle holding a sword in one claw and a book in the other.

'There's nothing else?' said the professor. 'That cannot be . . .'

Morozova shook her head.

'Go back three slides, one at a time,' said the scientist, a note of panic in his voice.

The projectionist did as he was asked. Fironov counted the slides back, squinting hard at each one as he did so.

'There is information missing,' he said, swallowing.

'Something important?' said Rossel.

Fironov's shoulders slumped. He took out a handkerchief and mopped his brow.

'Vital,' he said.

The last slide of the man with the thin white line above his eye came back round.

'Does anyone recognise him?' asked Colonel Zotov.

Everyone shook their heads.

But Rossel was lying.

As he looked up at the screen, he noticed Fironov and Nikitin were staring at him.

A phone rang. Colonel Zotov picked it up. A raised voice at the other end of the line gave an order. The colonel's back straightened as soon as he heard it.

'Yes, Comrade General,' he said. 'At the headquarters of the League. We will come at once.'

52

Lines of workers swaddled in thick coats battled the snow and wind as they trudged homeward up and down Nevsky Prospect. The two ZIS-50s that had rolled into the courtyard outside the safe house, complete with armed guards, drew to a halt on the road near the former cathedral. Nikitin parked his car directly behind them.

Rossel got out of the car and stood on the pavement next to the major. He took out some matches and cupped his hands to shield the thin flame from the wind.

As a dozen soldiers clambered down from the back of the trucks, Colonel Zotov and Fironov got out of the front of the first one. They waited for Rossel and Nikitin to join them.

'Birds of good omen,' said Colonel Zotov. Everyone followed the colonel's gaze. A flock of black dots was flying over the dome of the museum. At this distance, it was impossible to tell what species they were.

'We still have a modicum of good news for the general,' said Fironov. 'But . . .'

He left the rest unsaid. His meaning was understood.

'Men, stay here,' Colonel Zotov told his troops. 'We will be back shortly. Comrade Fironov, you have the photographs?'

'Yes, Comrade Colonel.'

'Very well. The four of us will go to see the general now. He will want the full story.'

Zotov led the way towards General Pletnev's personal headquarters in the Museum of Atheism. As they passed one of the two bronze statues that stood at the end of each encircling arm of the former cathedral, the GRU colonel pointed upwards.

'Marshal Kutuzov. A lucky fool. Claimed to have prayed to Our Lady of Kazan before defeating Napoleon.' Zotov snorted. 'Imagine telling Stalin you were depending on an ikon to beat the Fascists at Stalingrad or Seelow?'

They were still thirty metres away from the huge bronze doors when Colonel Zotov stopped to straighten his cap and check his uniform. Rossel almost walked straight into him and had to sidestep to the left to avoid the collision.

'Bad news is best delivered in sharp creases,' said the GRU officer. 'That way it always looks like it's somebody else's faul—'

His hands went to his throat. A thin red geyser bubbled up through his fingers. He took a hand away and examined the bloody palm of his right glove.

Rossel grabbed Zotov under the arms as he slumped to the ground. The statue of Kutuzov – the best cover they had – was only a few metres behind them. For a few seconds, Rossel dragged the colonel towards it. But then, realising he was dead, he left him and ducked behind it.

Pistol drawn, Nikitin appeared on the other side, crouching down and pushing Fironov to the ground. On Nevsky Prospect, the contingent of soldiers by the trucks were sharing cigarettes and talking among themselves, unaware their commanding officer had been hit. Nikitin began to yell at them, but they were busy laughing and stamping their feet. One of them dropped to his knees, stayed there for a moment, and toppled over. The others gazed incuriously for two or three seconds at the body of their comrade.

Then they leapt for cover.

A bullet zinged off the granite plinth on which Kutuzov stood. Another pinged off the statue itself. Rossel pressed himself into the stone while Nikitin yelled at Fironov to keep still. The scientist was shaking with fear. By now a passer-by – a middle-aged man – was shouting in panic, and people on Nevsky Prospect were beginning to notice, and to scatter. The soldiers were using their vehicles as cover and were scanning the cathedral for the shooter, rifles raised in futile defence. Nikitin yelled at them, too – 'Fan out, you idiots, get behind the museum, get under the field of fire, stay low!'

Fironov was pale and gasping for air. 'I can't stay here, I can't stay here . . .'

Rossel slapped the scientist hard across the cheek. His eyes widened in shock.

'Don't move, not a step. Stay here and keep your head down. Understand?' he said.

Fironov nodded.

'Good lad,' said Nikitin.

He turned to Rossel.

'Is it her?' he said.

'Who else is it going to be?' said Rossel.

The major rubbed his nose with his sleeve.

'Left and right?'

'No,' Rossel replied. 'If the sniper is on the roof, she can move fast to change the angle of fire. For both of us, the best chance is get to the colonnade; moving between each column; varying our pauses, no pattern. As soon as you hear the next shot, move.'

Nikitin nodded.

Seconds later a bullet zipped past. A soldier screamed.

'Now,' said Rossel.

As they leapt from the cover provided by the base of the statue, Rossel fixed his eyes on the huge circular portico to the left of the museum and began racing towards it. In his peripheral vison, he could see Nikitin just to his right, slightly behind him. To their left was the Griboyedova Canal.

A lucky bullet for him, he realised, was any that hit the major.

A lucky bullet for Nikitin is any that hits me.

He covered the final few metres and flung himself behind the steps leading up to the entrance on the canal's side. A curse told him Nikitin had also made it. Round the corner came one of the army trucks; three soldiers running alongside, using it as a shield.

The doors on this side were locked, possibly barricaded if the sniper had had enough time. But there were windows leading straight into the main hall. It was a way in, but, if they were slow in climbing through, it would be an easy place to get picked off, assuming the sniper had seen them and retreated inside to deal with the threat. Nikitin was too bulky to be quick, and Rossel was still nowhere near up to full strength. Both men were breathing hard. But it was the quickest route.

Rossel scanned the ground for something to smash the glass. There – a hubcap, battered out of shape. Something that had fallen off a bus or a tourist coach. He ran to pick it up and advanced back towards the window, carrying it as if it were the rusting shield of a down-at-heel knight. The thought reminded him that he had lied to Fironov, lied to them all, about the final slide. He had recognised the face on it. It had taken him another few minutes to place it in his memory. But then, with shock, Rossel realised he knew exactly who the Nazi with the duelling scar was.

Gripping the hubcap on both sides, he made two sharp stabbing motions. Two panes of glass, each about a third of a metre square, popped out of the frame and smashed against the stone floor within.

They peered into a storage room complete with a sink and an overflowing bin.

Two more thrusts, and two more panes dropped out.

A couple more blows took out the crossed wooden stanchions of the frame.

Nikitin began to haul himself inside. Rossel followed.

*

They pulled the main door of the storage room ajar and looked out into the shadowy hall of the museum. On the far wall, the grave face of a partisan – armed to the teeth and vowing destruction to the enemies of the Soviet Union – looked back. The partisan's eyes gave nothing away, but his palm was raised.

A warning. One they didn't have time for.

'I'll go first,' said Rossel. 'You wait half a minute and follow.'

'Follow where?'

'Pletnev's office. I think we can assume the sniper is not here to admire the exhibition.'

He pushed open the door and stepped out into the Museum of Atheism.

Cover was not the problem. There was plenty of it, thanks to the long double lines of columns that ran to the centre.

But the sniper had her choice of cover, too.

He weaved his way through the columns, trying to remember where the door that led to Pletnev's subterranean office was. The former sacristy.

Near the centre of the nave was the display of waxwork figures from the Spanish Inquisition – monks, conquistadores, Torquemada, the figure of a man being stretched on a rack and the hooded executioner – all looking just as he remembered them.

The layout came back to him. The staircase that led to Pletnev's office was off to the left. Not at the far end of the nave, but close by. He tapped the bird on his chest.

At last, a lucky break . . .

He pushed the door open. The stairs descended into darkness.

Surely, she could not have made it this far, this fast? Unless there is another way?

He went through and pulled the door behind him to blot out his silhouette.

No sound. No movement that he could discern.

There was a dim light at the bottom, and as he reached the end of the stairs he swept the space in front of him with his pistol. The door to the general's office was ajar. He pushed it a little wider with the barrel of his pistol.

Back turned, a cowled and hunched figure was sitting at Pletnev's desk.

Rossel stepped into the room.

'Comrade General?' he said.

Pletnev did not move.

Rossel crossed the room. He stepped behind the desk and reached out with his left hand to tap the seated figure on the shoulder.

Lifeless, the body in the chair slumped forward.

As it did so, the hood slipped off the side of its face, revealing a forlorn, brutal countenance with two neat holes in the side of its head.

Sergeant Grachev might have escaped the icy waters of the Moika.

But he had not, it seemed, got very much further.

'The gloom of the world is but a shadow, yet within our reach is joy,' said a voice behind him.

Rossel placed his pistol on the general's desk with care. He put his hands up and turned around.

Mila Kitsenko's skin was so pale it was almost translucent. Her eyes were green, wide and unblinking, filled with the certainty of faith. Like Grachev she was hooded, in a dark green cloak that looked well suited to her work. It gave her the appearance of a melancholic nun.

'The words of Savonarola,' said Kitsenko. She pointed at Grachev. 'I have read them on his display case so often that the sentence has become like a psalm to me. I have been here many times.'

She had the barrel of her Mosin–Nagant rifle pointed at Rossel's stomach. She was small, yet handled the weapon without apparent effort.

'You've been using the new metro system to move the bodies. One of them, I know, runs very near here. Slipping up silently behind your victims, pressing a pistol to their backs, walking them into the tunnels. But, once there, Akimov ran, I assume. So, with him, you had to use your rifle.'

She nodded.

The hunter must become the prey.

That, according to Major Firsova at the sniper school, is what Mila's father had taught her. To understand how a quarry moves, thinks, hides . . .

He raised his hands a little higher. 'The struggle against religion is the struggle for socialism,' he said. 'When I was young, I used to believe that.'

Kitsenko lifted the muzzle of her rifle.

'I still do.'

53

Rossel, hands still high, was walking in front.

Kitsenko ordered him back up the stairs and told him to halt next to a huge banner declaring the liberation of the proletariat from the shackles of religion.

On another wall, a piece of plywood proclaimed the words of Lenin in crimson paint: *Religion is one of the forms of spiritual oppression that weigh on the masses no matter where they are, crushed by eternal toil for others.*

They passed more display cases of objects Rossel had not yet seen. Medieval masks, more torture instruments, paintings of drunken monks and debauched nuns, caricatures of Jesus and the disciples in the style of Socialist Realism.

On the edge of the great central hall, in an alcove from where the famous ikon of Our Lady of Kazan had once looked down on her adoring worshippers, General Pletnev sat bound and gagged.

His eyes were closed, his head bowed. But he was alive.

Pletnev inhaled sharply through his nose and raised his head.

On the wall above him, in the space vacated by the ikon of Our Lady, was a photograph of someone else.

Another face Rossel recognised.

One of Babayan's shadows in the snow – the child the old priest had talked of at the very end of the railway line as they hauled their human steamroller through the wastelands. Alexei: the heir to the last tsar, the hope of the Romanov dynasty; murdered, along with his entire family, in the damp basement of the Ipatiev House in Yekaterinburg. Some of Babayan's words came back to him: 'God has raised these martyrs to his kingdom.'

Mila Kitsenko had raised Alexei, too. Inside Pletnev's museum. Inside his Kingdom of the Godless.

Pletnev's hands were tied behind his back and his waist was lashed to the back of the chair with some rough hemp. Kitsenko ordered Rossel to remove the gag. The general took several deep breaths, growing less pale with each one.

'Ah,' said the general. 'That is disappointing, I had my hopes pinned on you, Comrade Rossel. You have a quality I could have used at Seelow. Let's call it panache. But Mila always was a model of Soviet efficiency.'

There was no fear in the general's voice. He talked as if observing distant field movements through binoculars and then passing on orders to a subordinate.

'She has murdered six men, general,' said Rossel.

'At least. Mila believes in her cause. So did you, once. My enquires led me to understand you were, as a youth, a fervent member of the League. Someone who, given time and the right training, could have been one of our most zealous foot soldiers.'

'You have something of mine,' Kitsenko said to Rossel.

Rossel nodded and unbuttoned the top of his shirt, feeling for the locket.

He handed it to her. She took it and hung it on a hook just above the picture of Alexei.

She handed him a pair of handcuffs. With the barrel of her rifle she motioned him a few paces to the right, to a big water pipe that ran all the way from the floor to the distant ceiling. Without being asked, Rossel cuffed his right wrist to the pipe.

Kitsenko checked it.

'Sit,' she said, kicking a chair towards him. Rossel did so.

Then she turned and began to run, at pace, towards the back of the main hall – behind what once would have been the altar. She moved, Rossel noticed, with grace and economy, creating a sense of being ephemeral. As if, when slipping from one position to another on a battlefield, she might disappear.

*

Rossel and the general listened to the echo of Kitsenko's footsteps.

Rossel spoke first.

'I presume she's taking a position on the dome?' he said.

Pletnev nodded.

'There are stairs that lead to the roof,' he said. 'From up there she has a clear firing line to any point on Nevsky, plus points all around. For several hundred metres, at least.'

Rossel yanked his handcuffed arm a couple of times to test the heating pipe.

'Protocol 478 deals with counter-revolutionary insurrection,' said Pletnev. 'I'm assuming it has been authorised and that the museum is now surrounded. But if she gets a couple more shots away from up there it will keep the militia and MGB at bay for a while.'

'Time for what?'

Pletnev craned his neck towards the photograph of the tsarevich Alexei above his head.

'Isn't it obvious? We are to be martyred.'

'But she could have killed you at any time with just one shot from that rifle. Me too, for that matter.'

'Not close, not eye to eye, with each bullet a benediction. She started her little habit in the war, after her friends were killed. Now, I presume, it's the ritual to which she is addicted.'

Rossel gave another couple of half-hearted pulls at the water pipe.

Pletnev tutted.

'In the field, when nothing can be done, the best thing to do is often to do just that.'

'Major Firsova at the sniper school told me about them,' said Rossel. 'About her and her closest comrades. They called themselves the *troika*. She said they were the terror of the Germans at Stalingrad.'Pletnev nodded.

'All our snipers were. But Mila had her own unique calling card, if she got close enough to her victims. She would cut out their tongues. At first it was just a few Fascists. No one was really very bothered about that. But afterwards some of the men kept their distance, uncertain if she was a devil or a saint. Then she overheard a Red Army captain praying to Christ under his breath just before his platoon crossed a river for an assault. Later, he was found with his tongue missing and a quote from Lenin – "Paradise on Earth is more important than paradise in Heaven" – inside his throat. That was when I had to reassign her to another unit.'

Shots – one, then two more – heard; in the distance, but clear.

Answering fire. From more than one direction, and louder. The soldiers must have spread out, readying for an attack on the museum.

How can she hope to escape?

'Cut out their tongues? Words in their mouths?' Rossel said, meeting the general's gaze. 'So, you knew it was her all along? As soon as Nikitin told you about the scrolls?'

'Yes, Comrade Lieutenant Rossel. And I was meant to. Corpses left in places where I could not miss them, murdered in a particular way that I well understood. Mila was sending me a message.'

Lieutenant . . .

It was long time since anyone had called him that.

'A message about what?'

'About treachery. "How gentle is deception . . . for it defies perception." About the purity of faith our Marxist cause demands, and the price that must be paid by those who betray it.'

Rossel sniffed the air.

Smoke . . .

He looked up just as Kitsenko stepped out from behind the nearest column. Her rifle was slung over her back. She went over to Pletnev and examined his bonds. Then she stood and stroked the general's head.

'Stalingrad,' she whispered to him. 'Watching *The Mandrake* in your bunker as the shells rained down, seemingly unable to touch us. I have often thought of it.'

Rossel sniffed the air again. This time the smell of smoke was stronger.

'One hundred and seventy kills,' said Pletnev to Kitsenko. 'Not counting those you have assassinated since then for Comrade Beria, Mila. For the MGB. Am I right? Then, as now, you lived as a Valkyrie, as a chooser of the slain.'

The smoke was visible now, and it wasn't from a few candles.

Where the hell was Nikitin?

Kitsenko nodded.

'"When the last believer dies, so then does God himself." That's what we used to say to conclude every League meeting. That has always been my purpose.'

Pletnev smiled.

'Mine too. But if you think you've made some deal with Beria, Mila? That he'll help you restore the fortunes of the League? Then despite all you have done, you are still a child.'

Rossel could not see flames, but now he could hear them.

Kitsenko took a step back. Her face darkened. From somewhere in her jacket, she pulled out a large hunting knife and stepped towards the general. Rossel glanced up at the locket hanging above the picture of Alexei on the wall.

The hair in the locket, he remembered Bondar saying, was old.

Could it belong to the tsarevich?

'You worship the boy Alexei – is it that, Comrade Kitsenko?' Rossel said. 'You believe he directs your actions in some way.'

She stepped a little closer to Pletnev.

'It is his hair, yes.'

'A decent effort, Comrade Detective,' said Pletnev. 'But your bourgeois romanticism has blinded you to the truth. As a child in Yekaterinburg, Mila went on secret pilgrimages to the Ipatiev House, to visit the killing grounds of the Romanov family. But it was not Alexei she venerated.'

'Who, then?' said Rossel.

'The number inscribed on the locket, 1500, is the Party number of man called Yakov Yurovsky. The worker of a Bolshevik miracle. And a friend of her father. He cut off Alexei's hair as a souvenir. Later, he gave Mila some of it.'

'I've never heard of him.'

'Most have not. But when they executed Alexei, the boy sat bolt upright in a chair, a mute witness to the slaughter of his family. They stabbed and shot him but he wouldn't die. So Yurovsky finished him off with two bullets in the head. Mila has canonised Yurovsky as a Marxist saint.'

Mila now stood between the two men. With her left hand, she reached into her pocket and took out a scroll.

'On cloudless nights,' she said to Pletnev, 'through the sights of my rifle, playing across the faces of men who did not know they were about to die. Colonels poring over maps, captains peeping over trenches, sentries at their posts. In the small hours of the night, men let their minds turn to their deepest secrets. As I took aim, I felt I could read their thoughts. After we had been together for a little while, I could read yours, too, General.'

She placed the knife on a small table in front of Pletnev and unholstered the pistol at her hip.

'But at first, as we lay together in your bunker at Stalingrad, I believed you when you claimed to burn with Marxist purity. When you vowed to make the League of the Militant

Godless the true Soviet government once the war was over. The promises you made to me. All lies.'

The smoke was beginning to pour down the walls. Rossel felt the first heat of the fire. He could hear shouts from outside – an assault was imminent.

'Everything you claimed to be, you are not. You played the part of the atheist warrior monk to become leader of the League. You became leader of the League to gain political power. You play at being a man of the people, but think only of your own glory. Of becoming leader – you think this German bomb will give you that.'

Pletnev shook his head.

'Even now I think of the League,' he protested. 'Of the need to destroy every remaining church, synagogue and mosque. Do you think Beria will give you that? Not even Stalin himself will. Or why would he have reopened so many of them?'

At last . . .

Nikitin, his pistol drawn, was moving from column to column.

Rossel turned his head towards Kitsenko.

'Before you execute him, doesn't the general at least deserve to know what's written on his scroll?' he said.

She paused for a moment. But then marched – four quick steps – behind the general and, grabbing his brow with her free hand, pulled his head back. Pletnev grimaced, but did not cry out. She rammed the pistol into the general's temple and stared hard at Rossel.

'*Nikolai Alexandrovich, in view of your relatives' continuing attack on Soviet Russia, the Ural Executive Committee has decided to execute you,*' she said. 'That is what's written on the paper. Those were the last words Yurovsky read out before he executed the tsar and his family. Once those words were said, there could be no turning back. He was the man who ensured our glorious Revolution was unstoppable.'

Nikitin was moving through a cloud of grey smoke and black ashes.

Kitsenko coughed. She glanced up at the dome, smiling at the sight of the flames. She bent down, placed the pistol at a specific point on Pletnev's temple and craned her neck a little to stare into the general's face.

Pletnev's face remained a mask.

'Death holds no fear for me,' said Kitsenko. 'I know all her secrets.'

Nikitin fired. The retort boomed around the museum. In the same instant, the main door, only metres away, was smashed open. Firefighters, armed militia and soldiers began to stream into the building, shooting everywhere.

Rossel flinched as something hit his face. He raised his free hand and felt blood. A ricochet had grazed his cheek.

He looked around.

Kitsenko had vanished.

54

Nikitin raced towards Pletnev and started to undo his bindings. The general was coughing uncontrollably. Rossel's own chest was burning with the smoke. A soldier smashed at his handcuffs with a hammer, another used the butt of his rifle. More men tugged and twisted at the pipe, until somehow his hands were free and he was being pulled towards the main door, fresh air and the squeal of sirens.

Two soldiers hovered over the general and shouted for water.

It arrived in chipped tin bottles. Both the general and Rossel drank deep.

'Stay here and keep your head down,' said Pletnev as he doused and cleaned his face. 'My men will search the building and capture her.'

But Rossel was already on his feet and heading back inside. Straight for the stone staircase that led to the roof.

*

Even though he was breathing hard, he took the stairs two at a time. The higher he climbed, the denser the smoke. He reached the top and bent over, wheezing, sweating from his exertions but also the increasing heat. A dark vestibule had

doors leading out to the eastern and western quarter-circles.
Soldiers were ducking through both in ones and twos.

Left or right?

He chose right.

'She's there!'

A soldier was pointing towards the dome. 'We have her
cornered.'

The man turned to wave on his comrades.

A bullet whistled past his face, removing most of
one ear.

*

*A good sniper always knows the way out, knows where
her exit is.*

Kitsenko would have selected her position with care. To
get to that part of the roof, around the dome and above the
main building, you had to clamber over a wall. Which gave
a sniper an excellent view of the head of anyone coming
over. Staying in a crouch, he edged his way around, looking
for somewhere to place a boot and attempt the climb. The
wounded soldier clutched at his head and screamed a vow
of vengeance.

He had to get there first before Pletnev's men silenced
Kitsenko. For weeks she and Rossel had fought for the
same prize, for different masters. He wanted to know the
truth, even if the knowledge was fatal.

What did Beria want? *We could make a king of bombs,
with the right materials and design.*

How had Kitsenko tracked down her victims? What had
they known?

Rossel hoisted himself up, legs scrabbling for purchase, and landed in a heap on the other side, relieved to see a row of small parapets just big enough to shield his head and torso.

Risking a look, he saw orange flames tinged with green licking all around the windows of the cylindrical structure that supported the dome. On the other wall, soldiers were trying to join him but one fell back – *she must be on the far side of it*. Rifles were appearing above the wall, their owners firing wildly. The heat was growing. Keeping as close to the flames as he dared, he went halfway round the dome, anti-clockwise. There had been enough snow recently to cover the surface; Kitsenko's footprints were clear as she had moved from one shooting point to the next. Below, militia cars, fire engines and military trucks were jumbled all over the ground in front of the cathedral.

Heart pounding, he took two sharp breaths. For the first time, he missed the pistol Nikitin had given him.

She must be close, unless she had retreated to the farthest edge of the roof.

He tried to listen, to focus his mind above the sound of the shots. Kazan's dome towered above him.

Still no Kitsenko.

There . . .

The tip of a rifle barrel. On the far side of what looked like a large metal box, probably a water tank.

The barrel disappeared. Then the box was covered by drifting black smoke – the fire was spreading across the roof. He started crawling towards it but the roof felt hot.

What better way for her to make her point as an atheist than by burning down the house of God?

He reached the metal box.

She was on the other side, about two metres away – had to be; the only other way was down.

Water was trickling out of the bullet holes. He'd been right, it was a tank: the ice was falling off it in chunks and hissing as it hit the roof. The smoke was constant now, and the heat becoming unbearable.

He reached up.

Snow on the surface but the ice is melting.

Rossel took off his coat, reached up once more and dunked it into the freezing water. He dragged it back on again, buried his head inside it and took a lungful of air. Then, having counted to three, waiting for a moment when the shooting would subside, he launched himself through the flames and around the back of the tank, pulling up his greatcoat around his ears.

As Rossel emerged from the inferno, Kitsenko half-turned, her rifle still facing the soldiers.

Right hand reaching out for her weapon, left aiming to pull her over, Rossel hurled himself at her.

At the last moment she stepped backward. She was quick and Rossel caught her only a glancing blow. But he still managed to tear the rifle from her hands. He landed and looked up, his stomach turning as he saw she had a pistol in her hand.

How did I miss that?

As he rolled her shot went wide.

He kicked out, hit her knee hard. A second kick smashed into her thigh.

Kitsenko – left ankle hitting the balustrade, one hand seemingly groping for the setting sun – toppled over the side.

Rossel yelled her name and raced to the edge. But she had not fallen far. There was a thin sloping roof above the biggest doors to the cathedral and she was gripping its edge.

Kitsenko stared back up at him.

Twenty, maybe twenty-five metres below her feet were solid stone steps or the icy road. The fall would kill her.

Rossel dropped down and onto his stomach. They reached out to each other. Kitsenko let go with one hand, swung herself a fraction higher and grabbed Rossel by his left wrist.

A serene look drifted into her eyes. For her, death was a decision.

'Don't,' Rossel said. 'You don't have to . . .'

As if about to speak, Kitsenko opened her mouth. But she said nothing, only taking a breath as if to steady her nerves. As if her next kill was coming into view and she needed to be ready.

She blinked once. Twice. Then her right hand locked into his and he began to pull her up.

From the street below, a single shot rang out. He felt her fingers loosen.

Then, eyes still open and staring up at the fiery dome of the cathedral, Koshchei the Immortal slipped away.

55

The taste of the smoke was in his mouth, in his chest and stomach. His eyes were red and stinging. As the ZIS hit yet another pothole, Rossel clutched his stomach and thought about being sick. He had lost his soaking coat, but water had seeped through to his jacket and shirt. With the tarpaulin over the truck failing to keep out the wind, he was starting to shiver.

Next to him in the back of the truck sat the scientist Fironov and Nikitin. Opposite them were four GRU soldiers, two on each side. A fifth – a thin Central Asian with the sedate expression of Buddhist monk at prayer; the man who had fulfilled Pletnev's order to silence Mila Kitsenko – was cradling an automatic rifle.

Death solves all problems. Another saying of Stalin's the general seemed to have taken to heart.

Almost hysterical with relief that he had not been killed, Fironov had made straight for the general and informed him of the key details of the hydrogen bomb programme that had so recently come into his possession. Pletnev had insisted on seeing the evidence for himself, without delay.

After only ten minutes, the truck came to a halt opposite the GRU safe house. The Mongolian leapt out and pulled back the tarpaulin. Before getting out, Pletnev leaned forward and tapped Rossel's shoulder.

'Thank you, Lieutenant Rossel. I must say that.' He turned to Nikitin. 'And you, Comrade Major.'

Nikitin nodded. 'Happy to do my socialist duty, Comrade General.'

*

Upstairs, the professor fumbled over the slides and projector. With no need to argue over equations and diagrams with his fellow physicists, it took him not much more than fifteen minutes to talk the general through the Nazi design, and his conviction that they had hit upon the solution to building a hydrogen bomb.

Pletnev sat in silence throughout, registering no emotion at the final slide and the sudden mystery of the man with the scar.

Then he sat up.

'Commendable work, Professor. And now I must prepare for this evening's screening at the Young Pioneers' Palace,' he said. 'It is very important that I attend. I believe it is going to be something of a spectacle.'

Everyone in the room tensed. The general looked at each one of them in turn.

'Our Soviet Union grows weak. And corrupt. Comrade Stalin grows old while his courtiers squabble and fight and intrigue. It is, in short, like the last, decaying days of the Romanov era. The death throes of the *ancien regime*.'

He stood. 'But with this weapon, with this power, the Soviet Union need fear no one. So it is time.'

Rossel's mind tried to process what he was hearing.

No one would dare . . .

'And I will complete what I started in 1945,' said Pletnev, setting his cap straight. 'I shall teach a lesson that the German people will not forget and send a message that the world will be forced to hear.'

As Pletnev reached the door, he turned.

'Oh, one last thing. Is your additional hypothesis still true, Comrade Professor?'

'I'm sorry, Comrade General?' said Fironov.

'The theory you put to me on the steps of the museum. Your belief that Comrade Rossel knows a little more than he is letting on about the identity of this mysterious scarred man.'

Fironov reddened.

'Well, it was probably nothing. I simply observed . . .'

Nikitin took a pace forward.

'He does, Comrade General,' he said.

Rossel turned to stare at the major. Nikitin looked straight ahead.

'As I said to you earlier: Comrade Rossel, like everyone else, saw the photograph and the coat of arms on that final slide. He and I have seen the coat of arms before – above the doors to a mansion in the German town of Bayreuth. The house belonged to the Nazi physicist von Möllendorf – Baron Karl Friedrich von Möllendorf. I believe Rossel knows where to find him.'

Pletnev inspected his nails.

'How so, Comrade Major?'

'I was watching him when von Möllendorf's face was projected onto the screen,' said Nikitin. 'He stared at the image for longer than the rest of us, as if trying to remember something. I noticed a look of unexpected recognition. As an experienced interrogator, I've seen plenty of faces of people who are trying to conceal knowledge that might drop them in the shi . . . endanger them.'

Bastard.

Rossel jumped from his seat and threw himself at Nikitin. But the major parried his outstretched hands and smashed a fist into the side of his head.

Rossel hit the floor and stayed there.

'Congratulations, Comrade Major,' said Pletnev as he peered down at the prone figure. 'I knew I could depend on your loyalty.'

'Once again, I am honoured, Comrade General,' said Nikitin.

'Get up.' Pletnev stared down at Rossel as he issued the order.

Rossel rose, feeling his head.

'Have you indeed recognised this Fascist scientist?' said Pletnev. 'And do you know where he is?'

'Whether I decide to tell you very much depends on who you are, Comrade General,' answered Rossel.

Pletnev glowered at him.

'And who I am?'

'Either the fabled Hero of the Seelow Heights. Or the man Mila Kitsenko said she was hunting.'

'Ah.'

'And I think I already know the answer to that question.'

Pletnev jabbed a thumb over his shoulder and addressed one of his GRU agents.

'Arrest that man for counter-revolutionary activity – the burning of the Museum of Atheism at Kazan will begin the charges. Others will come later when I return from the Young Pioneers' Palace.'

The general glanced over his shoulder at Rossel. 'And Lieutenant? Major Nikitin will supervise your interrogation. I gather he has done so once before. And I have great faith in his abilities to make you cooperate.'

He turned and left with the major. Nikitin did not look back as he left the room.

56

Do, re, mi.

How long had it been?

A decade, perhaps even more? A decade since he and Nikitin had first set eyes on one another.

Do – the left little finger.

You can stop this, Nikitin had said. *All it takes is your confession.*

Re. The ring finger. Broken.

Mi. Then taken.

A diabolic scale that stopped only when he passed out, was revived, and lost consciousness again.

As Rossel held his hands up to his face, the general's voice rang in his ears.

Major Nikitin will supervise your interrogation.

How many fingers would he lose this time?

He kicked another chair across the room and cursed Nikitin, the general and his own stupidity again.

But mainly Nikitin.

How could he ever have trusted him?

Then he rested his hands on the table to regain his breath. Finally, his rage had blown itself out.

Having regained control of himself, he glanced all around the room.

There was no hope of escape. The windows were not merely covered, but the thick wooden boards were nailed into place. He had some matches in his pocket. But if he set fire to the furniture he was likely to burn himself to death.

Wandering into the small darkroom, with its enticing smell of chemicals, he dropped a match into a tray of red liquid. Nothing happened.

The door to the main room was locked from the outside and the GRU captain who had been left to guard him was armed with a PPSh submachine gun and a fierce loyalty to General Pletnev.

Rossel slumped down at the table in the middle of the room. The score was long gone, taken by the general's staff. Pletnev himself would be preparing for a congenial evening at the premiere of *Red Dawn-Red Dusk*.

All the Politburo would be there. Stalin was walking into Pletnev's trap.

But who cared which tyrant ruled the Soviet empire? Could Pletnev be any more brutal than the men who came before him?

At first a whisper, finally a never-ending scream.

He remembered the line about Mayakovsky's longing for suicide. The same, he knew, was true of murder.

And, most certainly, of revenge.

He and Nikitin, torturer and victim, reunited after years of redemption in war and in peace, had found a mutual enemy and formed an alliance. They had papered over the past, pushed it to the back of their minds.

Not any more.

He held up his broken fingers again. If only he could get out of here. Seize a gun or a knife. All he needed was one chance.

Anger took hold of him again, anger born of his own impotence. The Liesegang projector was within easy reach. He grabbed it and hurled it across the room and it crashed into the wall, its casing splitting open and shedding its metal guts all over the room. The sound was tremendous, shocking – out of all proportion to the size of the machine.

The door rattled open. The GRU captain who had been left to guard him surveyed the damage, one hand on his PPSh.

Rossel shrugged an insincere apology at the man, whose large frame filled the doorway, before resuming his inspection of the debris on the floor.

The soldier stood his ground.

Mostly the innards of the projector seemed to consist of lenses and bits of metal that held the lenses, plus screws and nuts. One disc of glass had bounced off the floor, rebounded off the wall and was still spinning on its circumference. Rossel and the guard tracked it as it reached the end of its journey and clattered to the floor.

It landed next to something dark.

Rossel took three quick paces and picked this other object up. It was the size of a large thick button and made of tarnished steel.

Just like the object Nikitin had unscrewed from the light-fitting in the Georgian restaurant Shemomechama.

A microphone.

Idle chit-chat. Coarse military humour. Coughs and belches.

And the basic facts, along with a great many details, of the Nazi nuclear weapons programme.

'See what this is, comrade?' Rossel said, holding it flat in the palm of his hand.

The GRU man did not move. But yes, he had seen it.

'A bug. They've been listening to every conversation in this room, probably for weeks. Months. Someone knows what General Pletnev has. Someone knows what he is going to do.'

He paused. Giving the man the time to fill the silence with his own panicked thoughts.

'So, it looks like you have a choice, comrade. Either you keep an eye on me and let your commanding officer walk into a trap. Or . . .'

With his PPSh raised, the captain stepped towards Rossel, left hand extended.

Before his fingers could close around the bug, Rossel flipped it skyward with his thumb.

The GRU agent's eyes followed it upward.

Rossel swung his right fist and hit him on the underside of his jaw.

The man's head jerked backwards. There was deafening roar as the magazine of his PPSh emptied into the ceiling, the finger of the already unconscious soldier locked around the trigger. Wood chips and plaster showered down on them both.

The firing stopped when the man's head hit the floor. His eyes blinked open and shut again.

Rossel bent down and began to unbutton the captain's coat.

57

In the evening gloom the streets seemed to fuse with Leningrad's canals, as if they too were flowing out to merge with the waters of the Gulf of Finland.

Rossel pushed the ZIS truck fast along the icy roads, heading for the Lieutenant Schmidt Bridge. He took the left turn onto Angliskaya Naberezhnaya at speed.

The fire at the Museum of Atheism was almost out, but Nevsky Prospect, he presumed, would be cordoned off up to there, so he needed to go around the edge of it.

The ZIS careered through Isaac's Square and down Voznesensky. Rossel looked into the sky away to his left. He thought he could see a thinning spiral of dark smoke drifting above and along the lights on Nevsky Prospect, but he could not be certain. He looked back at the road and got his bearings.

Left here.

But the cordoning off of Nevsky was having its effect on the flow of trams, buses, cars and pedestrians elsewhere. A sea of black and brown hats, heads, scarves, gloves and coats blocked their way. The traffic had slowed to less than walking pace. Rossel checked his watch.

Already 18.30.

He'd have to go on foot.

Leaving the ZIS in the middle of the road, he got out
and started pushing his way through the mass of bodies
along the Fontanka, towards the Anichkov Bridge. The
GRU coat, with its epaulettes, both kept him warm and
covered up his creased and still-damp suit. The captain's
cap kept the cold wind off his head, while the agent's stiff
identification card dug into his ribs.

In the evening cold, the people were whispering a refrain.
Rossel heard them in ones and twos, then in larger groups,
until it was taken up as a chant all along the canal. As if,
in hushed tones, the crowd was heralding the arrival of a
comet, or an imminent eclipse.

Stalin is coming.

*

In the distance, Rossel could see a large black horse rearing
up above the masses as if startled by a gunshot – one of the
four famous equine statues positioned at each end of the
Anichkov Bridge.

Rossel pushed past a grey-faced military veteran wearing his medals above a drinker's nose.

'Fuck you, comrade,' shouted the man, then stopping
himself when he saw Rossel's uniform. His wife began to
scold him for his bad language.

Rossel gave them a shrug and then wriggled past a
plump woman in a huge fur coat. A large huddle of excited
Young Pioneers now blocked his path.

The gate to a road leading off the Fontanka was shut and
guarded by a couple of corporals. Rossel walked towards

it and flashed his GRU captain's pass. The men saluted and opened the gate.

Free from the crowd, he picked up pace, until the Young Pioneers' Palace – formerly the Anichkov Palace – rose into view. It was a magnificent building covered with neoclassical pilasters and columns: one of Leningrad's many monolithic reminders of the three-hundred-year-old Romanov dynasty. Once the royal family's favourite home, the palace was the last place they had stayed before their fateful journey to the Ural Mountains.

Militia officers and soldiers were everywhere: holding back the crowds, cuffing anyone who showed too much enthusiasm for a glimpse of Comrade Stalin.

A shrill, impatient sound cut through the night air – the peeping of a horn.

All heads turned and more army and militia officers poured in, roughly separating the crowd and widening the road.

A black Packard limousine edged forward. In the passenger seat, Rossel could just make out a grey-haired man with a thin moustache and half-lens spectacles.

'In Stalin's court, every prince sleeps with his head on the block . . .'

Molotov, a stiff figure in the back, was looking thoughtful. A man unsure if he is returning to sainthood or the scaffold. Rossel was almost close enough to knock on the window. Instead, he turned his head away.

Something had changed.

Molotov was in disgrace. In near exile. Now he had returned.

Rossel pulled his shoulders back and, as if rehearsing for the May Day Parade, began marching towards the palace entrance.

Walk slow and with purpose, he thought, like everyone's waiting for me, not Comrade Stalin.

*

A line of black polished metal snaked from the palace as far as Nevsky Prospect – the cars of Party officials arriving late because of the disruption caused by the fire. Next to the outer gates were two large, whitewashed guardhouses. Always fresh paint for Stalin, Rossel thought.

Two soldiers stood to attention in each guardhouse, while four more were inspecting the credentials of the vehicles going in. They looked young. Brash. But also, he suspected, a little nervous.

Three giant red flags, each almost twenty metres tall, had been draped across the palace's façade. On each was printed the image of a man at the centre – Stalin; flanked by Beria and Pletnev. Stalin stared straight ahead while the other two regarded the Great Leader with open admiration. A perfect Soviet triptych.

The second part of the Young Pioneers motto – *Always prepared!* – was written in yellow letters on each flag. Rossel looked up at the huge image of Pletnev. His expression was firm-jawed and imperious – that of a man who believed he had just as much right to flutter on a flag as a hammer, sickle, swastika, crescent moon or cross.

Everywhere, senior officers from the Soviet armed forces stood around in small clusters, chatting before they went into the palace. High-ranking militia officers were here, too, but were firmly in the second tier of dignitaries. They kept themselves to themselves.

But something's wrong.

The entire Politburo – including Stalin himself – was converging in one place and the Ministry for State Security did not seem to be present.

Where were the blue-peaked caps of the MGB? They should have infested the place, projecting their own power in a setting where the projection of power was everything.

A phalanx of twenty men, dressed in black coats and grasping submachine guns, made a guard of honour as the cars of the Party officials rolled past them.

A woman with greying hair, wearing the uniform of a Young Pioneers teacher, was apologising for being delayed. 'They have blocked off half of Nevsky because of the fire. I have had to walk all the way from Palace Square.'

The guard she was talking to was tall, sleek and full of the self-importance a uniform often confers on those too immature to wear it. He scrutinised her pass while a second guard glared at her as she pleaded with them to hurry. Her Young Pioneers were waiting for her and would not know where to stand or when to shout hurrah for Comrade Stalin when he arrived.

She was let through.

'Documents, please.'

The middle-aged man in front of Rossel was also dressed in civilian clothes – some sort of *apparatchik* from one of the bureaus. He seemed nervous, stuttering his introduction and fumbling his papers. The brown hair oil he had plastered on his head was running down from under his *ushanka* and rolling down his left cheek. But, again, the guards said not a word, looking from ID document to face and back again. After a minute, he nodded. The man went in.

Rossel was next. Under his gloves, his palms sweated.

'Your documents, please.' The soldier glanced at the epaulettes and added. 'Comrade Captain.'

Rossel took out the GRU identity card. He handed it over but kept a grip on it as the soldier tried to take it.

He looked the youngster straight in the eye.

'You'd didn't see that?'

'See what?'

Rossel handed over his ID. As the soldier began to scrutinise it, Rossel pointed behind him.

'That last citizen,' he said. 'Nervous. Very. Why? And you missed something. You should have patted him down.'

'Missed something, Comrade Captain?'

'A shape under his coat. Could be nothing. But?'

The soldier went pale.

'I . . . I cannot leave my post, Comrade Captain,' he said.

Rossel took back his stolen pass before the guard could take another, closer look at the photograph.

'I'll let this go, comrade. On this occasion. Let me get after him. I will ensure that he is not about to cause any trouble.'

The youngster saluted.

'Thank you, Comrade Captain.'

Slipping the pass back into his pocket, Rossel walked through the gate.

'Not at all,' he said.

58

Inside the courtyard, a few final limousines were dropping off their passengers – more military dignitaries, weighed down with plump bellies and chestfuls of medals.

Rossel walked up a short gravel drive, interspersed with bleak winter flower beds blanketed in snow, to the main entrance.

On the steps of the building, in front of three symmetrical arched doorways, were more guards – GRU agents among them – standing to attention in greeting.

Trying a little too hard to look like these were the rarefied circles in which he belonged, Rossel strolled through the left-hand arch. He was in.

And somewhere, so were Nikitin and Defence Minister General Pletnev.

That was why there were no MGB officers, he realised. Pletnev had stationed his own men all over the Anichkov Palace. By tomorrow morning, Pletnev aimed to be in power. At that point, Nikitin would be untouchable.

It's now or never.

*

Everywhere there was the chinking of glasses, the salty aroma of caviar and smoked fish, and the murmur of overly polite, restrained conversation.

There was Molotov: not exactly surrounded by Party flunkies but not quite shunned, either. Then someone called his name in a loud voice – 'Vyacheslav Mikhailovich! What an honour!' – and General Pletnev was advancing with his arms outstretched, as if he was the host and this palace was his domain.

Rossel craned his neck to seek out Nikitin.

There he was, within touching distance of the general: sweating, shoulders hunched. As always, ready for a fight.

A grand marble staircase dominated the entrance hall. Chandeliers flecked with gold leaf hung from the stuccoed ceiling. Young Pioneers in their bright red-and-white uniforms and crisp scarves moved to and fro, serving plates of *blini* and glasses of champagne – French, not Soviet – on silver plates. All traces of the everyday activities of the Pioneers – sports classes, reading groups, lessons in Marxism – had been swept away. It was as though there had been no revolution, only a changing of the guard. The sense of history was palpable. If, at that moment, the dead tsar and his family could have materialised at the top of the stairs, all heads would bow down and Leningrad, cradle of Bolshevism, would become St Petersburg once more.

Khrushchev arrived, cracking jokes the second he walked through the doors, greeted by a fawning group of admirers. Trailing his habitual obscenities, he and his followers edged along the marble floor, a polished design of black-and-white squares. Molotov walked towards Khrushchev and the two fell into conversation in the midst of a group of generals, both men looking like chess pieces waiting to be moved. Molotov would be a worldly bishop. Khrushchev, Rossel thought, bald and bullet-headed, could never be anything other than a belligerent pawn.

They stepped onto the deep red carpet that ran up the stairs, towards the even grander room that hosted dramatic performances, propaganda concerts and film screenings to improve the young minds of the Pioneer movement. Arranged on either side of the staircase, like assembly lines of *matryoshka* dolls, were officers and minor Party members in a guard of honour.

On one side of the room was a table laid with a white linen cloth and silver salvers containing roast beef and pork. Rossel made his way towards it and slid one of the shorter knives into a pocket. The weapon of a labour camp prisoner.

Looking up, he could still see Nikitin standing at Pletnev's shoulder. He pushed past two militia officers and moved a little closer to them.

In Igarka, he had not found it within himself to kill.

This time, it would be different.

*

As he moved through the crowd, Rossel's eyes were fixed on the back of Nikitin's head. The major was still shadowing Pletnev but deep in conversation with a group of soldiers.

Rossel was close now. Only a few metres away.

He felt a firm tap on his shoulder. Without thinking, he turned around.

'Haven't we met, comrade?'

The man was dressed in a black suit, black tie and white shirt. His skin was the same deathly pale hue as when Rossel had encountered him before. Once in Moscow, and again on a moonlit night on the shores of Lake Ladoga. Through his pince-nez spectacles, Lavrentiy Beria was staring at him with bulging eyes in the manner of a royalist servant eyeing an unwelcome speck of dirt on an otherwise pristine linen table-cloth. Behind the lenses, his dark pupils were penetrating and predatory. Black ice on the surface of a fathomless pool.

'You look familiar,' said Beria, flashing an encouraging smile.

Rossel straightened and saluted.

'I don't think so, Comrade Minister.'

Beria was the most ruthless veteran of Stalin's eternal war on treason, counter-revolution, ideological deviancy and anti-Bolshevik thought. The man who had created the GULAG. Who ran his own operation to further develop the Soviet nuclear capability. And a merciless eliminator of anyone who placed obstacles in the way of his ambition.

As Rossel once had.

It was just over a year since he had uncovered Beria's twin vices of racketeering and rape, his victims a parade of young women and teenage girls. No matter that Senior Lieutenant Revol Rossel of the People's Militia had been looking for something else entirely.

Beria had enemies, too. And such indiscretions, however they came to light, were ammunition for them.

The minister took off his glasses, polished them with a handkerchief, and then replaced them. Under his coat, Rossel's hand closed around the knife.

'You're sure?' Beria said.

'Yes.'

'Name?'

'Captain Ivanov, Comrade Minister,' said Rossel, using the name on the identity card he had taken.

'Were my instructions not clear enough, Comrade Captain Ivanov?'

'Instructions?'

'You heard me. I issued instructions about the standards of dress for this evening to all Soviet officers, including GRU. Comrade Stalin is about to arrive and you look like you have been in a fight . . .'

Beria sniffed the air.

'. . . and you stink. Like an engine stoker.'

Beria clicked his fingers at an aide who was standing close by.

'Prokhorov. Get out your notepad and take this down.'

The man did as he was told.

'Ivanov. Captain. GRU. In disorderly dress and smelling like burnt toast . . .'

Beria reached up and tweaked Rossel's lapel. The minister's voice became soft, almost flirtatious.

'. . . is a cunt.'

'*Tak tochno*, Comrade Minister,' agreed the officer as he made the note with a flourish.

'Good.' Beria stared again Rossel's eyes. 'Now underline that last word.'

'Yes, Comrade Minister.' The man drew the line. 'Underlined.'

Beria turned to the aide.

'I wish to particularly impress upon you the necessity of placing that note in the centre of my desk tomorrow morning,' he said.

Then the minister gave a mocking salute and strolled away.

Rossel exhaled. Under the cap, with the epaulettes . . . the stolen uniform must have saved him. He began to walk across the lobby in an effort to lose himself in the crowd. But, unable to help himself, he looked over his shoulder, to see Beria staring at him once again.

This time in recognition. The look alone was enough to condemn him.

Beria turned to his aide Prokhorov, mouth open, ready to give an order.

But before he could do so, the crowd in the hall burst into applause. General Pletnev appeared halfway up the stairs. His dress uniform and medals gleamed. This was a different man to the one Rossel had first encountered in the museum. Someone who no longer felt the need to ride at the back of the parade. He radiated confidence and an unworldly sense of calm. Just as he must have done at Seelow, the general had the look of man who believed he could pluck bullets from the air.

Pletnev raised a hand for silence and the room obeyed. He gazed over the heads of the crowd to a cluster of musicians and a Young Pioneers choir, who had appeared to the left of the main doors. There was the woman who had preceded Rossel into the palace, her arms raised in preparation. She gave them a quick heave and the band started up – the Armenian composer Khachaturian's 'Poem about Stalin.'

The choir was in good voice:

Far and wide they sing
Songs of joy and labour;
Your name is always with us,
Like a banner, Comrade Stalin!

Behind them were another few rows of men and women, crammed into the grand hall to lend their vocal firepower to the later verses and fill out the faux-Oriental harmonies. After a few minutes, the cantata crashed to its end, rattling the chandeliers and bringing the conductor to convulsions.

A hush descended.

Men straightened their caps, women smoothed their skirts; every face adopted a fixed look of subservience. Even Beria, Khrushchev and Molotov straightened their backs.

But Pletnev didn't move a muscle.

The trap was set.

From outside came the roar of a motorcycle, then another drawing up next to it. From his vantage point, now half-hidden behind a fat column, Rossel could watch through the glass panes of the arched doors as four more outriders arrived, dismounted their bikes – low-slung Dnepr M-72s – and stood to attention. Next came two armoured cars, three ZIS trucks covered with tarpaulin, and finally a black America Packard limousine.

He heard everyone draw breath. A woman standing next to Khrushchev wobbled at the knees. The minister reached out a hand.

Standing just behind Pletnev, Nikitin was working his jaw underneath his scarred face.

Rossel took two steps forward. Then froze.

The snub end of a pistol was pressing into the small of his back.

'Don't move, comrade. Not so much as an eyelash.'

As the doors of the limousine were opened, a group of workers on the other side of the drive began to cheer, clap and shout – *Tovarishch Stalin zdyes', Tovarishch Stalin s nami* . . .

He is here, He is with us.

'Comrade Beria would like to see you again,' said the voice. Rossel realised who his captor was. Beria's aide, Prokhorov, who must have understood his boss's order, even though it had remained unheard.

A beautiful dark-haired woman, swathed in sable, began to sing a verse from *Zdravitsa*, the cantata Prokofiev had written for Stalin's sixtieth birthday.

> '*Your vision is our vision, O leader of the people!*
> *Your thoughts are our thoughts, indivisible!*
> *You are the banner flying from our mighty fortress!*
> *You are the flame that warms our spirit and our blood,*
> *O Stalin, Stalin!*'

It was only a short excerpt for soprano and harp, but no one had told the workers outside of this final performance and they drowned out the singing with their cheers until ordered to stop. Khrushchev was nodding along and grinning to someone in the crowd.

As they finished, a strange silence – the kind Rossel remembered from a battlefield just before a first shot was fired – settled upon the room.

One of the outriders took hold of the passenger door-handle and opened it. All heads in the room craned forward, in an impromptu competition to be the first to catch sight of the Great Leader.

After an agonising moment, a familiar figure – dressed in a white tunic, black boots and a military cap; left arm held close to his side in the familiar way – stepped out and onto the red carpet. Stalin turned to the distant crowd, and, standing with his back turned to the lobby, waved. Bulbs popped, photographers from *Pravda* and *Izvestia* fell to their knees to get a better angle.

Finally, Stalin turned and walked into the entrance hall of the Young Pioneers' Palace. Those nearest him were pushed back by armed bodyguards to make way for a little girl, about twelve years old, dressed in the uniform of the Pioneers and carrying a basket of flowers. She handed him a red rose and he patted her on the head.

Stalin took a moment to fasten it into his buttonhole.

As he did so, General Pletnev – vodka glass in hand, Nikitin by his side – descended the stairs. The crowd at the bottom parted, leaving them a path to the Soviet leader. Pletnev stopped a short distance away. When he spoke, his voice was soft and filled with reverence.

'Comrade Joseph Vissarionovich,' he began. 'As our father and mentor Lenin told us, there are decades when nothing happens and then there are weeks when decades do. On a battlefield, the same thing is true of minutes, of seconds, of moments. In them, history hangs low on the bough for those with the courage to take it. You have always been such a man.'

All around, Rossel could hear the metallic sound of submachine guns being cocked. More soldiers appeared,

417

forcing their way towards Pletnev and Stalin. The crowd broke out in gasps and stifled screams as the weapons were levelled straight at the head and body of the Great Leader.

But Stalin still seemed focused on the flower in his buttonhole.

'A toast,' said Pletnev, his voice now loud and firm. He raised his glass. 'To history!'

At that, Stalin looked up and smiled. General Pletnev looked into his eyes and took a sharp backward step. The glass shattered on the floor.

With a click of his fingers, Nikitin signalled to the soldiers standing closest to the leader. As one, they swung their weapons round and aimed at them directly at Pletnev's head.

Khrushchev stepped forward and pointed at the general.

'Arrest that man,' he said.

From nowhere – from out of the armoured cars, from the courtyard; but also from the crowd, from behind pillars and through doors – MGB officers swarmed into the building.

Pletnev watched them enter. Then he glanced around with an air of what seemed to be amusement. As if he were attending some Red Army training event for junior officers that had not quite gone to plan.

He nodded at Khrushchev. A battlefield general acknowledging the prowess of a respected opponent.

Moments later, with his arms held tight behind his back, a group of soldiers led him away.

Beria and Khrushchev were shaking hands: the former without much enthusiasm, the latter with gusto and a volley of what appeared to be instructions to his men.

Then Khrushchev turned to Major Nikitin, slapping him on the back. As shouts and scattered applause broke out, Rossel thought he could hear Khrushchev yelling congratulations. With a wink, the minister – just as he had at Lenfilm – made a series of exaggerated sweeping motions.

'Yes, as always, I'm the janitor, comrade,' he shouted to Nikitin. 'You, too, I think, no? It's just as I told you, comrade. Our glorious socialist revolution will always need peasants like us to clean up the shit . . .'

Rossel felt the pressure in the small of his back ease.

'What is going . . .' began Prokhorov.

Elbows slamming into the ribs of anyone close, Khrushchev pretended to sweep some more, his curses and laughter rising above the din – one of puzzled cries, demands for explanation, the yells of children, a choir being shouted at to give an encore, calls for more champagne – a din that did not quite mask the adjacent sound of gunfire that everyone pretended not to hear.

Just another basement execution in the name of Bolshevik rule, Rossel thought.

Left all alone, the Soviet leader had slumped into a gilded chair against a wall close to where Rossel was standing. His left arm, hanging stiff by his side, relaxed and straightened. He took a silk handkerchief from his pocket and began to mop at the sweat that was streaming down his brow.

As he did so, rouge and powder began to stain it.

Then, taking a deep breath to steady himself and standing to acknowledge the crowd, Boris Tarkovsky got to his feet and gave them all his deepest bow.

CODA

PRAVDA

Obituary

General Sviatoslav Pletnev – The Hero of the Heights

Dear Comrades,

Stalin's brother-in-arms and the most fervent of believers in Marx's cause, the great Hero of the Seelow Heights, a giant of the Communist Party and of the Soviet people, General Sviatoslav PLETNEV, no longer walks among us.

The Central Committee of the Communist Party of the Soviet Union, the USSR Council of Ministers and the Presidium of the USSR Supreme Soviet announce with profound sorrow to the Party and all working people of the Soviet Union that at 21.50 on 25 November, Sviatoslav Ivanovich Pletnev, Defence Minister, Soviet General and leader of the GRU, President of the League of Militant Godless, member of the Central Committee of the Communist Party of the Soviet Union, died after a short illness.

His name is dear beyond measure to our great Party, and to the working people of the world. Comrade General Pletnev helped to create the mighty League of Militant Godless. He was a leader of those who led our country to victory over fascism in the Great Patriotic War. His victory at the Seelow Heights means he will live forever in the glorious pantheon of socialist heroes. We echo here the sacred words of Comrade Stalin, the words which General Pletnev also used to turn the tide: 'Not one step back!'

The news of Comrade General Pletnev's death will bring profound pain to the hearts of the workers, collective farmers, intelligentsia and all the working people of our Motherland, to the hearts of the warriors of our glorious armed forces, to the hearts of millions of working people in all countries of the world. But let those counter-revolutionaries who lived in fear of his wrath feel no solace, for we will follow his example and root them out without mercy. Fear not, comrades, for the Central Committee has decreed in his honour to double our efforts, and hunt down with unceasing vigilance all those who hide within their breast a traitor's heart.

Long live the great and all-conquering teachings of Marx, Engels, Lenin and Stalin!

Long live our mighty Socialist Motherland!

Long live our heroic Soviet people!

Long live the great Communist Party of the Soviet Union!

Long live Comrade Stalin!

Central Committee of the Communist Party of the Soviet Union
USSR Council of Ministers Presidium of the Supreme Soviet

59

It had been a tense few hours as they embarked on the return leg of their journey from Igarka. Not even three weeks since they had left.

Rossel and Nikitin did not exchange a word. The third member of their party, the scientist Fironov, was trembling with anticipation of what they might find. He did not talk to them, instead scrawling calculations into a notebook.

Two hours into the flight north, Rossel finally spoke.

'Whose microphone was that? The one hidden in the projector, I mean,' he said.

Nikitin scratched his chin for a few seconds as he considered his reply.

'In the end,' he replied, 'it belonged to everyone who wanted Pletnev eliminated. MGB agents put it there, acting on Khrushchev's orders. But nothing happens in the MGB without Beria finding out sooner or later.'

'And Khrushchev did that because you told him to?'

Nikitin nodded, still not meeting Rossel's eye. 'After Pletnev gave me a job, I found out almost straightaway what his intentions were. I went to Khrushchev with a deal: my family's safety in return for everything I could find out about the general's plans.'

The plane lurched hard in a pocket of turbulence, making them both grab the seats in front of them.

'It turned out the general was already suspected of plotting to seize power by other members of the Politburo. Only Stalin refused to believe it.'

Out of the windows there was nothing to see but total darkness.

'So, a plan was hatched to trap Pletnev at the screening of *Red Dawn-Red Dusk,* right before the Party assembly,' Nikitin continued, 'to prove to Stalin that his favourite general was a traitor. They couldn't use Stalin himself, of course. But they quickly got hold of the next best thing. A convincing double.'

So Boris Tarkovsky had not been arrested by the MGB, thought Rossel. He had simply been recruited. Fadeyev, he presumed, had been in on the plan. His presence a ploy to convince any doubters that the arrest was real.

The plane's juddering appeared to have passed. Nikitin relaxed into his seat, relieved to be telling his story.

'And the general and his senior officers were taken to the basement of the Anichkov Palace and executed,' he said. 'Now there is talk of Tarkovsky playing our Great Leader in a Lenfilm production. Even whispers of the Order of Lenin.'

At Vorkuta, the three of them headed for the helicopter without delay. Just before they climbed in, Nikitin handed Rossel a couple of packs of cigarettes. Bulgarian, the good stuff.

Rossel opened a pack, lit two cigarettes and handed one over. By the time the bitter smoke had settled in the back of their throats and both had exhaled into the freezing northern air, a truce of sorts had been declared.

'Did Comrade Khrushchev live up to his end of your bargain?' Rossel asked as the blades began to turn.

But Nikitin had pulled his *ushanka* over his eyes and did not answer.

60

As the Mi-4's rotors stopped turning, Rossel and Nikitin clambered out of the helicopter and ducked down to shelter themselves from the driving wind and snow. The commandant of 105th Kilometre had ordered a large area cleared to make sure they could land, even in the bad weather.

Navigation had been simple. In places, the camp at 105th Kilometre was still burning, the flames visible from the air for miles. The prisoners had rioted, Nikitin had said. The guards had barred the gates and shot anyone who tried to get out. Inside the fence, the Thieves had gone on the rampage. The GULAG administrators in Vorkuta were in uproar.

Through the swirling snow, they could see that reports of the uprising had been accurate.

'Glad to be back?' said the major.

Rossel stared at the forlorn collection of huts set into the vast, barren snowscape, dwarfed by the endless blackness of the Siberian sky. Smoke trailed up like gnarled fingers from the walls and roofs of some of them. Others had been burnt to the ground.

'Not really,' he said.

The knifing wind fanned the fires, keeping them burning despite the blizzard. Under a guard tower to their left was a frozen pile of dead zeks: ten bodies or so deep, ten wide.

Up to a hundred corpses, thought Rossel, and counting.

Nikitin nodded towards the pile.

'Pletnev's new command?' he shouted.

Rossel nodded.

'Yes, a regiment of the damned.'

Dotted around them were the dark, heavy coats of the camp guards. Several had their rifles levelled at the perimeter fence.

Rossel walked across to the pile of bodies. Sticking out from the pile, half buried by his fellow inmates, was a face he recognised.

Babayan's eyes were open and staring skyward. As if the old priest was still searching for, and silently praying to, his God.

Rossel reached down and closed them.

'The rest, who knows?' he said. 'But not this man.'

*

Fifty metres away from the helicopter, the commandant was waiting to meet them. He was accompanied by a portly army colonel and a small group of soldiers.

Everyone except Rossel exchanged salutes.

'I think we have the men you're looking for, Comrade Professor Fironov,' the commandant said. 'Well, at least we have them cornered. The prisoners have been rioting for days. A dispute over rations. The malign influence of the criminal class. However, we now have the dogs cornered.'

'Good,' said Fironov in a clipped, bureaucratic tone.

429

Since his recent promotion – as recent as the previous day – the scientist was full of himself. After examining the information hidden in the microdots, Beria had transferred Fironov to the MGB and made him project leader of KB-11, the All-Russian Scientific Research Institute of Experimental Physics. All he had to do now was to find von Möllendorf and get him to reveal the last, vital details. That, Fironov had boasted, would enable the Soviet Union to build a bomb 'of unrivalled power'.

The commandant coughed as he pulled his coat tight around him.

'I regret to say a few of the German POWs have made a last stand with some of the Thieves,' he said.

'What?' shouted Fironov.

The Red Army colonel had tired of waiting and cut the debrief short. 'This way,' he said, striding off in the direction of the camp, bowing his head against the wind.

The rest of them followed, weaving a path through the guards.

'It took us nearly three days,' the colonel shouted over his shoulder, 'but we have almost quelled the insurrection.'

'Almost?' asked Rossel.

'A small group is holding out in the forge.'

The commandant picked up his pace, trying to keep up. 'About twenty Thieves and a few of the Germans,' he said. 'Led by two incorrigible criminals called Kuba and Medvedev. They have refused all offers to surrender peacefully.'

Rossel remembered the chant at morning roll call after Sobol had been murdered.

North, south, east and west, between the rising and the setting of the sun. Bitches, this will be your fate.

430

Even at the last, Kuba was refusing to be a Bitch.

The soldiers had driven trucks into the compound and arranged them in a defensive circle around the forge. In between the vehicles, they had built wooden barricades and wrapped them in barbed wire. The roof of the forge was on fire and the bodies of three men – one soldier, two zeks – were lying on the snow in between the building and the barricades. Too close to the Thieves for anyone to risk retrieving them.

A captain with a loudhailer was shouting out demands to the remaining prisoners.

'Today is your last day on earth, comrades. Unless you come out now – that's the choice you have to make . . .'

Rossel, Nikitin and the others stood close to a truck in the centre of the encirclement, about fifty metres away from the door to the forge.

'If it was up to me, I'd bake those *mudaki* like they were loaves of bread,' said the colonel.

'No,' said Fironov. 'We have orders from Comrade Beria. "Do what you like with the Russians, but the Fascists must be saved." The minister's order to me was very clear.'

As he spoke, the door of the forge was kicked open. A huge figure carrying a child-sized bundle in his arms walked out through the smoke and began to cross the snow. Behind them were two other Thieves with their arms raised. After that, a German with his hands in the air, followed by three more POWs.

Every single rifle was trained on the group.

The captain lowered his loudhailer. No one spoke. The wind was easing but the snow still fell.

Medvedev, the giant Thief, was now only a few metres away from where they were standing. He knelt and lay Kuba's body on the ground at Fironov's feet. A gift, it seemed, from the Thieves of Igarka to great Comrade Stalin, Tsar of all the East.

Kuba's head lolled at an angle. On his index finger, he was still wearing the brass washer he had slipped on the last time Rossel had seen him.

A line from the song of Kolka the Pickpocket rose in his head.

Tell them, Masha, that he don't thieve no longer . . .

A fitting elegy, Rossel thought, for the dead king of 105th Kilometre.

Medvedev stood up and stared at Rossel, recognising him.

'Greetings, Comrade Albatross. Being so short made Kuba too stubborn. And being too stubborn meant . . .'

Medvedev ran a finger across his own neck.

Fironov was growing impatient. He pointed at the German who had led his comrades out of the forge.

'This is him, I presume? Von Möllendorf. Are you sure, Rossel? He doesn't look much like the photograph . . .'

Rossel shook his head.

'No, that's not him,' he said. 'That's Walter.'

Walter, hands still raised, managed a thin smile that did not reach his eyes. In mangled Russian, he tried to tell Rossel that it was good to see him again.

'I'm here for Baron Karl Friedrich von Möllendorf,' said Fironov. 'The nuclear physicist. Where is he? He's not dead, is he?'

Walter thought for a moment.

'I could do with a cigarette,' he said.

Rossel handed him one. Nikitin took out a lighter and lit it.

Walter turned round and pointed to the forge.

'He's in there,' he said.

Fironov grabbed the loudhailer from the captain. 'Von Möllendorf,' he yelled. 'Baron Karl Friedrich von Möllendorf. Please show yourself, please come out, you will not be harmed.'

All eyes fixed on the door to the building. After a minute, a figure began to emerge through the smoke. Turning and twisting as if dancing a solitary reel, it moved towards them.

The moment Tsar Suka saw Rossel, he smiled.

'*Der Musikmann*,' he said. '*Der Musikmann*.'

Behind him, the roof of the forge collapsed, throwing sparks high into the night sky.

Fironov's hand fell to his side, the loudhailer slipped into the snow.

Then the Third Reich's most dangerous physicist, the man who had once known too much, began to sing a Wagnerian leitmotif. The same leitmotif that appeared in *Götterdämmerung*, at the exact point the microdots had been positioned.

It was the closest his shattered mind would ever get to comprehending the Nazi plans for the H-bomb. Let alone completing them.

Rossel stepped forward and shook von Möllendorf's hand.

'Yes,' he said. 'That's me.'

61

On the opposite side of Nevsky Prospect, the House of Books had disappeared.

All six storeys were covered by a huge red and yellow banner, on which was written the slogan of the League of Militant Godless: "The struggle against religion is the struggle for socialism." As if the Party had reduced all human knowledge to those few words.

Leningrad was a city in mourning. Rossel stood with Natalia Ivaskova not far from the scorched stones of Kazan Cathedral. The museum was wrapped in its own covering, a dowdy tarpaulin, as workers tried to save the dome.

A vast procession of black was moving in eerie silence down Nevsky Prospect. It would travel all the way to the Alexander Nevsky Monastery – a passing homage to another great Russian military figure – before transport by military vehicle to the Piskaryovskoye Cemetery. In death, it seemed, General Pletnev did indeed command an even greater army than he had in life.

Rossel looked over at his other companion. Anna Drugova had been freed from the camps along with the rest of her family, who had taken up residence once more in their old apartment. Nikitin, now with renewed influence, had been persuaded to intercede with Minister Khrushchev.

But the girl had not come to pay her respects to General Pletnev.

The three of them had been standing there for forty minutes and still the tanks, armoured cars, soldiers, Young Pioneers and lines of MGB and GRU crawled past. In the distance, they could just make out the ranks of members of the League of Militant Godless – a hundred deep, each carrying huge garlands of red and white flowers and greenery – as if even the forests of Karelia had come to pay their respects.

Rossel felt the city's collective sigh – soft, low and sorrowful. The mourners had caught their first glimpse of the general's coffin: drawn by six white horses and placed on a simple cart made, according to *Pravda*, from the shattered pieces of a giant Ukrainian cross.

A woman to Rossel's right broke into sobs. A big Cossack in front him took out a handkerchief and dabbed at his cheek.

As Pletnev's coffin drew parallel with them, the crowd cried out, moaned, exhorted – '*Narodny geroi sredi nas;* The people's hero is among us!'

And then – at first one lone voice, then another, and another – 'Not one step back, not one step back!' . . . Until the noise was so loud it scared into the air a flock of crows from the dome of the cathedral. Some old women, Rossel noticed, crossed themselves. One, near him, was even whispering an Orthodox prayer . . . Just as Marshal Kutuzov had once done to the Blessed Virgin of Kazan before his victory against Napoleon.

Rossel, Natalia and Anna were too far back to see, but the Soviet press had revealed that on top of the coffin rested

Pletnev's military cap, a copy of *Das Kapital* and – a great honour bestowed at the last moment to the military man and scholar – Stalin's own copy of *The Prince* by Niccolò Machiavelli, said to contain personal annotations, underlinings and jottings in the margins. 'The old bastard's lost none of his sense of humour,' Khrushchev had apparently remarked, grinning.

On a simple podium a hundred metres further down Nevsky, the leading members of the Politburo – Beria, Malenkov, Molotov and Khrushchev – had assembled. Rossel looked out for Nikitin. There he was, as promised; at the bottom of the platform, but close to Khrushchev.

And standing behind the major were his wife, his son Dima and his daughter Svetlana. As Rossel watched, Nikitin gave his wife a discreet kiss and patted his children on their heads.

According to *Pravda*, Stalin himself would meet his 'much-loved comrade-in-arms' at the cemetery. Where he would watch them inter the general in a temporary glass sarcophagus and then lay the first brick in what was intended to be a mausoleum and place of communist pilgrimage, with Pletnev's body on permanent display.

As Pletnev's coffin reached the members of the Politburo, it slowed. A volley of shots was fired into the air by specially selected members of the Red Army who had fought at the Seelow Heights. As the sound died away, the coffin began to move on.

'It is time,' Rossel said to Natalia. They retreated a few paces to the gardens in front of the cathedral, away from the lingering mourners.

The former dancer stopped and bent down to open the violin case she had been carrying. Then she offered Rossel his old instrument, along with the bow. But instead of taking it, he pointed with his crooked fingers towards Anna, who took both violin and bow from Natalia.

'Thank you for coming today,' said Rossel to Natalia, as Anna tucked the violin under her neck, getting used to the feel of it.

'I had hoped you would call,' she said. Then she leaned in and kissed him on the cheek.

Anna began to play.

The girl was brutally thin. Under her fur hat, her once lustrous hair was brittle and even flecked with grey. Her eyes were tinged with the regret of those who had seen too much.

Rossel held up Vustin's manuscript to 'Fugue No 13', written in the composer's own neat hand on the back of a prisoner's death warrant.

'Pianissimo,' he said. 'And slow, so slow . . . That's how I'd play it.'

The girl began to move the bow across the strings. She was no Oistrakh. Uncertain. Unpolished. But, for this recital, Anna possessed something much more important than talent – understanding.

For to do justice to Alexander Vustin's *Song of Lost Souls* you had to have first been one of them.

Rossel took Natalia's hand in his left and tapped his chest twice with his right. His own prayer to a god of sorts that he knew would most likely go unanswered.

As they watched on, the end of the procession went by: two huge trucks with rockets on them and a last troop of Young Pioneers.

437

As he listened, Rossel could see another army marching behind them – the day's labour gangs setting off in the direction of the railway lines. The ghosts of the gulag, trudging through Igarka. An endless line of forlorn pilgrims marching out to meet saints they no longer worshipped.

All of Babayan's shadows in the snow.

Acknowledgements

Of the many books we have read to understand more about the machinations of Stalin's regime, perhaps our most important resources were Simon Sebag Montefiore's *The Court of the Red Tsar* and Robert Conquest's *Stalin: A Biography*. For detail of the labour camp system we turned repeatedly to Anna Applebaum's *Gulag*, as well as the website of the human rights organisation Memorial and (especially for maps and images) the Czech website Gulag.cz. But the most valuable insights into the brutality and lawlessness of the Soviet labour camps came from Varlam Shalamov's extraordinary *Kolyma Tales* – harrowing but mesmerising.

If Danzig Baldaev's series of books entitled *Russian Criminal Tattoo Encyclopaedia* was inspirational for Revol Rossel's first outing in *City of Ghosts*, his *Drawings From The Gulag* was handy for this novel, even if one has to look at much of its contents with one eye closed. Mark Galeotti's *The Vory* is another excellent guide to the world of the Thieves.

On the German side, *Tales From Spandau: Nazi Criminals and the Cold War*, by Norman J.W. Goda, was invaluable, and not only for the prison regulations in the appendix. Joachim Fest's *Speer: The Final Verdict*, was also instructive. We found a very large *Luft-Navigationskarte in Merkatorprojektion* – and many similar maps – in the British Library in London, which enabled us to pinpoint Bayreuth after some playing around with reference systems. Misha Aster's *The Reich's Orchestra* was also useful.

We are extremely grateful to Tony Comer, the former departmental historian at GCHQ, the UK government's communications and cyber intelligence service, who reviewed Halder's cipher and the thinking behind it, and suggested certain modifications and improvements.

We must also express our gratitude to Dr Eugene Shwageraus of the Cambridge Nuclear Energy Centre for patiently talking us through the basic elements of nuclear fission (pun intended) and the development of the hydrogen bomb. He also pointed us in the direction of *Dark Sun: The Making of the Hydrogen Bomb* by Richard Rhodes – as did Tom Plant of the Royal United Services Institute, who further suggested a look at the *Los Alamos Primer* by Robert Serber, the introductory lectures for scientists working on the Manhattan Project.

Despite the above research, and much more in other books and on the internet, this is a work of fiction. We have been wilfully inconsistent in sticking to the facts or applying what we have learned. In all cases, the mistakes, deliberate or otherwise, are ours alone.

On the transliteration of Russian: sometimes we have relied on the system used by most English-speaking students of the language; at other times we have followed generally accepted spellings as found in the guidebooks or on the internet in order not to confuse our readers. Where we have been sure of our ground, we have used the names of streets and places that were in use during the Soviet era (many have been changed since 1991).

Finally, huge thanks to Giles Milburn, Liane-Louise Smith and the team at Madeleine Milburn, and Jon Elek and Rosa Schierenberg at Welbeck, for their unwavering support, patience and encouragement. We could not have wished for finer counsellors and representatives.

About the Author

Ben Creed is the pseudonym for Chris Rickaby and Barney Thompson, two writers who met on the Curtis Brown creative writing course.

Chris, from Newcastle upon Tyne, found his way into advertising as a copywriter and, after working for different agencies, started his own. He has written and produced various TV programmes for ITV and Five, and some award-winning experimental fiction.

Before deciding to pursue a career as a journalist, Barney spent two years studying under the legendary conducting professor Ilya Musin at the St Petersburg Conservatory. He has worked at The Times and the Financial Times, where he was legal correspondent, and is now an editor, writer and speechwriter at UNHCR, the UN Refugee Agency.

Their first book, *City of Ghosts*, was nominated for the Crime Writers' Association Gold Dagger for best crime novel of the year.